Veterinary Disaster Medicine

Working Animals

T0272302

Veterinary Disaster Medicine

Working Animals

Wayne E. Wingfield, MS, DVM
Sherrie L. Nash, MS, DVM
Sally B. Palmer, DVM
Jerry J. Upp, DVM, EMT

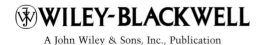

A John Wiley & Sons, Inc., Publication

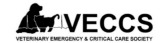

VETERINARY EMERGENCY & CRITICAL CARE SOCIETY

Edition first published 2009
© 2009 Wayne E. Wingfield

Blackwell Publishing was acquired by John Wiley & Sons in February 2007. Blackwell's
publishing program has been merged with Wiley's global Scientific, Technical, and Medical
business to form Wiley-Blackwell.

Editorial Office
2121 State Avenue, Ames, Iowa 50014-8300, USA

For details of our global editorial offices, for customer services, and for information about how
to apply for permission to reuse the copyright material in this book, please see our website at
www.wiley.com/wiley-blackwell.

Authorization to photocopy items for internal or personal use, or the internal or personal use of
specific clients, is granted by Blackwell Publishing, provided that the base fee is paid directly to
the Copyright Clearance Center, 222 Rosewood Drive, Danvers, MA 01923. For those
organizations that have been granted a photocopy license by CCC, a separate system of
payments has been arranged. The fee codes for users of the Transactional Reporting Service are
ISBN-13: 978-0-8138-1017-1/2009.

Designations used by companies to distinguish their products are often claimed as trademarks.
All brand names and product names used in this book are trade names, service marks,
trademarks or registered trademarks of their respective owners. The publisher is not associated
with any product or vendor mentioned in this book. This publication is designed to provide
accurate and authoritative information in regard to the subject matter covered. It is sold on the
understanding that the publisher is not engaged in rendering professional services. If professional
advice or other expert assistance is required, the services of a competent professional should be
sought.

Disclaimer
The contents of this work are intended to further general scientific research, understanding, and
discussion only and are not intended to and should not be relied upon as recommending or
promoting a specific method, diagnosis, or treatment by practitioners for any particular patient.
The publisher and the authors make no representations or warranties with respect to the
accuracy or completeness of the contents of this work and specifically disclaim all warranties,
including without limitation any implied warranties of fitness for a particular purpose. In view
of ongoing research, equipment modifications, changes in governmental regulations, and the
constant flow of information relating to the use of medicines, equipment, and devices, the reader
is urged to review and evaluate the information provided in the package insert or instructions
for each medicine, equipment, or device for, among other things, any changes in the instructions
or indication of usage and for added warnings and precautions. Readers should consult with a
specialist where appropriate. The fact that an organization or Website is referred to in this work
as a citation and/or a potential source of further information does not mean that the author or
the publisher endorses the information the organization or Website may provide or
recommendations it may make. Further, readers should be aware that Internet Websites listed in
this work may have changed or disappeared between when this work was written and when it is
read. No warranty may be created or extended by any promotional statements for this work.
Neither the publisher nor the author shall be liable for any damages arising herefrom.

Library of Congress Cataloging-in-Publication Data

Veterinary disaster medicine : working animals / Wayne E. Wingfield . . . [et al.].
    p. ; cm.
  Includes bibliographical references and index.
    ISBN 978-0-8138-1017-1 (spiral bound : alk. paper)   1. Veterinary emergencies.   2. Service
dogs–Wounds and injuries–Treatment.   3. Horses–Wounds and injuries–Treatment.   4. First
aid for animals.   I. Wingfield, Wayne E.
    [DNLM: 1. Emergencies–veterinary.   2. Disasters.   3. Dogs–injuries.   4. First
Aid–veterinary.   5. Horses–injuries.   SF 778 V5857 2008]
    SF778.V48 2008
    636.089′60252–dc22

                                                                    2008035482

A catalog record for this book is available from the U.S. Library of Congress.

Set in 9 on 11.5 pt Sabon by SNP Best-set Typesetter Ltd., Hong Kong

Printed in Singapore by Markono Print Media Pte Ltd

1 2009

Dedication

To Dr. John Anderson, the Father of Veterinary Disaster Medicine, who led the way. To our teammates who trained, deployed, and worked so hard. To the animal owners, search-and-rescue, first responders, and EMS personnel who accepted us. To the four-legged disaster victims who appreciated our knowledge and skills. This book is for all of you.
WEW

I would like to dedicate this book to my four-legged friends who have taught me so much along the way. My pets taught me patience and acceptance as a child. To the many patients and their caretakers I have met in my journey as a veterinarian; they have taught me kindness, perseverance, humility, and a sense of humor. I want to thank my husband, Bob, for his patience, willingness, and assistance that allowed me to help my patients and others in need, especially when it was not always at a convenient time. I also thank my family for the support and understanding they have given me throughout the years.
SLN

To all the unsung heroes.
SBP

I would like to dedicate this book to my late father, Randy, who left this world way too prematurely; to my mother, Pauline, who got me through the tough years; and to my wife, Stephanie, and kids, Kristen, Megan, and Kyle, who support me in my disaster preparedness no matter how long I am away from home.
JJU

Contents

Contributors

Wayne E. Wingfield, MS, DVM
Diplomate, American College of
  Veterinary Surgeons; Diplomate,
  American College of Veterinary
  Emergency and Critical Care
Emeritus Professor, Emergency and
  Critical Care Medicine, Department of
  Clinical Sciences and Veterinary
  Teaching Hospital, College of
  Veterinary Medicine and Biomedical
  Sciences, Colorado State University
and
Veterinary Medical Officer and Squad
  Leader, National Medical Response
  Team—Central USA, National Disaster
  Medical System

Sherrie L. Nash, MS, DVM
Owner/Veterinarian, Animal Care Clinic,
  Harlowton, MT
and
Veterinary Medical Officer, National
  Veterinary Response Team 4—
  National Disaster Medical System

Sally B. Palmer, DVM
Owner/Veterinarian, Palmer's Animal
  Wellness Services, PLLC, Denver, CO
and
Veterinary Medical Officer, National
  Medical Response Team—Central
  USA, National Disaster Medical
  System

Jerry J. Upp, DVM, EMT
Owner/Veterinarian, Midtown Animal
  Hospital PC, Gering, NE
and
Veterinary Medical Officer, Deputy
  Commander and Squad Leader,
  National Veterinary Response Team 4,
  National Disaster Medical System

Introduction

Working animals are injured or killed in disasters as frequently as are humans. With this in mind, the purpose of this veterinary disaster medicine book is to acquaint individuals with the requirement for training and to provide a ready resource in preparation for assisting working animals that become victims of a disaster.

This book was written with the able assistance of experienced veterinarians who have deployed to numerous disasters. Too often in the past, we have been faced with reading through volumes of information in an attempt to extract key information. To help solve this problem, the authors of this book used their experience and expertise to develop key information in an outline format. This provides the veterinarian, veterinary technician, search-and-rescue personnel, and emergency medical services individuals a ready source of important information. This guide is not intended as a traditional textbook. Rather, it is designed to provide factual information for the reader and to stimulate further learning and discussion. In preparing this book, we have attempted to take a middle ground between oversimplification and overcomplication, to broaden our readership. Undoubtedly, veterinarians and veterinary technicians practice first aid skills daily. With specialization in veterinary medicine, a specialist in treating small animals often needs a quick refresher on treating horses. This also applies to the equine specialist, who often finds a quick review of canine medicine to be useful. Of necessity, there is jargon in the text material that must be integrated into one's vocabulary in order to facilitate interaction. Additionally, we have included some information on species other than the dog and horse; this was done as a response to our experiences in responding to disasters. It is unusual to see only dogs and horses. We have provided at least a small amount of information on other species in case the need arises. Information directed at humans is also included. Since humans are often the handlers, they, too, may be at risk, and it is important to know what level of risk humans may be assuming.

The authors of this book are truly appreciative of your interest in helping animals in need. We are also indebted to the animals from which we have learned during our life-long experiences. Every animal has taught us something, and it is only proper that we now start to return our debt by training and applying our knowledge to become better prepared for assisting working animals in future disasters.

Wayne E. Wingfield, MS, DVM
Sherrie L. Nash, MS, DVM
Sally B. Palmer, DVM
Jerry J. Upp, DVM, EMT

Introduction

Veterinary Disaster Medicine

Working Animals

CHAPTER 1
FIRST AID FOR WORKING DOGS

Wayne E. Wingfield, MS, DVM

On deployment to a disaster scene that may include working dogs, it is important to obtain information relevant to potential hazards that the dogs may encounter. One hazard is the environmental temperature in which they may be working, so one must be prepared to treat hyperthermia or hypothermia. Another hazard is the chemicals present in a building that a dog may step through, breathe, or ingest during a search, so one must know how to counteract the chemicals. Drinking contaminated water during a search may also be a hazard. Knowledge of the hazards that may be faced will increase the handler's ability to avoid a problem and will prepare the veterinary unit to care for the dogs.

Veterinarians and veterinary technicians practice first aid daily. A review of first aid for dogs will be most useful for veterinarians and technicians who predominantly see large animals in their daily routine; for all other first responders, this chapter will provide information on the basics of canine first aid.

1. First Aid for Working Dogs

1.1. Presentation of a Sick or Injured Dog

1.1.1. *History:* When presented with a sick or injured animal, try to gain as much history and information from the handler as possible. Above and beyond an initial observation, find out the following information:

I. Where did the illness/injury occur? This is important so others can be warned of a potential hazard.
II. When did the illness/injury occur? The duration of an illness/injury often guides treatment by the veterinarian.
III. What happened to the dog? This may help guide others to the detection of unseen hazards.

1.1.2. Standard medical questions

I. Coughing, sneezing (Bloody? Purulent? Foreign debris? Productive? Nonproductive?)
II. Vomiting (Color? Frequency? Bloody? Coffee-grounds color? Foreign debris? Bile? Food?)

3

III.   Diarrhea (Straining? Mucoid? Color? Foreign debris? Volume? Blood?)
IV.   Lethargy? Anorexia? Depression?
V.   Increased/decreased urination? (Normal urinary output for dogs is ≈0.5–1 ml/lb/hr body weight/hr [1.1–2.2 ml/kg/hr].)
VI.   What is the dog's body weight? (Used for drug dosing and fluid administration.)
VII.   Any abnormal behaviors noted?
VIII.   Any abnormal bleeding noted?
IX.   Did the dog ingest anything that might be toxic?

1.2. Handling

1.2.1.   Safety is paramount. You must take into consideration your own safety, the safety of other people assisting, and the safety of the dog.

1.2.2.   The three main risks of injury are being bitten, scratched, or hit in the face by the head of a thrashing dog. A normally gentle or well-trained dog may bite, paw, or thrash when injured due to pain and anxiety.

1.2.3.   Muzzles (Figs. 1.1–1.2)
   I.   A muzzled dog should never be left unattended.
   II.   If a dog is in respiratory distress or heat stress, the ONLY type of muzzle that may be used is a wire-cage muzzle.

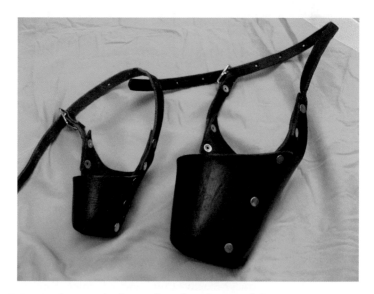

Figure 1.1.   Leather muzzles for small- and medium-sized dogs.

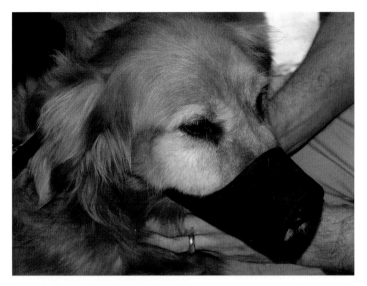

Figure 1.2. Cloth muzzle on a large-breed dog.

III. Cloth muzzles are available; proper sizing is important. A "field" muzzle may be fashioned out of 2- to 4-inch roll gauze (Figs. 1.3–1.6) or with a quick-release knot (preferably two on big dogs).

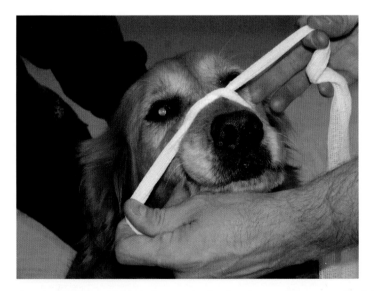

Figure 1.3. Gauze being used to tie the muzzle of a dog. Notice one person is firmly holding the dog while a rescuer first wraps the gauze around the muzzle and then ties a half-hitch knot on top of the muzzle.

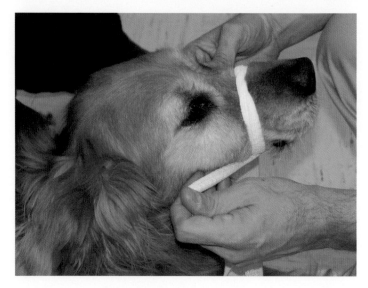

Figure 1.4. The gauze is next wrapped down and around the muzzle with a second half-hitch knot now tied underneath the muzzle.

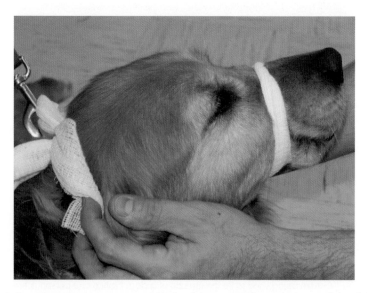

Figure 1.5. The gauze is now secured behind the occipital protuberance of the skull and a bow-knot is tied in case the muzzle needs to be promptly removed should the dog begin to vomit.

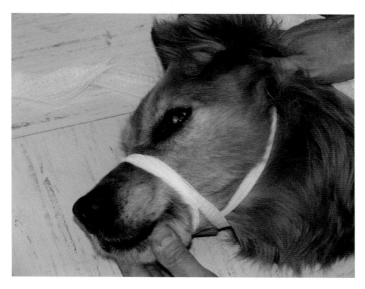

Figure 1.6. Gauze muzzle is now securely in place.

IV. A cloth or "field" muzzle must be removed immediately if an animal vomits or develops signs of respiratory distress or heat stress.

1.2.4. Restraining methods

I. Restraint pole(s) may be used to gain control of a dog (Fig. 1.7).

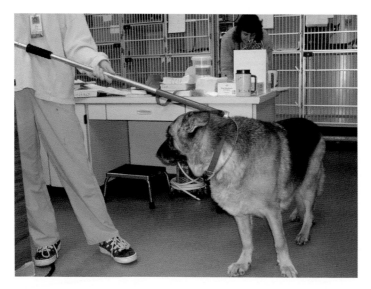

Figure 1.7. Catch-pole applied around the neck of a dog. With this pole the dog can be controlled and kept away from the rescuer, thus preventing personal injury.

II. To control the head: Stand, facing the same direction as the dog and to the side and slightly behind the dog. Grasp the loose skin on either side of the neck (Fig. 1.8).

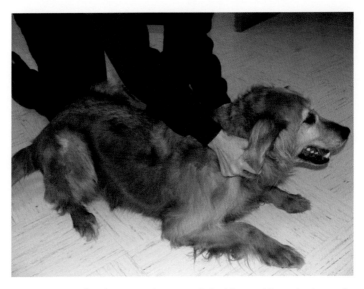

Figure 1.8. Restraint of a dog is easily accomplished by grabbing the loose skin on either side of the neck and remaining behind the dog in order to prevent being bitten.

III.   To restrain a dog in lateral position: Position yourself on the dorsal (back) side of the dog. Place one arm over the neck of the dog and hold the forearm of the down leg. Place your other arm over the lumbar/abdominal region and hold the tibial region of the down leg (Fig. 1.9).

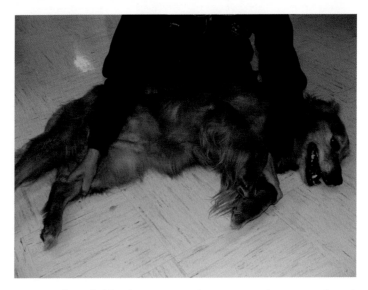

Figure 1.9. In order to hold a dog in a recumbent position, the rescuer places him/herself over the back. The rescuer then grabs a downside forelimb and hind limb. The forearm and elbow are applied to the dog's neck to further control the dog's movement.

1.3. **Vital Signs** (Table 1.1)

Table 1.1. The Canine Physical Examination.

Physical Parameter	Technique	Expected Results
Temperature	Rectal	100°–102.5°F
Pulse rate	Femoral arterial pulse, inner thigh	60–160 bpm
Heart rate	Auscultate the heart over the left fourth intercostal space	60–160 bpm, synchronous with the heart
Respiration lungs	Auscultate both right and left side. Observe breathing pattern.	Clear lung sounds. 15–30 breaths/minute. Panting is likely normal. No respiratory effort or distress.
Hydration	Feel mucous membranes (gums); pinch skin over the thorax.	Moist mucous membranes; skin snaps back.
Mucous membranes	Check color and capillary refill time (CRT)	Pink and CRT <2 seconds
Eyes	Clear cornea and anterior chamber, pupillary light response (PLR), conjunctiva, nictitating membrane, ophthalmoscopic retinal exam.	Clear, no discharge. PLR present in both eyes; nictitating membrane is flat and nonbulging; conjunctiva should be white with no evidence of excessive redness.
Ears	Visual exam, odor? Otoscopic examination.	No discharge or malodor. Tympanic membrane is intact.
Nose	Visual inspection. Place feather or microscopic slide under each nostril.	Minimal serous (clear) discharge; symmetrical airflow from each nostril.
Oral cavity	Lift lips; check teeth/gums. Open mouth; check tongue.	No blood or pain. Gag reflex is present. Licks nose after open mouth is closed.
Peripheral lymph nodes	Palpate parotid, submandibular, prescapular, axillary, and popliteal lymph nodes.	Small, nonpainful, or nonpalpable.
Abdomen	Observe. Palpate spleen (left), intestines, and urinary bladder.	Symmetrical, not distended, no retching, nonpainful.
Urogenital	Female: Vulva, mammary glands

Male: Prepuce, penis, scrotum. Lubricated, gloved finger, prostate. | No swelling, discharge, pain, wounds, or blood. |
Rectal/perineum	Observe area. Lubricated, gloved finger.	No swelling, wounds, pain, or blood.
Musculoskeletal	Observe gait and posture. Palpate any abnormalities.	No lameness, swelling, or stiffness.
Neurological	Mental state, cranial nerves, spinal pain, limb reflexes? Observation. Handler's comments.	Bright, alert, responsive to commands, visual, no spinal pain, normal cranial peripheral nerve reflexes.

1.3.1. Temperature (T)

I.   101.5°F (38.6°C) is "textbook" normal. A normal temperature may be within the range of 100°–102.5°F (37.7°–39.1°C).

II.   A rectal thermometer is most accurate, but an ear thermometer may be accurate as well if proper technique is used.

1.3.2. Pulse/heart rate (P/HR)—At rest

I.   Large- and giant-breed dogs: 60–100 bpm

II.   Medium-breed dogs: 90–110 bpm

III.   Small-breed dogs: 100–120 bpm

IV.   Relatively accessible arteries to assess pulse rate and strength:
   A.   Femoral artery—Generally easiest to find (Figs. 1.10 and 1.11).
   B.   Dorsal pedal artery—May be difficult to palpate. Can be helpful in assessing perfusion of the distal limb.

1.3.3. Respiratory rate (R or RR)—At rest

I.   15–30 bpm

II.   A normal, but significantly increased, resting respiratory rate (i.e., panting) may occur from anxiety or as a means of temperature control.

1.3.4. Mucous membrane (MM) color

I.   Normal: pink

II.   Subjective assessment of perfusion, oxygenation, shock, and homeostasis.

III.   Animals with partial or complete gray or black pigmentation of their gums can confound assessment of MM color. Mucosa of vulvar lips or prepuce can also be checked.

1.3.5. Capillary refill time (CRT)

I.   Normal: <2 seconds

II.   Press gum with finger and blanche to white. Remove finger and observe time for pink color to return (Fig. 1.12).

1.3.6. Blood pressure (BP)

I.   Hypotension: <90 mm Hg systolic (i.e., mean <60 mm Hg)

II.   Hypertension: currently defined as >180 mm Hg systolic; >100 mm Hg diastolic.

III.   Measuring BP out in the field is more problematic in animals than in people. The compact, easily used sphygmomanometer cuff unit for humans does not work on dogs. Patient cooperation can also be an issue. In the field hospital setting, the use of noninvasive BP monitors using Doppler or oscillometric technology is very practical for animals. Invasive (direct) BP measurement is best reserved for use in a critical care unit or surgical setting.

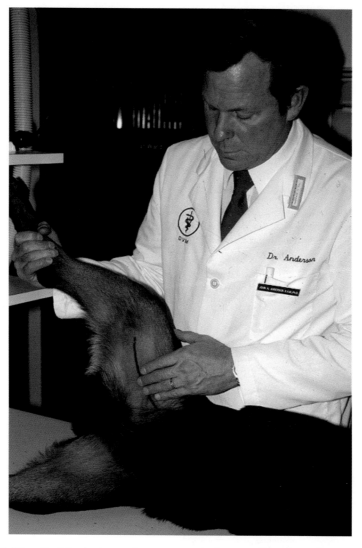

Figure 1.10. Dr. John Anderson demonstrating the location of the femoral artery on a dog. This is the best place to obtain a pulse rate and pressure in the dog.

1.4. Antiseptics and Flushing Agents

1.4.1. Saline solution: physiologic saline solution (PSS), 0.9% NaCl
   I. Best choice if a joint or medullary cavity of bone is exposed.

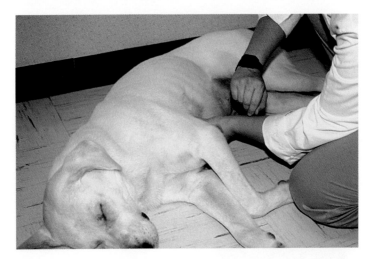

Figure 1.11. One can easily palpate the apex beat of the heart on the left side and at approximately intercostal space 6–7 at the costochondral junction. If an arrhythmia is noted, simultaneously palpate the heart beat and femoral pulse. The heart and pulse rate should be the same.

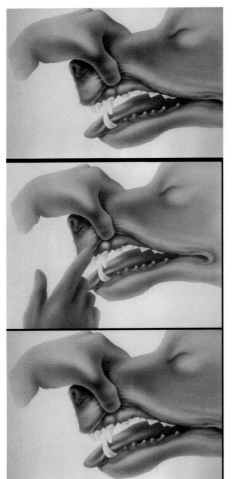

Figure 1.12. Capillary refill time in the dog is observed by gently lifting the lip; using an index finger, the gums are pressed to blanch out an area; and upon releasing the finger, begin counting the number of seconds it takes to reperfuse the area previously blanched by the index finger. A normal capillary refill time in a dog is less than 2 seconds.

1.4.2. Chlorhexidine solution 2%
I. Must be diluted with water. (Dilute to pale-blue color.)

1.4.3. Povidone-iodine (Betadine) solution
I. Must be diluted with water. (Dilute to iced tea color.)

1.4.4. Hydrogen peroxide (H_2O_2)
I. Best choice for puncture wounds
II. Should not be used repeatedly as an antiseptic as it is damaging to healthy tissue.

1.4.5. Do NOT use scrub agents (i.e., chlorhexidine scrub or Betadine scrub) on wounds as these are detergents.

1.5. Antimicrobial Ointments (e.g., Neosporin, Triple Antibiotic, Novalsan Ointment)

1.5.1. Antimicrobial ointments may be applied to wounds initially to decrease bacterial contamination or control infection, but once a wound is considered clean, ointments should no longer be used.

1.5.2. Antimicrobial ointments should not be used if the wound will be sutured or if a wound will require more definitive treatment imminently.

1.5.3. Antimicrobial ointments should not be used if a joint or medullary bone is exposed.

1.6. Bandaging Principles

1.6.1. In terms of first aid, the purpose of a bandage is to control hemorrhage, prevent further contamination of the wound, and provide comfort in stabilizing the wound until definitive medical treatment can be obtained.

1.6.2. First-aid bandage components
I. Stirrups (1-inch white tape)
II. Telfa (± sterile) no-stick pad
III. Cast padding, Soft Kling, roll cotton
IV. Roll gauze–conforming (2- to 4-inch)
V. Vet Wrap (2- or 4-inch)
VI. Elastikon (2- to 4-inch)

1.6.3. Wrap each layer of a bandage in the same direction (Figs. 1.13–1.17).

1.6.4. Bandages on limbs should not be placed so as to create a tourniquet effect.

1.6.5. Body-wrap bandages should not restrict the dog's ability to breathe, and the caregiver should recognize temperature and humidity considerations and the increased risk of heat stroke.

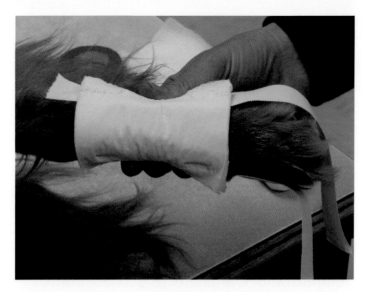

Figure 1.13. Application of a bandage on the distal forelimb begins with placement of two tape strips applied on the medial and lateral sides of the limb. A gauze pad is being applied over the wound.

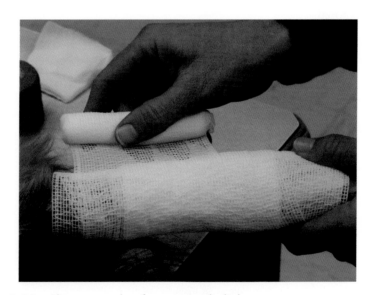

Figure 1.14. Kling gauze is best for wrapping the limb.

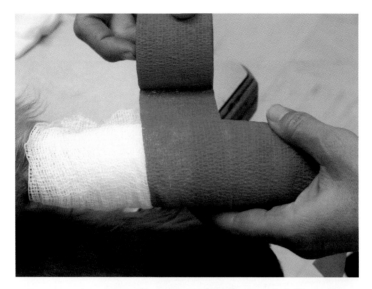

Figure 1.15. Once the gauze is applied, an elasticized product like VetWrap is used to secure the gauze.

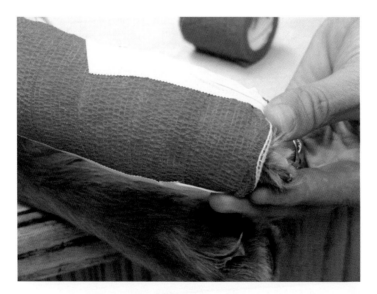

Figure 1.16. It is important to leave the digits out of the bandage. This not only provides the dog better traction but also allows examination of the toes to note if the bandage might be too tight. If the two middle digits are spread apart under a bandage, it is very likely the bandage is too tight and should be loosened immediately.

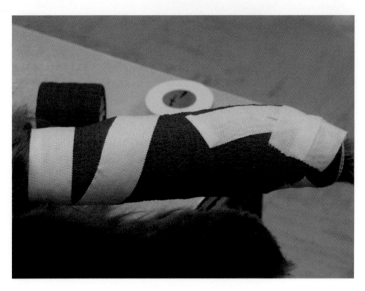

Figure 1.17. Adhesive tape is wrapped around the VetWrap in order to further secure the bandage.

1.6.6. Unless a bandage is being applied specifically for a wound to digit 3 or 4, these digit nails should be visible when bandaging a limb. This allows assessment of swelling and perfusion of the bandaged limb (Figs. 1.18–1.20).

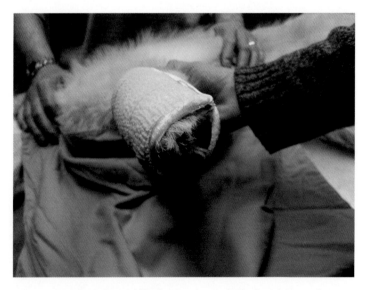

Figure 1.18. Notice how the middle digits are outside the bandage and are in apposition to each other. This is how the toes should look if the bandage is not too tight.

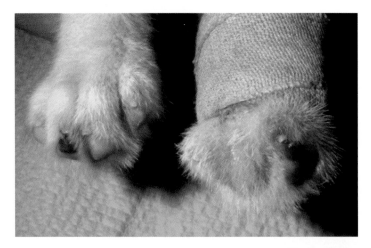

Figure 1.19. Should the bandage be applied too tightly, the middle two digits will separate and should be promptly removed and then reapplied.

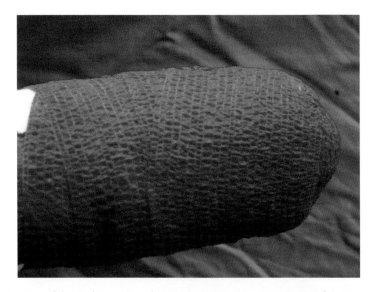

Figure 1.20. If the pads are injured, it is sometimes necessary to cover the entire extremity with a bandage.

1.6.7. When applying a bandage to a limb, the use of stirrups will help keep the bandage in place (Figs. 1.21).

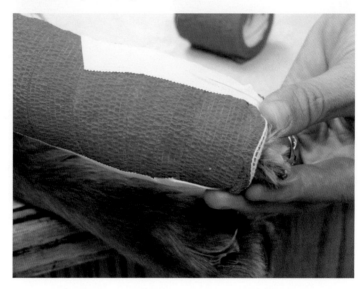

Figure 1.21. The final step in applying a bandage is to take the tape stirrups and extend them up over the bandage. This will help secure the bandage and prevent the dog from easily removing it.

1.6.8. The carpal pad/accessory carpal bone is a potential pressure point. First-aid bandages do not have to be too concerned with this point, but "definitive" bandages should be modified with "donut hole" padding to protect against pressure necrosis (Fig. 1.22).

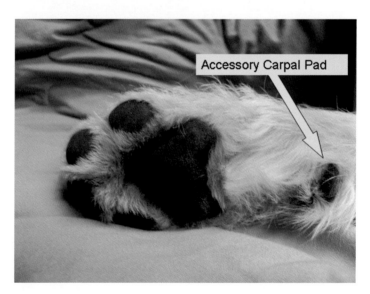

Figure 1.22. When applying a bandage to the distal forelimb, be aware of the location of the accessory carpal pad (*blue arrow*). It is located on the caudal aspect of the lower limb.

1.6.9. Except for initial hemorrhage control, puncture wounds should not be bandaged.

1.6.10. Wet bandages should be changed as soon as possible.

1.7. Emergency Conditions Affecting Working Dogs

1.7.1. Shock

I. *Shock* is defined as abnormal tissue perfusion leading to abnormal cellular metabolism. There are many causes of shock which have led to the following etiological classification:

    A. Hypovolemic shock (dehydration)

    B. Cardiogenic shock (heart diseases and arrhythmias)

    C. Traumatic shock (hit by a car, kicked by a horse)

    D. Septic shock (parvovirus enteritis, pyometritis, gastric dilatation–volvulus)

II. The classic signs of an animal in shock include the presence of a weak pulse; pale MM (gums); increased heart, pulse, and RR; and cold extremities (feet and ears) (Fig. 1.23).

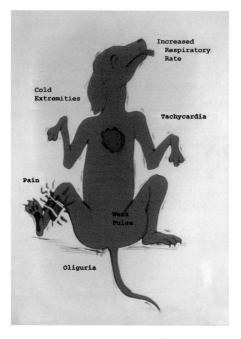

Figure 1.23. Common clinical findings in a dog suffering from shock include weak pulse, pain, tachycardia, cold extremities, oliguria, and an increase in respiratory rate.

    A.   Tachycardia—heart rate >160 bpm

    B.   Hypotension—pallor, CRT >3 seconds, weak pulses

    C.   Tachypnea—>30 bpm

    D.   Hypothermia—temperature <98°F

    E.   Weakness, restlessness, depression, mental confusion

    F.   Reduced urinary output—<0.5–1 ml/lb/hr

    G.   Coma, dilation of pupils

  III. First aid management of shock involves the following actions:

    A.   Be careful!! The pet is often in pain, possibly excited, and may bite or claw you.

    B.   Check the airway and be sure the animal is breathing.

    C.   Apply a pressure bandage to any obvious hemorrhage

    D.   Keep the animal warm and try to calm the animal.

    E.   If there is evidence of a central neurological injury, immobilize the pet on a solid surface such as a piece of plywood. Be very careful when moving the animal!

    F.   If a fracture involves a lower part of the extremity, apply a temporary splint.

  IV. Transport the animal to a veterinarian's hospital as soon and quickly as possible.

    A.   Treatment will begin with the use of crystalloid fluids (Normosol-R, Ringer's lactate, 0.9% sodium chloride).

      1.   The initial dosage one should be prepared to administer intravenously (IV) is calculated using the following formula: ml = BW (lb) × 40 ml/hr (≈90 ml/kg/hr).

    B.   Corticosteroids continue to be controversial but are often administered IV after at least 25% of the crystalloids have been given.

      1.   Dexamethasone sodium phosphate: 1–4 mg/kg IV one time.

    C.   Sodium bicarbonate is rarely required in the treatment of shock in the dog unless the cause of the shock is associated with ingestion of agents such as ethylene glycol (antifreeze), raisins, or wood alcohol.

    D.   Depending on the amount of blood lost, it is sometimes useful to administer either whole blood or blood substitute products.

      1.   The amount of blood to be administered is usually based upon the following formula: for each 1% rise in packed cell volume (hematocrit) you want to achieve, it will require 1 ml/lb body weight of whole blood.

        a.   Sample calculation: If the 75-pound dog's packed cell volume is currently 15% and you want to raise that value to 30%, it will require 1 ml/1 lb to raise the PCV by 1%. To raise the PCV 15%, it will require 15 ml/lb. The dog weighs 75 pounds, and therefore it will require a transfusion of 1125 ml of whole blood.

1.7.2. Neurological Injuries

  I. Neurological injuries to a working dog most commonly affect either the spinal cord or the brain.

  II. Clues to the presence of such injuries are often seen by observing the appearance of the dog.

A. The three motor postures of most significant concern are as follows (Fig. 1.24):

    1. Shiff-Sherrington posture: Severe spinal cord injury located between the second thoracic and third lumbar vertebra.

        a. Extensor rigidity in the front limbs and flaccid paralysis of the rear limbs (Fig. 1.24A).

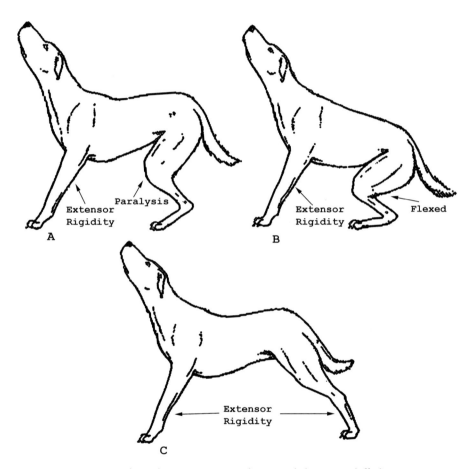

Figure 1.24. Neurological postures seen in the injured dog. **A,** Schiff-Sherrington motor posture suggesting a severe spinal cord injury located between T2 and L5 vertebrae. The dog will show upper motor neuron signs, with extensor rigidity of the forelimbs and flaccid paralysis of the rear limbs, and usually there is no sensation of pain when squeezing the toes of the rear limb. Generally, this has a grave prognosis. **B,** Decerebellate motor posture with the front limbs extended, the head thrown back (opisthotonus), and the rear limbs flexed. This usually suggests an injury to the cerebellum and carries a fair prognosis for recovery. **C,** Decerebrate motor posture with extensor rigidity in the forelimb and hind limb and opisthotonus. This posture generally carries a grave prognosis.

    2. Decerebrate rigidity: Head injury but usually has a favorable outcome.

        a. Extensor rigidity in the front limbs and rear limbs are flexed (Fig. 1.24B).

    3. Decerebellate rigidity: Severe brain injury with a very grave prognosis.

        a. Extensor rigidity in the front and rear limbs (Fig. 1.24C).

III. First aid care would involve the following:

    A. Carefully transport the dog to a veterinary hospital as quickly as possible.

    B. With a spinal cord injury, place the animal on a back board, sheet of plywood, or other mobile solid surface (i.e., door). Tape the animal to the surface so it is unable to move and transport to the nearest veterinary hospital.

1.7.3. Hypoglycemia

I. Hypoglycemia may result when the blood glucose is abnormally low.

    A. Normal blood glucose for a dog = 70–140 mg/dl.

    B. Hypoglycemia results when the blood glucose is <60 mg/dl.

II. Clinical signs of hypoglycemia

    A. Weakness, incoordination, confusion, collapse

    B. Muscle tremors

    C. Seizures

    D. Hyperthermia or hypothermia

III. Treatment

    A. 50% dextrose given at a dosage of 0.5–1.0 ml/lb slowly IV. If possible, dilute the 50% solution to at least a 10% solution to avoid phlebitis following administration of a hypertonic solution (50% dextrose).

    B. Intravenous fluids: 5% dextrose in water or Normosol-R + 5% dextrose or Ringer's lactate + 5% dextrose.

        1. Calculate the volume required by using the following formula:

        $ml = (BW_{kg} \times 30) + 70$.

            a. Sample calculation: How much fluid should a 75-pound (34-kg) dog receive? $ml = (34 \times 30) + 70$ or ≈ 1093 ml over 24 hours.

    C. Diazepam may be needed to control seizures.

        1. Intravenous dosage: 1 mg/kg to effect.

        2. Per rectum dosage: 1–2 mg/kg to effect and a maximum dosage of 40 mg.

IV. Control body temperature with cooling or warming as needed.

IV. Beware of cerebral edema with seizures.

    A. Dexamethasone sodium phosphate: 1–4 mg/lb IV.

    B. Mannitol: 0.25 g/kg IV.

1.7.4. Gastric dilatation-volvulus (canine bloat)

I. Gastric dilatation-volvulus (GDV) is a peracute condition predominantly affecting large-breed, deep-chested dogs. It results from an abnormal, acute accumulation of air in the dog's stomach. The source of this air is believed to be from abnormal swallowing of air (aerophagia) (Fig. 1.25).

    A. Diet has been implicated in the etiology of canine bloat but thus far there is no evidence to support this theory.

    B. Most clinically affected GDV dogs have gas-filled stomachs, and analysis of the gas has shown it to be consistent with room air.

    C. GDV appears most commonly in the nervous and hyperactive dogs.

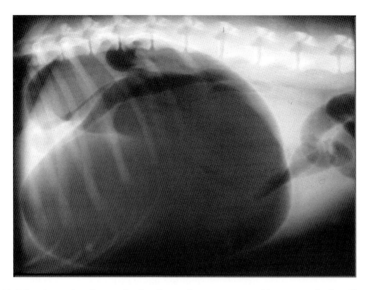

Figure 1.25. Lateral radiograph of a dog with acute gastric dilatation-volvulus. The air-filled stomach now fills most of the abdominal cavity. Notice the twisting of the stomach whereby the pylorus is now dorsal to its normal ventral position within the abdomen. The rotated stomach impinges on both the caudal vena cava and portal vein, leading to severe shock.

II. Clinical signs of GDV in the working dog.
  A. The classic picture of a GDV dog is described with the following three characteristics:
    1. Retching with the inability to vomit ("dry-heaves").
    2. Abdominal distention with tympany.
      a. Using one's index finger and thumping on the right side near the last rib will result in a very tympanic (drum-like) sound.
    3. The inability to pass an orogastric tube.
      a. Passing an orogastric tube relieves the gaseous accumulations, but failure to pass a stomach tube does not rule out the presence of gastric volvulus (twisting of the esophagus and stomach).
  B. The GDV dog will exhibit abdominal discomfort, will often pace about, and will whine due to pain.
  C. There are usually clinical signs of shock with the HR and P being elevated and pulse pressure being decreased.
  D. The CRT is quite variable. If the dog is in the hyperdynamic phase of shock, the CRT will be accelerated or normal. If the shock is hypodynamic, the CRT will be prolonged or normal.
  E. When viewed over the dog's back looking forward, the abdomen tends to protrude unevenly to the right.
III. Treatment of GDV
  A. Emergency treatment involves the following:
    1. Gastric decompression
      a. Most commonly involves the passage of a large bore (colt-sized) orogastric tube.

- Measure the length of the tube by measuring from the tip of the dog's nose to the last rib. Make a mark on the tube to alert you when the stomach has been reached.
  - Use a roll of 2-inch tape inserted behind the canine teeth to pass the tube and prevent the dog from biting down.
- As the tube is passed, never push the tube too vigorously as this might result in a ruptured esophagus.
- If obstruction is encountered, stop and either let a more experienced person pass the tube or, as an alternative, you may need to trocarize the stomach through the abdominal wall.
  - Using a 10- to 14-gauge, 1.5-inch, sterile hypodermic needle, first percuss the abdomen on the right side. You are seeking an area that is quite resonant. If you do not have a resonant sound, it may be due to the fact the spleen has also rotated with the stomach. Do NOT trocarize through the spleen!
  - Once you have found that resonant area (usually located on the right and at the lower half of the abdomen), quickly insert the needle all the way to the hub. Foul-smelling gas will escape the needle. Leave the needle in place, and as the stomach decompresses, gently press upon the cranial abdomen to release even more gas.
  - Once you have trocarized the stomach, it is usually possible to now pass the orogastric tube.

B. Shock therapy is begun by inserting a large-bore (16- to 18-gauge) catheter in either the cephalic or lateral saphenous vein.

 1. Begin crystalloid administration at a rate of 40 ml/lb/hr ($\approx$90 ml/kg/hr).

C. Transport the dog quickly to a veterinary hospital.

D. Do not think the stomach has rotated back to its normal position even though you were able to pass the stomach tube.

E. Definitive treatment for GDV requires a veterinary surgeon.

 1. Treatment of shock
 2. Surgical replacement of the stomach to its normal position.
 3. Surgical prevention of future rotation of the stomach.

1.7.5. Heat stroke/hyperthermia

I. This refers to an extremely high core body temperature >105°F/40.6°C that occurs when excess heat, generated by body metabolism, exercise, and/or environmental conditions, exceeds the body's ability to dissipate that heat.

II. Heat loss can occur by convection (air currents), conduction, radiation, or evaporation.

III. Dogs do not sweat (except through their pads) so this method of evaporative cooling is not available to them. Dogs pant and drool to cool themselves by evaporation, and vessels on the skin and periphery dilate to cool by radiation and convection.

IV. Core temperatures >106°F are harmful to cellular metabolism. At core temperatures above 109°F, things fall apart biochemically: oxidative phosphorylation is uncoupled, cell membrane function is impaired, and critical enzymes are denatured. Organ failure may occur (because of this cell death) even after the core temperature has returned to normal.

    A. Early signs of hyperthermia
      1. Rapid panting
      2. Rapid HR
      3. Bounding P
      4. Bright-red and dry MM (gums)
      5. CRT <0.5 second
    B. Later signs
      1. Profound depression
      2. Unable to stand
      3. Weak pulse
      4. Pale/ashen MM
      5. Vomiting/diarrhea
    C. Terminal signs
      1. Shallow respirations
      2. Seizures
      3. Coma
      4. Death
  V. First aid treatment for hyperthermia
    A. Transport to or create a cooler environment (e.g., shade, air-conditioned car, etc.)
    B. Ideally, soak hair coat with COOL water (55°–65°F), or place in COOL water (55°–65°F) bath.
      1. Do NOT use ice baths or cold (35°–40°F) water baths as this promotes skin vessel constriction, which impairs heat loss and induces shivering, which increases heat production.
    C. Any water (e.g., water bottle, etc.) cooler than ≈90°F can be used, with fanning, to aid in cooling.
    D. Moving air over the dog will help with evaporative and convection cooling (e.g., fanning).
    E. Cool packs applied to large vessel areas (inguinal, axillary, and jugular) will cool blood returning to the body core. Towels soaked in cool/cold water and changed frequently can be used.
    F. An extreme measure is to use a syringe to give a cool (65°–75°F) water enema (20–40 ml). This must be done with care, so as not to damage the rectum.
    G. When body temperature drops to 103°F, stop active cooling. Continue to monitor core body temperature as it may continue to decline and warming procedures may be indicated.
    H. The goal is to reduce the core body temperature to approximately 102°F in 30–60 minutes.
    I. Transport to definitive medical care ASAP.

1.7.6. Hypothermia and frostbite

  I. Degrees of hypothermia
    A. Mild is 86°–90°F and can be withstood for 24–36 hours
    B. Moderate is 72°–77°F, and animal may survive for 4–24 hours
    C. Severe is <60°F with a maximum survival of 5–6 hours.
    D. Frostbite when body temperature is <93°F.

II.   Clinical signs
   A.   Diminished consciousness
   B.   Low BP (weak/absent pulses)
   C.   Bradycardia
   D.   Shallow, infrequent respirations
   E.   Dilated pupils
   F.   Delayed, diminished reflexes
   G.   Shivering
   H.   Increased muscle tone without shivering (T < 90°F)
   I.   Cyanotic/pale body part
   J.   Anesthesia (no pain sensation) of frozen body part
III.   Treatment
   A.   Airway, oxygen
   B.   Warm IV solutions to 104°–109°F.
      1.   Use extreme caution in delivering IV fluids while the animal is
      hypothermic.
      2.   Most commonly, the volume to be administered starts at a rate of
      10 ml/lb/hr.
   C.   Active/passive rewarming
      1.   Mild hypothermia: Remove from cold, wrap with blankets, warm water
      bottles.
      2.   Moderate: Warm water bottles, heating pads, ± warm water immersion
      (careful not to burn skin).
      3.   Severe: Use active rewarming techniques.
         a.   Continuous warm IV fluids.
         b.   Warm peritoneal dialysis.
         c.   Warm water enema.
         d.   Warm water gastric lavage.
      4.   Frostbitten areas: Remove from the cold, provide rapid rewarming with
      immersion in warm water (102°–104°F), apply warm compresses, prevent
      refreezing, do not rub affected digits.
   D.   Supportive care
      1.   Analgesics (morphine, oxymorphone, butorphanol [Torbugesic],
      buprenorphine [Buprenex])
      2.   Antibiotics—penicillin, cephalexin
      3.   Local injury wound care
   E.   Patient monitoring
      1.   Body temperature (avoid hyperthermia).
      2.   Urine output (maintain >1 ml/lb/hr).
      3.   Blood chemistry values may be useful.
      4.   Pneumonia is a common complication.

1.8. Common Injuries

1.8.1. Lacerations
I.   First aid principles
   A.   Quickly assess the wound for depth, severity, and structures (i.e., tendons,
   joints, nerves, vessels) involved.
   B.   Control hemorrhage with direct pressure or pressure bandage. (If unable
   to achieve some degree of hemostasis, continue direct pressure or apply

pressure bandage, if possible, and seek definitive medical treatment as soon as possible.)

C.   Clean and flush the wound with PSS, dilute chlorhexidine solution, dilute Betadine solution, or hydrogen peroxide.

D.   Blot dry

E.   Apply an antimicrobial ointment if definitive assessment and treatment will be delayed.

F.   Apply a bandage.

G.   Obtain definitive medical assessment and treatment.

H.   Antibiotics and/or anti-inflammatory drugs may be indicated.

II.   Lacerations may involve major arteries, veins, nerves, tendons, etc. If these structures are involved, the primary concern will be to control hemorrhage (via direct pressure or pressure bandage) and seek definitive medical treatment as soon as possible.

1.8.2.   Pad lacerations

I.   Normal appearance of dog pads (Fig. 1.26).

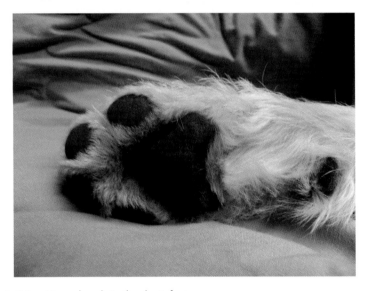

Figure 1.26.   Normal pads in the dog's foot.

II.   Most pad lacerations are best managed by bandaging and second-intention healing (granulation).

III.   If a digit or metacarpal/metatarsal pad laceration requires sutures, a splint will also have to be applied. However, these lacerations should be bandaged until definitive suturing can be done.

IV.   First aid for pad lacerations

A.   Remove gross contamination (glass, metal, gravel)

B.   Flush with PSS, dilute chlorhexidine solution, dilute betadine solution, or hydrogen peroxide.

C.   Blot dry.

D.   Apply antimicrobial ointment.

E.   Apply bandage covering the entire foot: stirrups, Telfa, Soft Kling or cast padding, gauze, Vet Wrap, Elastikon (Fig. 1.27).

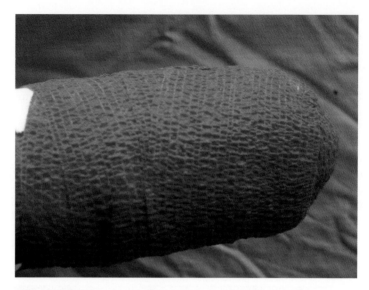

Figure 1.27. Bandaging a foot pad injury requires that the entire foot be covered by the bandage.

    F. Bandages should be changed daily initially, and then may be changed every 2–4 days.

1.8.3. Limb lacerations

  I. First aid for limb lacerations:
    A. Many of these lacerations are best managed definitively by suturing, so field first aid is primarily to control hemorrhage, decrease contamination, and approximate tissue edges.
    B. Flush with PSS, dilute chlorhexidine solution, dilute Betadine solution, or hydrogen peroxide. If a joint is exposed, PSS should be used.
    C. Blot dry.
    D. If a wound is heavily contaminated, and definitive treatment will be delayed, apply an antimicrobial ointment. Do NOT apply if joint is exposed.
    E. Generally, lacerations distal to the elbow and stifle (knee) are amenable to bandaging.
    F. Apply bandage: stirrups, Telfa, Soft Kling or cast padding, gauze, Vet Wrap, Elastikon top and foot.
    G. Apply bandage from toes (leaving nails of digits 3 and 4 visible) to ≈2 inches above the laceration (Fig. 1.28).

1.8.4. Head and face lacerations

  I. First aid for head and face lacerations:
    A. Many of these lacerations are best managed definitively by suturing, so field first aid is primarily to control hemorrhage and decrease contamination.
    B. Hemorrhage is often best controlled with direct pressure using 4 × 4 gauze sponges, pads, towels, etc. and hand pressure, as applying an effective pressure bandage in this region can be difficult.
    C. Flush with PSS, dilute chlorhexidine solution, dilute betadine solution, or hydrogen peroxide. Use caution with solutions around eyes.

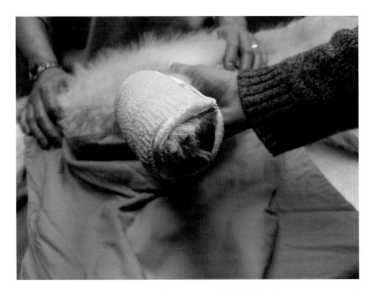

Figure 1.28. If possible, keep the toes free to provide the dog better traction and to provide you the opportunity to observe the toes to detect swelling when an excessively tight bandage is applied.

D. If a wound is heavily contaminated and definitive treatment will be delayed, apply an antimicrobial ointment.
E. Bandage if possible.
F. If the ears are not wounded, they should be free of the bandages (Figs. 1.29–1.32).

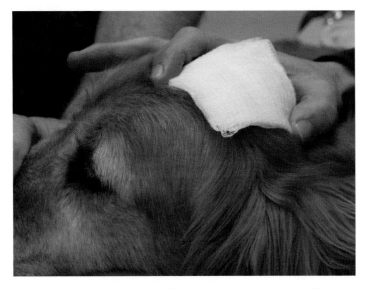

Figure 1.29. Wounds on the dog's head are covered with a gauze/Telfa bandage.

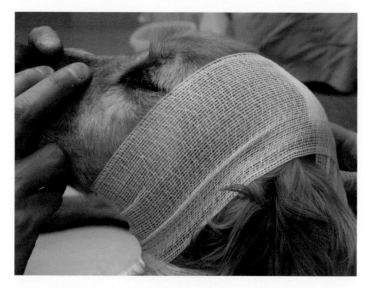

Figure 1.30. Kling™ gauze is wrapped around the head to hold the gauze/telfa pad in place.

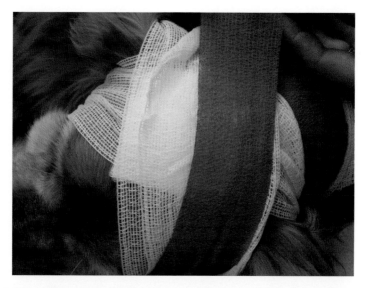

Figure 1.31. Wrapping the head in a crisscross fashion will allow the ear flaps to be free. Following the application of the Kling bandage, VetWrap is used to hold it in place.

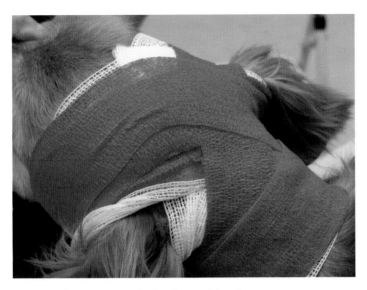

Figure 1.32. Final appearance of a head wound bandage.

1.8.5. Neck and trunk lacerations
I. First aid for neck and trunk lacerations:
   A. Many of these lacerations are best managed definitively by suturing, so field first aid is primarily to control hemorrhage and decrease contamination.
   B. Flush with PSS, dilute chlorhexidine solution, dilute betadine solution, or hydrogen peroxide.
   C. If a wound is heavily contaminated, and definitive treatment will be delayed, apply an antimicrobial ointment.
   D. Bandages must be applied with attention to airway, swallowing, venous return, breathing, and heat stress.

1.8.6. Puncture wounds
I. There are two primary considerations in the assessment of puncture wounds. The first addresses immediate, life-threatening hemodynamic issues (bleeding, cardiac tamponade, tension pneumothorax). The second, and more common, relates to potential morbidity associated with bacterial infection, both anaerobic and aerobic.
II. If one suspects a puncture wound has penetrated into the chest cavity, abdominal cavity, or pelvic canal, definitive medical care should be obtained immediately.
III. If the wound can be addressed in the field, clip the hair from the site of the wound, if possible. This will facilitate future wound site identification for definitive treatment.
IV. Gently probe a puncture wound with a sterile blunt instrument or moistened sterile cotton swab to assess depth, direction of track, and presence of foreign body.
V. Use a syringe (NO needle) or apply antiseptic solution to a sterile cotton swab to flush and cleanse wound.

VI.   Hydrogen peroxide is the best initial flushing/cleansing agent for puncture wounds. Subsequent flushing should be done with dilute chlorhexidine solution or dilute Betadine solution.

VII.   The goal of treatment is to promote drainage, decrease the risk of developing an anaerobic environment, and encourage second-intention healing from the deep tissues outward. To this end:

    A.   Antimicrobial ointments should NOT be applied to puncture wounds.

    B.   Puncture wounds should NOT be bandaged.

    C.   Puncture wounds should NOT be sutured.

    D.   Surface crusts should be removed and the track flushed.

VIII.   Obtain definitive medical care as antibiotics and anti-inflammatory agents are indicated.

1.8.7.   Torn nails

I.   Torn nails are very painful and will continue to be painful until the torn horn is removed.

II.   First aid for a torn nail:

    A.   Flush with or soak in antiseptic solution. Dilute chlorhexidine solution or dilute Betadine solution is best.

    B.   Reduce torn horn to normal anatomic position if possible.

    C.   Bandage paw.

    D.   Obtain definitive medical treatment for debridement of nail.

    E.   Antibiotics and anti-inflammatory agents may be indicated.

1.8.8.   Broken toes

I.   Broken toes are extremely painful. Definitive treatment options include coaptation, internal fixation, or amputation.

II.   First aid for a broken toe is primarily to prevent unnecessary motion in the area and obtain definitive treatment as soon as possible. In terms of first aid, generally speaking, this means doing nothing.

    A.   Applying a splint or bandage to the paw area will often cause more pain and discomfort for the dog.

    B.   Dogs are able to ambulate on three legs and this effectively protects the affected paw.

    C.   If it is not possible for the dog to ambulate on three legs (e.g., through building rubble, across water, other injuries present), it is best to carry the dog.

1.8.9.   Eye injuries

I.   All eye injuries should have definitive medical evaluation and treatment as soon as possible. (Irritation or foreign body removal that resolves 100% with PSS flushing may be the exception to this rule.)

II.   When examining eyes, avoid facing the dog into direct sunlight.

III.   There are various eye ointments available.

    A.   Ointments should NOT be used until a dog is through working.

    B.   Ointments containing steroids should NOT be used until a definitive ophthalmic evaluation has been done.

1.8.10.   Eye Irritation and conjunctivitis

I.   The most common eye problem is irritation and conjunctivitis.

II.   Eye irritation can be minimized by periodic flushing across the eye and under the eyelids with PSS.

1.8.11.   Ocular foreign bodies

I.   Foreign bodies trapped under the eyelids are treated by flushing with PSS in combination with judicious use of a moistened cotton swab/gauze sponge.

II.   Dogs have a third eyelid (the nictitating membrane) that comes "up" from the ventral medial canthus to cover the eye and offer another layer of protection. Topical anesthetic is required to examine under and clear foreign bodies from behind the nictitating membrane.

Suggested Reading

Wingfield, W. E. *Veterinary Emergency Medicine Secrets*. Philadelphia, Hanley and Belfus, 2001.

Wingfield, W. E., M. R. Raffe. *The Veterinary ICU Book*. Jackson Hole, WY, Teton New Media, 2002.

CHAPTER 2
FIRST AID FOR WORKING HORSES

Sally B. Palmer, DVM

Situations may arise in a preresponse staging or disaster/emergency response where a working horse will require medical attention and a veterinarian familiar with equine care is not readily available. In this setting, small animal or nonequine livestock veterinarians, veterinary technicians, or human medical personnel such as physicians, nurses, physician assistants, paramedics, or emergency medical technicians may be called on to administer first aid until more definitive equine veterinary care is obtained. This chapter aims to help those familiar with medicine use their skills and knowledge to stabilize and provide treatment for an unfamiliar patient—the horse.

2. First Aid for Working Horses

2.1. Handling

2.1.1. When handling any animal, *safety* is paramount. You must take into consideration your safety, the safety of the people assisting you, the safety of bystanders, and the safety of the horse. Evaluate the area and minimize hazards before addressing the horse. Decrease the number of bystanders, clear away obstacles, or move to a quieter, more secure location if possible.

2.1.2. The main risks of injury to personnel are being kicked, struck (kicked with a front limb), stepped on, jumped on, knocked down, or bitten. To minimize these risks, it is important to communicate your intentions and expectations verbally to your assistant(s) and to any bystanders who could be injured and to communicate by touch and demeanor with the horse.

2.1.3. The horse should be held by a capable assistant rather than tied, and this assistant assumes a critical role in securing everyone's safety. The assistant holding the horse should be on the same side of the horse as the medic. If the medic changes sides, the assistant should also change sides. Ideally, everyone, including bystanders, should be on the same side of the horse. Because this is not always practical, it is the medic's and assistant's responsibility to maintain an awareness of bystanders and to warn them to move out of a danger zone.

2.2. Physical Restraint

2.2.1.   Most horses with which you are presented will have on a halter (and lead rope) or bridle (and reins). When holding the lead rope or reins, do NOT loop the excess lead rope or reins around your hand (Fig. 2.1). Rather, fold or flake the excess in your hand (Fig. 2.2). This will allow you to let out some slack if needed while minimizing the risk of serious injury to your hands.

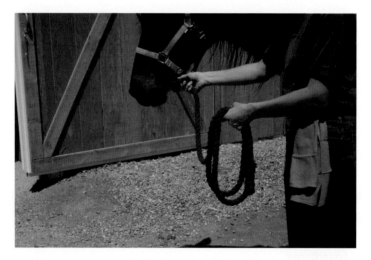

Figure 2.1   The *incorrect* way to hold a lead. Do not loop the excess lead around your hand as this increases the risk of serious injury.

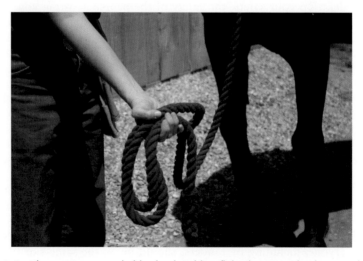

Figure 2.2   The *correct* way to hold a lead. Fold or flake the excess lead in your hand.

2.2.2. Stud Chains (Stallion Chains)

I. Stud chains are a type of lead rope with approximately 20 inches (50 cm) of small-link chain on the clip end (Fig. 2.3). This lead rope is attached to the halter in various configurations (over the nose, across the gum, or in the mouth) to allow the handler a more severe method of control (Figs. 2.4 and 2.5). In experienced hands, stud chains can be effective. In inexperienced hands, they can be dangerous.

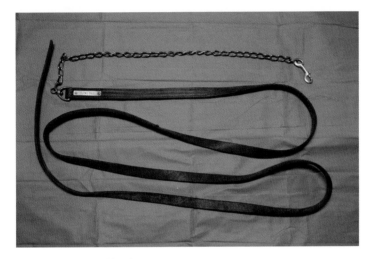

Figure 2.3 Stud chain and lead.

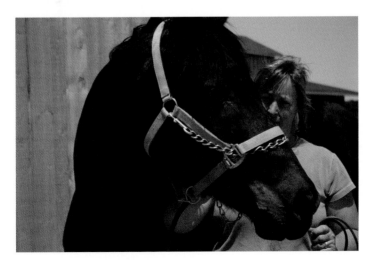

Figure 2.4 Stud chain over the nose.

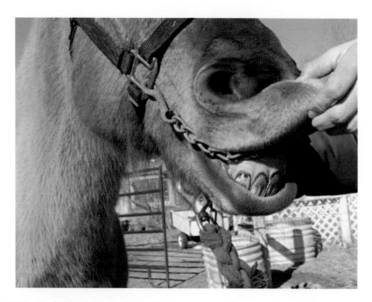

Figure 2.5 Stud chain across the gums.

2.2.3. Twitches

I.   A twitch can be a very helpful aid in restraining a horse for examination or treatment (Fig. 2.6). They are applied to the upper lip of a horse as a method of acupressure and distraction (Figs. 2.7 and 2.8). It has been suggested that this acupressure triggers the release of endorphins.

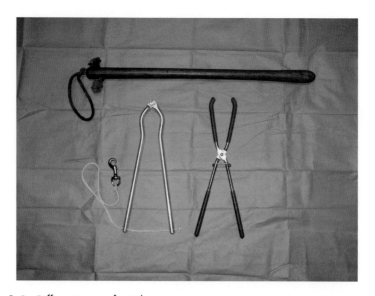

Figure 2.6 Different types of twitches.

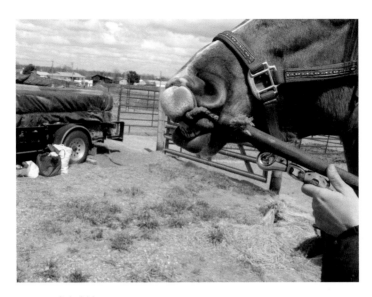

Figure 2.7 Twitch held by an assistant.

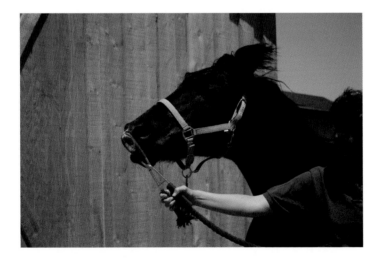

Figure 2.8 Self-holding twitch.

II.   The person handling the twitch must stay to the side of the horse and apply the twitch with "Goldilocks pressure"—not too much and not too little—to be effective. As with stud chains, twitches are best used by an experienced assistant as they can cause injury to the horse if excessive pressure is applied, and they should not be used for extended periods of time. The handler is also at risk of being struck by the horse or handle of the twitch.

III.   Ear twitches and neck twitches are handholds that should not be used.

2.2.4. Ropes

I.   The use of ropes to "incapacitate" a leg or restrict its motion is not an appropriate method of physical restraint in a first aid or disaster setting; as such, scotch hobbling, tying a leg up, single side line, etc. should not be used for restraint.

2.3. Chemical Restraint

2.3.1. Chemical sedation is the cornerstone of restraint for horses.

2.3.2. These drugs are much more effective when the patient is calm; in an excited or high-anxiety state, the horse will frequently override the sedative effects of these drugs. Minimizing commotion, removing the horse from a chaotic area, or simply allowing him to calm down before examining him can help make the use of sedatives more rewarding.

2.3.3. Do NOT become complacent around a sedated horse. A tranquilized or sedated horse can suddenly jump, bite, kick, or strike with lightning speed.

2.3.4. Drugs commonly used for sedation and chemical restraint are listed in Appendix A (p. 76).

2.4. Vital Signs (Table 2.1)

Table 2.1. Expected Normal Values for the Resting Healthy Horse.

Horses	Value
Rectal Temperature	
Foals during first few days	Up to 102.7°F (39.3°C)
Foals to 4th year	99.5°F–101.3°F (37.5°–38.5°C)
Horses, Adult	99.5°F–101.3°F (37.5°–38.5°C)
Horses, over 5 years	99.5°F–101.4°F (37.5°–38.0°C)
Pulse/Heart Rate	
Foals, Newborn	128 bpm
Foals, 1–2 days	100–120 bpm
Foals, <2 weeks	80–120 bpm
Foals, 3–6 months	64–76 bpm
Foals, >6–12 months	48–72 bpm
Foals, 1–2 years	40–56 bpm
Adult Horses	
Stallions	28–32 bpm
Geldings	33–39 bpm
Mares	40–56 bpm
Respiratory Rate	
Foals	14–15 bpm
Horses, adult	9–10 bpm

2.4.1. Temperature (T)

I.   Normal temperature is 99° to 100.5°F (37.2° to 38°C).

II.   A rectal thermometer is most accurate and should be lubricated to ease insertion. One should hold on to the thermometer or attach a lanyard to it that can be clipped to the tail to prevent the thermometer from being sucked into the rectum (Fig. 2.9).

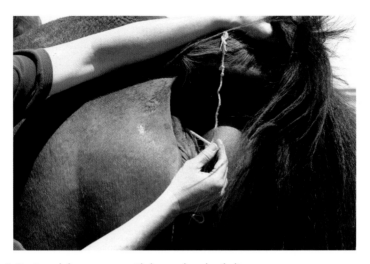

Figure 2.9   Rectal thermometer with lanyard and tail clip.

2.4.2. Pulse/heart rate (P/HR)

I.   Normal resting HR is in the range of 35 to 45 beats per minute (bpm).

II.   To obtain HR in a standing horse, the heart is most easily auscultated on the left thoracic wall just caudal to the long head of the triceps brachii muscle and elbow (Fig. 2.10).

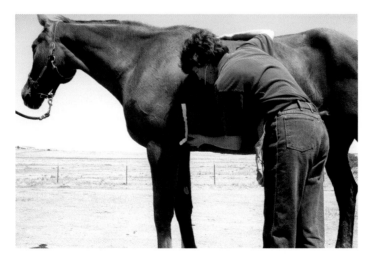

Figure 2.10   Auscultation of the heart on the left thoracic wall. The long head of the triceps muscle and elbow are marked with tape.

III. Readily accessible arteries to assess P rate and P pressure include the facial artery (Fig. 2.11), the transverse facial artery (Fig. 2.12), and the medial and lateral digital arteries (Figs. 2.13 and 2.14).

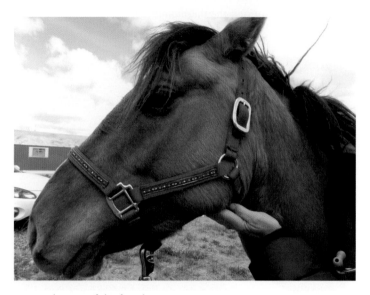

Figure 2.11 Palpation of the facial artery.

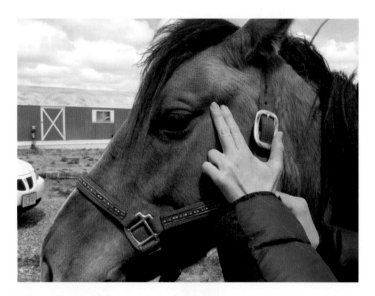

Figure 2.12 Palpation of the transverse facial artery.

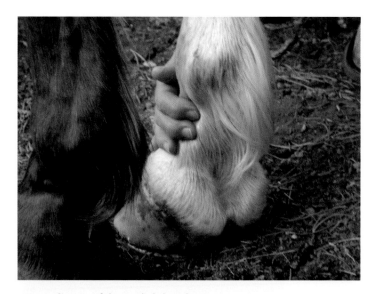

Figure 2.13 Palpation of the medial digital artery.

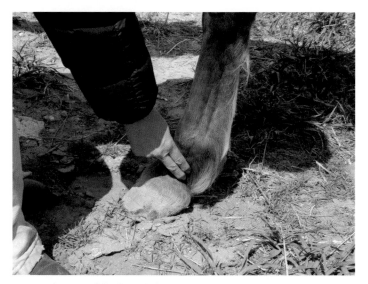

Figure 2.14 Palpation of the lateral digital artery.

2.4.3. Respiratory rate (RR)
I.   Normal resting RR is in the range of 10 to 14 breaths per minute

2.4.4. Mucous membranes (MM)
I.   Normal MM are pink and moist.
II.   The gums are the easiest location to assess MM (Fig. 2.15). MM color aids in the subjective assessment of perfusion, oxygenation, and shock. Pale, cyanotic, hyperemic, injected, or muddy MM suggest cardiovascular and/or respiratory pathology.

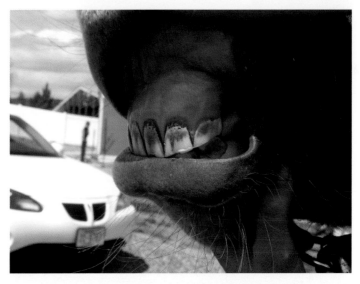

Figure 2.15 A horse's gums are used to assess mucous membrane color and capillary refill time.

2.4.5. Capillary refill time (CRT)
I.   Normal CRT is 1 to 2 seconds.
II.   CRT aids in the subjective assessment of perfusion and shock. To assess CRT, press your finger into the gum to blanch it white and then remove your finger and observe the time for color to return.

2.4.6. Blood pressure (BP)
I.   Objective BP measurement on horses in the field is not practical. Pulse quality and pressure are a subjective indication of BP.

2.4.7. Intestinal motility
I.   Gut motility can be subjectively assessed by auscultation of the upper (dorsal flank) and lower (ventral flank) quadrant on both the left and right side of the horse, noting the quantity and quality of borborygmi (bowel sounds) (Figs. 2.16 and 2.17). Normal gut sounds resemble distant rumbling thunder, at a frequency of approximately 2 to 3 per minute, with intermittent gurgling.

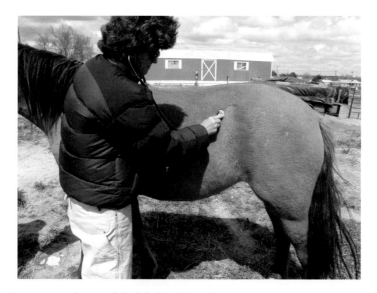

Figure 2.16 Auscultation of the left dorsal quadrant.

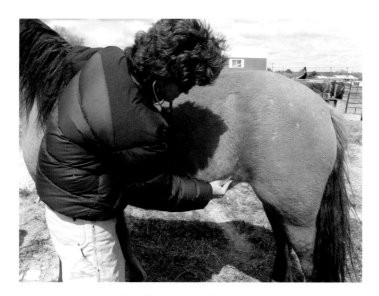

Figure 2.17 Auscultation of the left ventral quadrant.

2.5.   First Aid Wound Care Principles

2.5.1.   Wound infection is a serious complication that contributes significantly to delayed wound healing. Appropriate first aid can help decrease this risk. Wound cleansing, lavage, antiseptics, antimicrobial ointments, and, where appropriate, bandaging can decrease contamination and facilitate wound healing. When feasible, using the basic aseptic techniques of hand washing and/or wearing gloves can help minimize additional contamination.

2.5.2.   Irrigation and antiseptic agents
  I.   There are many irrigation and antiseptic agents available. For some injuries (e. g., a laceration of the pectoralis muscles), many of these agents would be a viable choice, but for other injuries (e.g., an eyelid laceration), particular agents may be preferred and others possibly contraindicated (Table 2.2).

Table 2.2.   Wound Irrigation and Antiseptic Agents.

	Water	Crystalloid Fluids	Chlorhexidine Diacetate, 2% Solution*	Povidone-Iodine, 10% Solution*	Hydrogen Peroxide
Further dilution required			Yes (Water)	Yes (Water or saline)	No
External soft tissues	Yes	Yes	Yes	Yes	
Simple puncture wound		Yes	Yes	Yes	Yes
Eye/ocular adnexa	Yes	Yes	No	Yes	No
Bone		Yes	Yes	Yes	No
Exposed joint		Yes	No	Yes	No
Cautions	Imbibe tissues		Imbibe tissues	Imbibe tissues	Limit use to 1–2×

*These are "solutions"; do not use "scrub" agents.

  A.   Irrigation agents delivered at an oblique angle under pressure between 7 and 15 pounds per square inch (PSI) are most effective at cleansing wounds and decreasing bacterial load. This pressure lavage can be accomplished using a 35-ml or 60-ml syringe with a 19-gauge needle and is superior to irrigation with a bulb syringe. For added safety to both horse and medic in the first aid setting, a 35-ml or 60-ml syringe with an 18-gauge Angiocath (stylet removed) can be used to deliver pressure lavage. Care must be taken not to drive contaminates into the tissues and to stop the irrigation before tissue swelling or imbibition occurs.
  II.   Water
  A.   Water can be used on external surfaces to remove gross contamination such as dirt, gravel, plant material, etc. Because of water's hypotonicity, care must be

taken to avoid overuse and tissue imbibition. It is a good choice for removal of large amounts of gross contamination or contamination from a large area, following with a more detailed decontamination of the wound(s) with an isotonic irrigation solution and/or appropriate antiseptic.

B.   Water delivered via a hose at the appropriate flow with a nozzle (or thumb) can provide the fluid pressure that aids in the removal of debris. Some horses are not conditioned to being sprayed with a hose and may become quite excited. Directing the hose stream to the ground adjacent to the horse and then moving it onto the horse's hoof and leg and on up to the trunk, neck, head, or rump if needed may greatly decrease the horse's anxiety.

III.   Saline solution, Normosol-R, lactated Ringer's

A.   These commonly used sterile crystalloid fluids can also be used for wound lavage and irrigation, thereby maximizing the flexibility of a limited cache inventory.

B.   Saline solution (physiologic saline solution [PSS], 0.9% NaCl) is a good choice if a wound will require copious amounts of lavage to remove dirt, gravel, plant material, or other debris. As it is nearly isotonic (plasma osmolality = 300, versus 0.9% NaCl = 308), a large volume can be used to aid in the removal of foreign debris. Once this gross contamination level has been diminished, an antiseptic agent may be used to further decrease the number of microorganisms.

C.   For use on or around the eye, PSS is very good as an eyewash.

D.   Normosol-R, a buffered polyionic solution with pH 7.4, is a preferred choice for irrigation when a joint is involved; however, saline solution (pH 5.7) and lactated Ringer's solution (pH 6.7) are also acceptable choices for lavage.

IV.   Chlorhexidine diacetate solution 2%

A.   Chlorhexidine diacetate solution 2% is an antiseptic solution that has a good spectrum of activity against many gram-positive bacteria, including *Staphylococcus aureus*, and some gram-negative bacteria, including *Escherichia coli*. It maintains good activity in the presence of organic matter and has good residual activity.

B.   This 2% stock solution should be diluted in water to avoid damaging tissues. Although the dilution recommendation as stated on the label is 1 oz or 2 T or 30 ml/gallon (3785 ml) of water (a ≈0.02% solution or ≈1:125 dilution), 25 ml chlorhexidine diacetate 2%/1000 ml water (a 0.05% solution or 1:40 dilution) has been recommended as a superior wound lavage for dogs and humans and is the recommended dilution for wounds on horses as well. Concentrations stronger than 1:40 are detrimental to tissues.

C.   When chlorhexidine solution is diluted with saline, precipitates form that do not compromise its antiseptic properties or wound healing. However, because of these precipitates, it is suggested that water be the preferred diluent.

D.   Chlorhexidine diacetate solution is an excellent antiseptic that decreases bacterial concentrations on the surface of soft tissues and bone, but it has its limitations: it should NOT be used in or around the eyes and is not suitable for joint lavage.

V.   Povidone-iodine solution (10%) (Betadine Solution)

A.   Povidone-iodine solutions (10%) are a tamed iodine solution containing 1.0% iodine combined with a carrier and are NOT to be confused with tincture of iodine (7%), which contains 7% elemental iodine.

B.   Povidone-iodine solution (10%) should be diluted in water or saline to an "iced tea/weak iced tea" color. This dilution with water (or saline) releases the iodine, thereby increasing its antiseptic properties. Failure to dilute this solution is not only more irritating to tissues but also less effective.

C.   There are two main areas where povidone-iodine solution is the antiseptic of choice and **chlorhexidine or hydrogen peroxide is contraindicated: the eyes and joints**.

1.   Povidone-iodine solution diluted with saline solution to a "weak iced tea" color is an effective antiseptic of the eye and eyelids that is not irritating to the conjunctiva or eyelids.

2.   Antiseptics are generally contraindicated in joint lavage as they are damaging to the articular cartilage and synovial membranes; however, a dilute 0.2% (1:50 dilution) of povidone-iodine solution 10% can be used in through-and-through lavage, and thus is the preferred antiseptic if a wound exposes a joint.

VI.   Hydrogen peroxide (H_2O_2)

A.   Catalase is an enzyme present in most cells, with the exception of some anaerobic bacteria, which catalyzes the decomposition of hydrogen peroxide. When hydrogen peroxide solution comes in contact with catalase on wound surfaces, oxygen is released, which has a germicidal effect. In addition, this effervescent action mechanically helps remove contamination. Although not effective on bacterial spores, the release of oxygen does create a less hospitable environment for anaerobic bacteria.

B.   Hydrogen peroxide's mode of action makes it a good choice for the initial treatment of simple puncture wounds that do not involve a joint or tendon sheath.

C.   Hydrogen peroxide should not be used repeatedly as it injures capillary beds and is damaging to healthy tissues.

VII.   Dakin's solution 0.5% (sodium hypochlorite solution):

A.   Dakin's solution 0.5% is a 1:10 dilution of stock laundry bleach; it is more commonly used in human medicine.

B.   The 0.5% solution should be further diluted to one-half to one-quarter strength. Its bactericidal action results from the release of chlorine and oxygen, but Dakin's solution is cytotoxic to fibroblasts.

C.   Clinical application is limited to dissolving necrotic tissue and is not recommended as a topical disinfectant for wound lavage.

VIII.   **Precaution:** Of particular note, the antiseptics discussed above are "solutions"; **do not use "scrub" antiseptic agents** (i.e., chlorhexidine *scrub* or Betadine *scrub*) on wounds as these are detergents for use on intact skin in which the normal protective barriers are in place. Detergents and alcohols are damaging to tissues exposed in wounds.

2.6. Antimicrobial Ointments

2.6.1.   There are a variety of over-the-counter and prescription antimicrobial ointments and creams that are applied to wounds to decrease bacterial contamination or control infection. They should not be used if a wound will receive more definitive treatment *imminently* because of the difficulty in clearing them from the tissues, and they should not be used on exposed joints. During the healing process, once a wound is considered "clean," these ointments and creams should be discontinued.

I. A limited inventory of first aid antimicrobial ointments or creams for horses should include the following:

    A. Ointments of a larger "bulk" quantity—for example, povidone-iodine ointment 1-lb container, chlorhexidine ointment 1-lb container, or triple antibiotic ointment such as Neosporin in 1-oz tubes.

    B. Ophthalmic preparations—for example, Triple Antibiotic Ophthalmic Ointment (neomycin/polymyxin B/bacitracin) or Triple Antibiotic Ophthalmic Solution (neomycin/polymyxin B/gramicidin) or Ciprofloxacin Ophthalmic Ointment or Solution (Ciloxin).

        1. As a guideline, ophthalmic ointments will contain the word "ophthalmic" (or some variation thereof: "ocu", "opti") in the product name or label and only ophthalmic preparations should be used in or around the eye.

        2. Some ophthalmic preparations combine antibiotics and corticosteroids. Corticosteroids are contraindicated when corneal wounds or ulcers are present, so it is important to read the label and understand the contents of ophthalmic preparations. In a *limited* first aid cache, it would be preferable to carry ophthalmic antimicrobial ointments without corticosteroids as they can be used in a variety of situations without the risks associated with misuse of corticosteroid-containing products.

2.7. First Aid Bandaging Principles

2.7.1. There are a variety of bandaging protocols, techniques, and preferences that are acceptable within the medical axiom of "above all, do no harm." Understanding the purpose of various layers and types of bandage materials and the anatomical pitfalls of bandaging horses can help minimize adverse effects from bandaging. In terms of first aid, the purpose of a bandage is to control hemorrhage, prevent further contamination of a wound, and provide comfort in stabilizing a wound until definitive medical treatment can be obtained.

2.7.2. First aid bandage components (Fig. 2.18) include:

I. Tape stirrups (2-inch [5 cm] white or Elastikon tape)

II. No-stick pads (Telfa)

III. Roll cotton, 1 lb

IV. 4- to 6-inch (10- to 15-cm) conforming roll gauze (Conform, Soft Kling, Kerlix)

V. 4-inch (10-cm) adhesive elastic wrap (VetWrap, Coban, PetFlex, Flex-Wrap)

VI. 3- to 4-inch (7- to 10-cm) Elastikon Tape

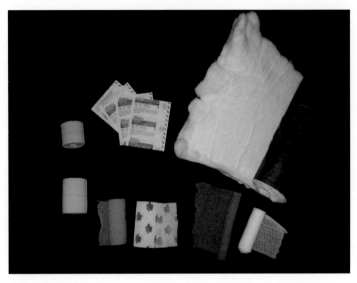

Figure 2.18 Bandage components (clockwise from top left): 2-inch Elastikon tape, no stick pads, roll cotton, conforming roll gauze, VetWrap, 4-inch Elastikon tape.

2.7.3. Leg bandaging

  I. If a wound does not prohibit tape stirrups from being used, for example, a circumferential degloving injury, they can help prevent a bandage from sliding down. Two strips of 2-inch white tape or Elastikon tape are placed on opposite sides of the limb and extend approximately 6 inches (15 cm) beyond what will be the bottom of the bandage (Fig. 2.19). This extension will be doubled back onto

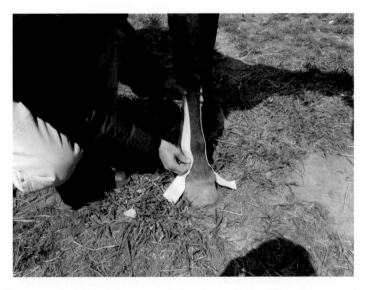

Figure 2.19 Two-inch tape stirrups applied to the medial and lateral aspects of the lower limb.

the bandage and incorporated into the bandage on the (outer) rolled gauze layer or the VetWrap layer, thus creating the tape stirrup that helps hold the bandage in place.

II.   No-stick pads (Telfa) are placed over the wound (Fig. 2.20). No-stick pads prevent the exposed tissues of a wound from adhering to the dressing and help prevent the disruption of any clot formation.

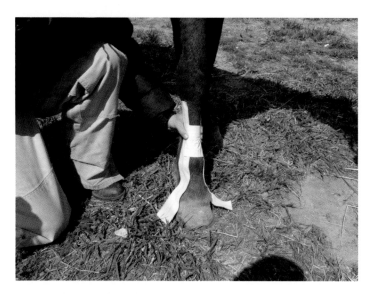

Figure 2.20   Application of a no-stick Telfa pad over the wound.

III.   Some prefer to wrap conforming roll gauze as the next bandage layer to hold the no-stick pad in place. Because of the risk of wrapping this layer too tightly, having a crease or fold present that can become a pressure point, or having it shift from bandage motion and inadvertently creating a tourniquet type effect, it is preferred to place rolled cotton as the next layer (Fig. 2.21). The rolled cotton will hold the no-stick pad in place, conforms well, and provides cushioning. This bulky layer allows the subsequent layers to be applied fairly tightly while minimizing the risk of crushing or constricting the tissues leading to compromised circulation.

IV.   After the rolled cotton layer, 4- to 6-inch (10- to 15-cm) conforming roll gauze is used to compact and hold the rolled cotton layer in place. One should wrap this moderately tight layer *from distal to proximal* (Fig. 2.22). In doing so, bandage compression is applied in the direction of venous and lymphatic return, helping to minimize the "trapping" of return circulatory flow.

   A.   The tape stirrups can be folded back against either this layer or the next layer (Fig. 2.23).

V.   Adhesive elastic wrap (VetWrap, Coban, PetFlex) is the outer layer, again wrapping moderately tight, *from distal to proximal*. This layer affords the bandage some protection from the elements and debris (Fig. 2.24).

   A.   As an alternative, a reuseable elastic wrap such as an ACE Bandage, may be used for this layer. These reusable wraps do not have the mild adhesive

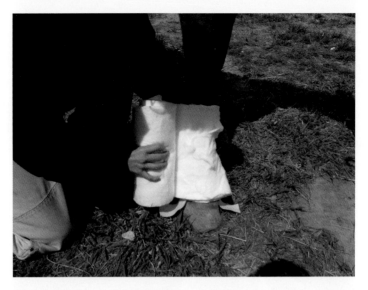

Figure 2.21 Rolled cotton layer. All layers are wrapped in the same direction: counterclockwise on left-side legs, and clockwise on right-side legs.

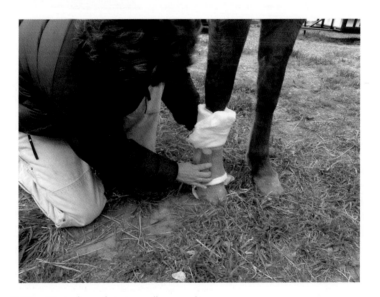

Figure 2.22 Six-inch conforming roll gauze layer.

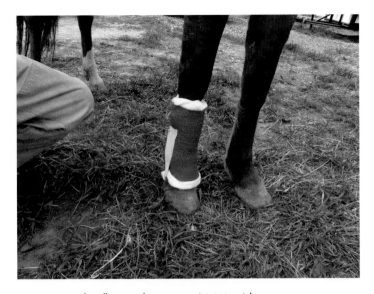

Figure 2.23   Four-inch adhesive elastic wrap (VetWrap) layer.

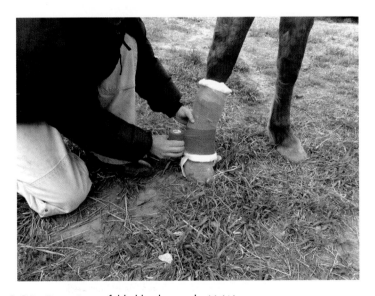

Figure 2.24   Tape stirrups folded back onto the VetWrap.

property that VetWrap, Coban, etc. have and therefore have a tendency to slide down. Folding the tape stirrups back onto this layer and taping the top and bottom of the bandage will help counter this slipping, but these reusable elastic bandage wraps need extra monitoring.

VI. The conforming roll gauze and elastic wrap layers should not exceed the top or bottom edges of the rolled cotton (Figs. 2.22 and 2.24).

VII. Three-inch (7-cm) or 4-inch (10-cm) Elastikon tape is used at the top and bottom of the bandage extending from the bandage onto the skin/hair as a seal to keep debris from getting in under the bandage and also to hold the tape stirrup ends in place on the VetWrap layer (Fig. 2.25).

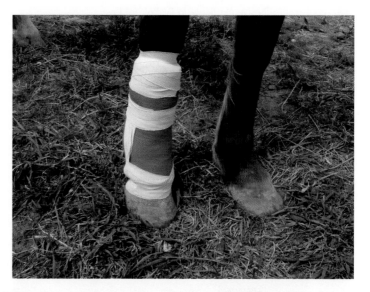

Figure 2.25 Three-inch Elastikon tape at the top and bottom keeps debris from getting under the bandage, and another strip holds the tape stirrups in place.

VIII. Each layer of a bandage should be wrapped in the same direction (Figs. 2.21, 2.22, and 2.24). To avoid causing tendonitis in the lower legs, commonly referred to as a "bowed tendon," the direction of wrap should be counterclockwise on the left-side legs and clockwise on the right-side legs (i.e., cranial [front] → lateral [outside] aspect → caudal [back] aspect → medial [inside] → cranial [front] → etc.) (Figs. 2.21, 2.22, and 2.24).

IX. When bandaging the carpus ("knee") of a horse, the accessory carpal bone is at risk to develop pressure necrosis (Figs. 2.26 and 2.27). To prevent this, a "donut hole" should be cut into the bandage over the accessory carpal bone (Fig. 2.28A + B).

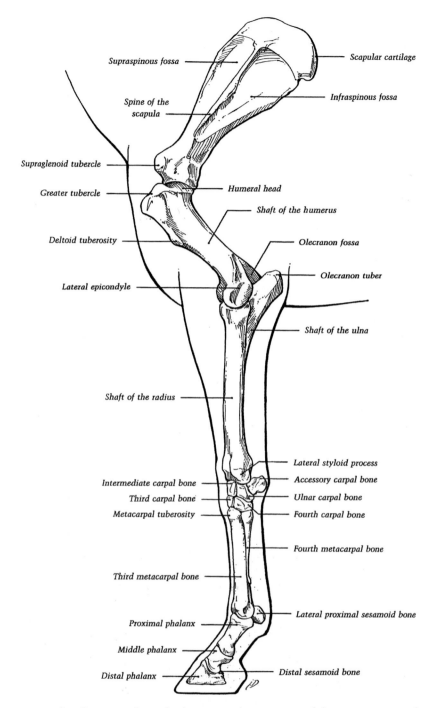

Supraspinous fossa

Scapular cartilage

Spine of the
scapula

Infraspinous fossa

Supraglenoid tubercle

Humeral head

Greater tubercle

Shaft of the humerus

Deltoid tuberosity

Olecranon fossa

Olecranon tuber

Lateral epicondyle

Shaft of the ulna

Shaft of the radius

Lateral styloid process

Intermediate carpal bone

Accessory carpal bone

Third carpal bone

Ulnar carpal bone

Metacarpal tuberosity

Fourth carpal bone

Fourth metacarpal bone

Third metacarpal bone

Lateral proximal sesamoid bone

Proximal phalanx

Middle phalanx

Distal phalanx

Distal sesamoid bone

Figure 2.26 This illustration shows the location and prominence of the accessory carpal bone. (From *Adams' Lameness In Horses, 4th ed.* 1987 by Ted Stashak, courtesy of Blackwell Publishing.)

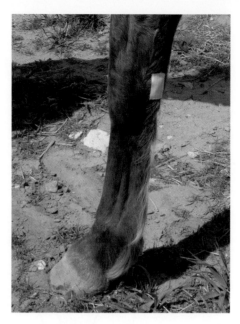

Figure 2.27 The tape marks the location of the accessory carpal bone on the front limb of this horse.

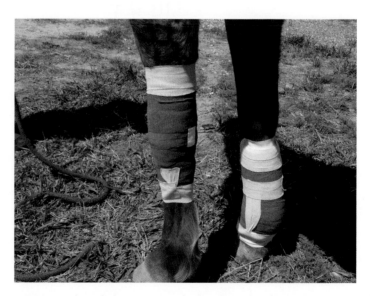

Figure 2.28A. A "donut hole" is cut into the bandage over the accessory carpal bone to relieve any point pressure and prevent pressure necrosis from developing.

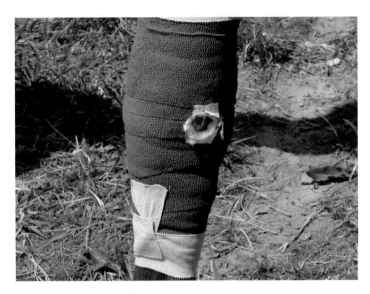

Figure 2.28B. Closer view of donut hole.

X.   When bandaging heel bulb lacerations, it is best to incorporate the whole hoof into the bandage. A disposable baby diaper can be used in place of roll cotton and fits nicely around the foot (Fig. 2.29). As an additional layer added to the outside, duct tape crisscrossed in strips to cover the bottom of the bandage will make it more durable and decrease water on the ground from soaking into the bandage (Fig. 2.30).

XI.   After a bandage is placed on the hock of a horse, it is not uncommon for its first step to result in a "peeing on a fire hydrant" pose with the hyperflexion of the hock and exaggerated abduction of the hip. It appears as if it may fall over; however, within two or three steps, the horse tends to normalize the gait. While it is rather dramatic, there is no cause for concern.

XII.   As a guideline, bandages should be changed daily to every 3 days depending on need, and wet bandages should be changed as soon as possible to avoid maceration of tissues.

XIII.   Except for initial hemorrhage control, puncture wounds should not be bandaged. Puncture wounds are best managed by allowing them to heal via secondary intention from the deeper tissues outward. Bandaging a puncture wound may decrease drainage, encourage a crust to form, and seal in exudate and contamination thereby increasing the risk for infection.

2.8.   First Aid for Common Injuries and Conditions

2.8.1.   Lacerations and abrasions

I.   Quickly assess lacerations and abrasions for depth, severity, and involved structures including tendons, joints, nerves, vessels, or ocular (eye) injury.

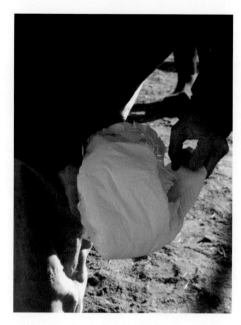

Figure 2.29 A disposable baby diaper can be used in place of roll cotton when bandaging the hoof and/or heel bulbs.

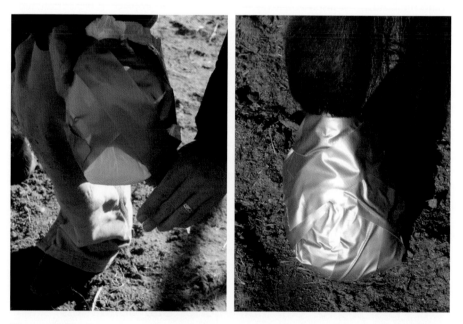

Figure 2.30 Duct tape crisscrossed in strips to cover the bottom of a hoof bandage will make it more durable and decrease water on the ground from soaking into the bandage.

II.   Control hemorrhage with direct pressure, bandage, or pressure bandage.
   A.   A pressure bandage places padding (gauze sponges, lap sponges or towels, sanitary napkins/menstrual pads, etc.) over the hemorrhaging area to create additional compression or pressure on that area. Its purpose is to control hemorrhage and as such is a temporary bandage. If unable to achieve some degree of hemostasis, continue direct pressure, apply a pressure bandage, or add pressure bandaging to a bandage in place and seek definitive veterinary medical treatment as soon as possible.
III.   When bleeding has been controlled, clean the wound with an appropriate lavage and/or antiseptic agent.
   A.   Saline or dilute povidone-iodine solutions are indicated if eyes or joints are involved.
IV.   Dry the wound area by blotting and not wiping to avoid disruption of clots.
V.   Apply an antimicrobial ointment if definitive assessment and treatment will be delayed, but do not apply antimicrobial ointments to exposed joints.
VI.   Place a bandage on amenable areas to minimize further hemorrhage, contamination, and help stabilize the wound from further trauma.
VII.   Lacerations and abrasions in areas of the equine body that are difficult or impractical to bandage include the upper limbs, trunk, rump, neck, head, and face.
   A.   First aid for lacerations and abrasions in these areas is directed at controlling hemorrhage and decreasing wound contamination with irrigation and antiseptic solutions.
   B.   The same principles apply to these wounds as to those that can be bandaged in terms of application of antimicrobial ointments and creams; if more definitive treatment of a wound will be delayed, antimicrobial ointments or creams should be applied.
   C.   Vaseline or an insect-repellent ointment (Swat) may be placed on the skin/ hair dependent to or below a wound as a protective barrier against wound drainage and serum scald and to reduce insect attack. Antimicrobial ointments may also be used for this purpose until less-expensive options become available.
VIII.   For wounds of the head and face where the eyes or eyelids could come in contact with an antiseptic solution and/or ointment, povidone-iodine solution and an ophthalmic antimicrobial ointment are the preferred choice.
IX.   Clipping the hair from around a wound and wound edges will help decrease contamination but may be impractical in the first aid setting and is better addressed during more definitive care. Care must be taken not to allow the clipped hair to fall into the wound, and to this end, packing the wound with gauze sponges and water-soluble KY Jelly before clipping can help minimize this contamination. Some horses are not familiar with clippers and may startle at the sound and/or feel of them. It is important to remember this for safety's sake, but with patience, most horses will accept being clipped.
X.   For all lacerations, obtain definitive veterinary medical care as soon as possible. Additional assessment and treatment including the possibility of primary closure, and timely administration of antibiotics, nonsteroidal anti-inflammatory drugs (NSAIDs), and a tetanus vaccination booster may be indicated.

2.8.2.   Puncture wounds
   I.   There are two primary considerations in the assessment of puncture wounds. The first addresses immediate, life-threatening hemodynamic issues such as

bleeding, tamponade, and tension pneumothorax. The second, and more common, relates to potential morbidity associated with bacterial infection, both anaerobic and aerobic.

II. If one suspects a puncture wound has penetrated into the jugular furrow (Fig. 2.31), chest cavity, abdominal cavity, or pelvic canal, definitive veterinary medical care should be obtained immediately.

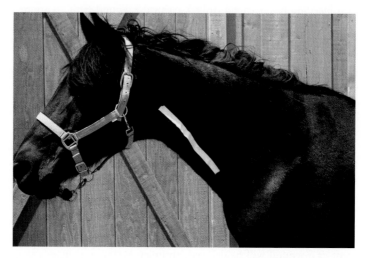

Figure 2.31 Important anatomical structures such as the carotid artery, jugular vein, esophagus, trachea, and vagosympathetic trunk all run in the area of the jugular furrow, marked by white tape.

III. For those puncture wounds that can be addressed in the field, cleanse the surface area of the wound with an antiseptic solution to decrease the contamination that could be carried into the wound on exploration.

A. Gently probe the puncture with a sterile blunt instrument or moistened sterile cotton swab to assess depth, direction of track, and presence of a foreign body.

B. Use a syringe alone or with an Angiocath (stylet removed) to deliver antiseptic solution into the wound. Antiseptic solution applied to a sterile cotton swab can also be used to cleanse the wound.

C. If the puncture wound does not involve a joint or tendon sheath, hydrogen peroxide is a good choice for the initial irrigation and cleansing as the release of oxygen makes for a less favorable anaerobic environment and its effervescent property helps clear debris. Because of the harmful effects to healthy tissues, subsequent antiseptic flushing should be done with chlorhexidine diacetate solution or povidone-iodine solution.

D. If a puncture wound does, or might, involve a joint or tendon sheath, Normosol-R, 0.9% NaCl, or lactated Ringer's sterile crystalloid fluids are the irrigation agents of choice. Because of the risk of developing septic arthritis or septic tenosynovitis from a puncture wound involving these structures, definitive veterinary medical care should be obtained as soon as possible.

IV. The goal of treating uncomplicated puncture wounds is to promote drainage, decrease the risk of developing an anaerobic environment, and encourage second intention healing from the deep tissues outward. To this end, antimicrobial ointments should not be applied, puncture wounds should not be bandaged, and they should not be sutured. Continued care includes gently removing surface crusts and irrigating the track with an appropriate antiseptic solution.

V. Obtaining definitive veterinary medical care for puncture wounds is recommended as systemic antibiotics, anti-inflammatory agents, and a tetanus vaccination booster are indicated.

2.9. Fractures

2.9.1. Fractures in horses are devastating and frequently life-ending injuries. Horses with spinal fractures or skull fractures resulting in catastrophic neurological damage, severe fractures (comminuted fractures, badly contaminated open fractures, severe joint involvement, fractures resulting in nerve or vascular compromise, etc.), or multiple limb fractures should be humanely euthanized (see Chapter 10).

I. An isolated limb fracture may be amenable to treatment, and first aid is directed at stabilizing the injured bone to prevent further damage.

2.9.2. When placing a bandage or splint to support a fracture, the joint above and below the affected bone should be immobilized. Failure to do so increases the risk of creating more damage and trauma due to the fulcrum effect of the splint or bandage on the fracture site. In a first aid setting, this realistically limits the areas amenable to bandaging or splinting for fracture stabilization to the lower limbs, distal to the carpus ("knee") and hock.

2.9.3. A Robert Jones bandage or a Robert Jones bandage incorporating some sort of rigid splint material can be used for first aid fracture stabilization. A Robert Jones bandage uses the same bandaging principles previously discussed with significantly *more* roll cotton being used in that layer. Because a limb fracture compromises load bearing stability this bandage has to provide additional support. This abundant layer of cotton is the key to a successful Robert Jones bandage.

I. The incorporation of rigid splint material if readily available, for example, rebar or a 3- to 4-inch (7- to 10-cm)–diameter PVC half pipe, also helps to decrease the flexibility of a bandage but does not replace the necessity of a healthy cotton layer.

II. Splint material is placed outside of the (outer) conforming roll gauze, and an additional layer of roll gauze is used to hold the splint material in place, followed by the VetWrap and Elastikon layers.

III. If this bandage/splint involves the carpus ("knee"), a donut hole should be cut into the bandage over the accessory carpal bone.

2.10. Lameness

2.10.1. Any discussion of lameness can snowball into something encompassing volumes of text that makes *War and Peace* look like an abridged short story; I like to call it the Big Bang Theory of Lameness. For the purposes of this chapter, the discussion of lameness in the working horse in a first aid setting will be very limited. I refer the reader to *Adams' Lameness in Horses*, 5th ed by Ted S. Stashak, DVM, MS, for an excellent treatise on lameness.

2.10.2.   Diagnosing the cause of lameness can be challenging, often necessitating the use of nerve blocks and imaging such as radiographs and/or ultrasound. Assessing lameness in an austere first aid setting relies on history and physical examination.

I.   Information from the handler that may be helpful includes the following:
   A.   How old is the horse?
      1.   Older horses may have arthritis or other chronic lameness conditions that may be exacerbated with increased exercise/work.
         a.   Examples of these conditions include high ringbone (arthritis of the pastern joint [proximal interphalangeal (P1-P2) joint]) or low ringbone (arthritis of the coffin joint [distal interphalangeal (P2-P3) joint]) and "navicular disease," also referred to as caudal heel syndrome, involving degeneration of the navicular bone and/or inflammation of the navicular bursa in the foot.
   B.   Has the horse had any lameness problems in the past?
      1.   For example, tendon injuries take a prolonged period of time to recover from fully. A tendon injury from months or even years previous may be at risk for reinjury.
   C.   Has the horse been shod (new horseshoes applied) or trimmed recently?
      1.   It is not uncommon for the nail of a shoe to be misplaced into the sensitive tissues. Even when repositioned correctly, the traumatized area can develop into an abscess.
      2.   A recent trimming or shoeing may result in changing the balance of a foot. Anyone who has changed footwear from a frequently worn well-fitted supportive athletic shoe to a rarely worn dress shoe (high heels) can empathize.
   D.   When was the lameness noticed first?
      1.   Lameness that develops during exercise/work suggests a more acute injury such as a ligament, tendon, or fracture injury. Lameness that becomes apparent after the horse is rested suggests a more chronic condition that has been inflamed with increased use.
   E.   Has the lameness improved or worsened since first noticed?
      1.   Some mild arthritic conditions may improve during exercise/work, while other soft tissue injuries may worsen with exercise/work.
   F.   Is more than one leg involved?
      1.   Acute traumatic injuries such as sprains (the stretching or tearing of ligaments) and strains (the stretching or tearing of tendons) generally affect a single limb. Other conditions, such as laminitis, tend to affect either both front feet or all four feet. Navicular disease affects both front feet but may present as a single-leg lameness or a shifting leg lameness depending upon which foot hurts the most at a given time.

G.   In what activities has the horse been engaged during the past week?

    1.   For example, a horse run on asphalt may develop a painful inflammatory condition of the feet from the repetitive concussive forces called (concussion) laminitis—commonly referred to as "road founder." A horse working in mud may strain tendons causing tendonitis; a horse working search and rescue in the mountains may sustain a puncture wound of the sole resulting in a sole abscess.

H.   Did the horse sustain any known trauma?

    1.   For example, did he slip or trip, or go down in any way? Was he struck by any objects or did he collide with any obstacles?

I.   Has the horse received any medication that may alter the appearance of the lameness?

    1.   For example, NSAIDs may alleviate inflammation and signs of pain that could change the results of a lameness exam, or support a conclusion based on response to the drug.

II.   It is helpful to describe which limb(s) is (are) affected and the severity of lameness. Various grading scales have been described using 0–4, 1–4, 0–5, mild/moderate/severe, etc. By convention, "0" means no lameness present, and the highest number "4" or "5" means non–weight-bearing lameness, with the numbers in between correlating to progressively worse or more noticeable lameness.

A.   The American Association of Equine Practitioners (AAEP) has established a lameness scale of 0–5.

    1.   0—Lameness not perceptible under any circumstances.

    2.   1—Difficult to observe and not consistently apparent.

    3.   2—Difficult to observe at a walk or when trotting in a straight line, but consistently apparent under certain circumstances.

    4.   3—Consistently observable at a trot under all circumstances.

    5.   4—Obvious at a walk.

    6.   5—Minimal weight bearing or inability to move.

III.   Which scale is used is not as critical as communicating which scale is being used to describe the lameness. To convey this information, the numerator is the subjective assessment of the lameness, and the denominator is the maximum number for that scale. For example: LF (left, front leg) grade 2/4 lame, or RH (right, hind leg) grade 3/5 lame, or RF (right, front leg) grade 4/4 lame, or LF grade 3/5 and RF grade 1/5 lame.

IV.   Observe the horse for any obvious swellings, blemishes, or deformities.

V.   Palpate the limbs and back for any signs of swelling, tenderness, heat, or pulse quality changes.

VI.   Flex and extend individual joints to assess pain or a worsening of the lameness after stressing the joint.

VII.   Palpate the flexor tendons and suspensory ligament individually while bearing weight and not bearing weight on the limb (Figs. 2.32 and 2.33).

VIII.   Clean the sole of the foot of all mud, dirt, gravel, and debris (Fig. 2.34).

IX.   Use hoof testers to assess for tenderness in the foot (Fig. 2.35).

2.10.3.   Following is a brief listing of types of lameness that may be encountered in the working horse:

    I.   Laminitis:

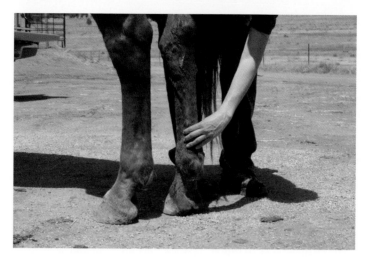

Figure 2.32 Palpation, while weight bearing, of the superficial and deep digital flexor tendons and the suspensory ligament on the plantar aspect of the right hind limb.

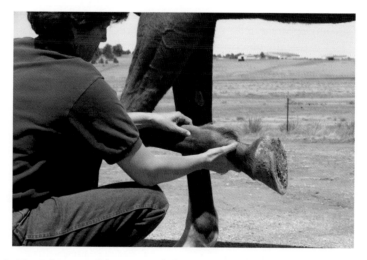

Figure 2.33 Palpation, while non–weight bearing, of the superficial and deep digital flexor tendons and the suspensory ligament on the palmar aspect of the left front limb.

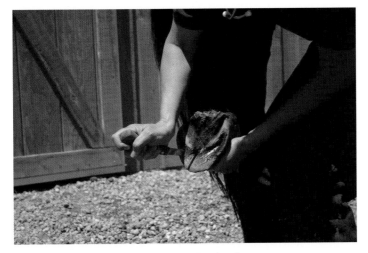

Figure 2.34 Clean the sole of the foot with a hoof pick.

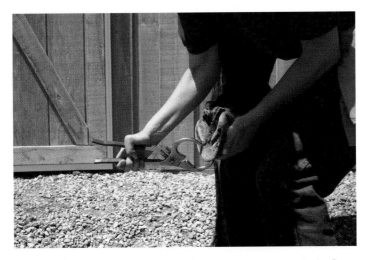

Figure 2.35 Hoof testers are used to assess for areas of tenderness in the foot.

A.   A much simplified explanation of the sensitive laminae of the foot is that this interdigitating very vascular and nerve-rich layer lies between the outer horny hoof wall and the bone within the hoof called the coffin bone (P3) and helps to secure the coffin bone to the hoof wall. Inflammation of this layer is termed laminitis, or the common term, founder. The actual disease process is much more complicated involving decreased capillary perfusion, arteriovenous shunting, coagulopathies, and ischemic necrosis of the laminae.

B.   Some predisposing factors leading to laminitis have been identified, but our understanding of the pathogenesis of these is not complete.

   1.   Three etiologies of laminitis that a working horse may be exposed to are:

     a.   Cold water founder, which can be seen when an overheated horse ingests a large amount of cold water. To minimize this risk, horses should be offered only small amounts of water until they have cooled down sufficiently.

     b.   Concussion founder or road founder occurs from the repetitive trauma to the feet from working on a hard surface such as a paved road, tarmac, or compacted gravel road. Avoiding faster gaits on these surfaces, especially galloping or running can help minimize the risk of road founder.

     c.   Laminitis may develop as a result of decreased or non–weight-bearing lameness in the contralateral limb. The great race horse Barbaro fell victim to this following his fracture and fracture repair. Horses at risk should have a support wrap(s) placed on the sound leg(s) and should be kept in a well-bedded or, if possible, soft sand stall.

   2.   Other causes of laminitis include ingestion of too much grain (grain founder), ingestion of lush green pasture (grass founder), endometritis (postparturient laminitis), laminitis from a drug reaction, or systemic infection.

C.   Clinical signs of laminitis include the appearance of "walking on eggshells," standing with the back feet farther forward under the horse in an attempt to decrease the weight on the front feet, heat detectable over the whole hoof wall, and bounding pulses in the medial and lateral digital arteries (Figs. 2.13 and 2.14). This is an extremely painful condition so other signs of pain may also be seen such as increased respiration, muscle tremors, and anxiety.

D.   Laminitis is a medical emergency, so definitive veterinary medical care should be obtained as soon as possible.

   1.   First aid treatment is to provide analgesia, decrease inflammation, and reduce the hypertensive cycle.

     a.   An NSAID that also provides pain relief is phenylbutazone (2 g IV slowly). The injectable form of phenylbutazone *must* be given IV as extravasation injury is quite damaging to tissues.

     b.   Acepromazine maleate injection (0.044–0.088 mg/kg [2–4 mg/100 lb body weight] IV slowly, or IM) is a neuroleptic tranquilizer that has no analgesic properties but does decrease anxiety and causes a drop in blood pressure via central and peripheral alpha-adrenergic actions. Because of this, acepromazine should NOT be used in stallions (intact male horses) due to the risk of priapism (persistent abnormal erection of the penis).

II.   Tendonitis (inflammation of a tendon)/desmitis (inflammation of a ligament)

A.   Tendonitis, commonly referred to as a bowed tendon, and desmitis occur in the lower limbs and usually involve the superficial digital flexor tendon, the deep digital flexor tendon, or the suspensory ligament.

B.   These structures become inflamed as a result of forces that overstretch or eccentrically overload the fibers such as occurs when a foot is planted while turning (or slipping). Tendonitis can also result from blunt trauma to the area such as being kicked or struck, and tendonitis can develop from an overly tight bandage, or a bandage that pulls the tendons out of their normal alignment.

C.   Clinical signs of tendonitis/desmitis include varying degrees of lameness from grade 2/5 with a very mild strain to grade 5/5 with complete rupture, tenderness to palpation of the individual structures (Figs. 2.32 and 2.33), and a swelling or "bowing" of the tissues on the palmar/plantar aspect of the lower limb (Fig. 2.36).

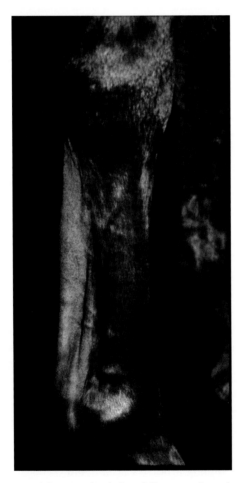

Figure 2.36 Tendonitis of the superficial digital flexor tendon ("bowed tendon"). (Photograph courtesy of Dean A. Hendrickson, DVM, MS; Diplomate, American College of Veterinary Surgeons; Professor of Surgery, Large Animal; Chief of Staff, Colorado State University.)

    D. First aid treatment for tendonitis/desmitis is directed at decreasing inflammation, providing analgesia, and supporting the injured tendon or ligament.

       1. Phenylbutazone (2 g IV slowly) is a good anti-inflammatory choice that provides pain relief by reducing the inflammation. (Phenylbutazone is also available in an oral formulation and may be used as well at the same dose 2 g PO.)

       2. Cold water hosing (hydrotherapy) or application of cold packs (wrapped in a towel rather than directly against the skin) to the affected palmar/plantar area can help decrease edema and further inflammation. As noted before, not all horses are accustomed to water hoses. Start with the hose directed at the ground adjacent to the affected limb and then move the water on to the hoof and leg.

       3. Bandaging the limb will help support the injured tendons. Since bandaging has been known to cause tendonitis, care must be taken not to worsen the condition. These bandages should be changed daily to allow assessment of the injury and for hydrotherapy, or any time there is suspicion the bandage could be doing more harm than good.

       4. As discussed in the previous section on laminitis, placing a support wrap on the contralateral limb may be indicated.

2.11. First Aid for the Eye

2.11.1. In addition to obvious injury or trauma to the eye and surrounding structures, blepherospasm, third eyelid elevation, epiphora, hyperemia, edema, and photophobia are all signs suggestive of eye injury, inflammation, or infection. Because many different eye problems can present with these same signs, all eye problems should have definitive medical evaluation and treatment as soon as possible.

2.11.2. Other than the "normal" superior (dorsal) and inferior (ventral) eyelids, horses have an additional eyelid called the nictitating membrane or third eyelid (Fig. 2.37). This third eyelid comes "up" from the medial canthus and functions to help protect the cornea, reshape the tear film, and provide some lacrimal activity, and it also has reticuloendothelial activity. Its movement is passive in that when the globe retracts into the socket it puts pressure on the postorbital fat, which in turn puts pressure on the gland of the third eyelid, which in turn moves the third eyelid across the eye.

    I. A painful eye is frequently retracted into the socket so sustained elevation of the third eyelid is an important sign of possible eye irritation, inflammation, or injury.

2.11.3. When examining a horse's eyes, avoid facing him into direct sunlight. Moving to a shaded area to decrease the brightness and glare can be helpful.

    I. PSS, 0.09% NaCl, or plain water can be used for irrigation. The only acceptable antiseptic solution is diluted povidone-iodine solution. As previously

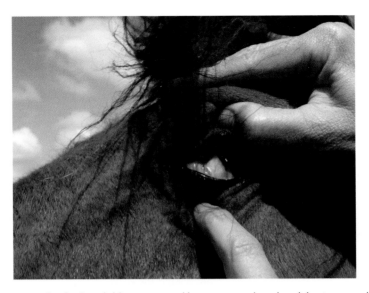

Figure 2.37 The third eyelid becomes readily apparent when the globe is retropulsed into the socket.

discussed, povidone-iodine solution 10% diluted with saline solution to a "weak tea/iced tea" color (approximately a 1:50 dilution) is an effective antiseptic for the eye and eyelids that is not irritating to the conjunctiva or eyelids.
II.   Ophthalmic ointments or drops containing corticosteroids or NSAIDs are contraindicated for certain conditions and injuries and as such should NOT be used until a definitive ophthalmic exam has been performed.
  A.   Ophthalmic ointments temporarily blur vision and so should not be used until a horse is through working.

2.11.4. Conjunctivitis
I.   Conjunctivitis is the most common eye disease in all species. Working horses exposed to increased dust, debris, air particulates, riot control agents, etc., are at risk for developing noninfectious conjunctivitis.
II.   Clinical signs include blepherospasm, elevation of the third eyelid, excessive lacrimation, epiphora, hyperemia of the conjunctiva, and edema of the conjunctiva.
III.   Periodic irrigation across the eye and under the eyelids with PSS to flush irritants can help prevent or decrease the severity of conjunctivitis. Pressure lavage is not indicated, so a plain 35-ml syringe without needle or Angiocath works well.
IV.   If a *thorough* ophthalmic exam supports the diagnosis of conjunctivitis (with NO corneal damage), then the use of a corticosteroid ophthalmic preparation is indicated.
  A.   Ketorolac tromethamine 0.5% ophthalmic solution (Acular) is a nonsteroidal anti-inflammatory ophthalmic preparation frequently used in human medicine for seasonal allergic conjunctivitis. It may be used in horses to control ocular inflammation (again, those with NO corneal damage) but its use should

be closely monitored. If corneal damage is present, topical ophthalmic NSAIDs may delay corneal healing. While they do not potentiate the enzymatic (collagenase) destruction of the corneal stroma as do corticosteroids, anecdotally they have been implicated as a rare cause of liquefactive stromal necrosis.

2.11.5. Horses are prone to develop anterior uveitis, so what may appear as signs suggestive of mild irritation can actually be more serious; underscoring the premise that all eye problems should have a definitive veterinary medical evaluation.

2.11.6. Ocular foreign bodies
I.   Foreign bodies trapped under the eyelids present with blepherospasm, third eyelid elevation, and excessive lacrimation.
II.   Foreign bodies are treated by irrigation with (PSS) or water in combination with judicious use of a moistened cotton swab or gauze sponge.
III.   Topical anesthetic drops such as proparacaine or lidocaine 2% are required to examine and clear foreign bodies from behind the third eyelid.

2.11.7. Corneal injuries
I.   In terms of first aid, the most important thing about corneal injuries is to recognize that there is one and to seek definitive veterinary medical care as soon as possible.
II.   Corticosteroid ophthalmic preparations are **CONTRAINDICATED** if a corneal injury is present. As previously discussed, topical nonsteroidal anti-inflammatory ophthalmic preparations must be used with extreme caution and can be considered contraindicated for corneal injuries as well.
III.   Systemically administered NSAIDs are effective in relieving ocular discomfort and should be given when corneal injuries or anterior uveitis are present.
   A.   Flunixin meglumine (Banamine) (1.1 mg/kg PO or IV every 24 hours) works well in horses and may be the drug of choice for acute uveitis. Although flunixin meglumine injectable is labeled for IM injection as well as IV, I recommend the IV route of administration is recommended because of the potential tissue reaction at the site of injection in the muscle.
   B.   Phenylbutazone (1–2 g PO or IV slowly) or ketoprofen (2.2 mg/kg IV every 24 hours) is a systemically administered NSAID alternative to flunixin meglumine (Banamine).

2.11.8. Thermal injuries
I.   Thermal injuries resulting from fire or explosions may affect the eyelids, conjunctiva, cornea, and uveal tract.
II.   First aid treatment is directed toward copious irrigation with water followed by the application of a topical antibiotic ophthalmic ointment. An ointment is used preferentially to antibiotic drops or solutions to decrease the risk of adhesions forming between the eyelids and eyeball (synblepharon).
   A.   Systemic NSAIDs should be given as soon as possible. Options include:
      1.   Flunixin meglumine (Banamine) (1.1 mg/kg IV), which may be the NSAID drug of choice for ocular discomfort.
      2.   Phenylbutazone (1–2 g IV slowly)
      3.   Ketoprofen (2.2 mg/kg IV)

2.12. Heat Exhaustion and Heat Stroke

2.12.1. Hyperthermia is an increase in core body temperature above normal that can progress to heat exhaustion or heat stroke.

2.12.2. With heat exhaustion and heat stroke, these extremely high core body temperatures >105°F (40.6°C) occur when excess heat, generated by body metabolism, exercise, and/or environmental conditions, exceeds the body's ability to dissipate that heat.

2.12.3. Heat loss occurs by convection (air currents), conduction, radiation, or evaporation. When the body's compensatory mechanisms are overwhelmed, heat exhaustion progresses to heat stroke in which clinically significant tissue damage occurs, frequently involving the brain, liver, kidneys, muscles, and hemolymphatic system.

2.12.4. Horses have a very large muscle mass that can generate tremendous amounts of heat during exercise. They can become quickly and severely dehydrated from both sweating and moisture loss associated with increased respiration.

2.12.5. A guideline, *Heat Exhaustion/Heat Stroke Risk Index*, can be estimated by taking the summation of the air temperature and relative humidity:
   <130—A horse can most likely cool himself.
   130–150—It becomes difficult for a horse to cool himself.
   >180—A horse's cooling system is ineffectual; even with significant sweating, there is minimal cooling effect.

This index is just a guideline and common sense must prevail when assessing heat exhaustion and heat stroke risk.

2.12.6. Working horses operating in an environment where they are at risk for developing heat exhaustion/heat stroke should have their body temperatures monitored periodically throughout their shift and upon completion of a shift. Guidelines should be established where a horse will be pulled from service if his temperature rises above a certain threshold (i.e., before heat exhaustion occurs) and basic treatment for reducing body temperature is implemented. On hot humid days when the risk of developing heat problems is high, protocols should be in place where horses are periodically cooled down prophylactically.

2.12.7. Clinical signs of heat exhaustion include increased or profuse sweating, increased heart rate, flared nostrils, and increased respiratory rate. **Horses CANNOT breathe through their mouths**, so they will not open-mouth pant like a dog. Progressively worsening signs include stumbling, weakness, depression, dry skin from having lost their ability to sweat, and spasmodic jerking of the diaphragm and flanks referred to as "thumps." Poor prognostic signs of heat stroke are collapse, seizure, and coma.

2.12.8. First aid treatment for hyperthermia is directed toward lowering the core body temperature. While obtaining more definitive veterinary medical treatment is vital, implementing measures to lower core body temperature should NOT be delayed.

  I.   The goal is to reduce the core body temperature to approximately 102°F (38.9°C) in 30–60 minutes.

  II.   Move the horse to a cooler environment that also provides good air flow, such as into the shade of a building, tree, awning, or tent canopy. Tarps can be rigged to provide shade, and misting can be very helpful.

  III.   Apply **COOL**, 60°–65°F (15°–18°C), water to the legs, chest, face, head, and neck to facilitate heat loss by conduction and evaporation. A hose is ideal for this, but it can also be done with a bucket of water and sponge, or using bottled water if nothing else is available. Avoid the large loin and rump muscle groups as this relatively cold water can cause vasoconstriction, leading to further damage in these muscles.

  A.   Do **NOT** use ice baths or cold, 35°–45°F (2°–7°C), water baths as this promotes skin vessel constriction, which impairs heat loss and induces shivering resulting in increased heat production.

  IV.   In addition to the application of cool water, moving air over the horse by fanning or use of an electric fan will help with evaporative cooling.

  V.   Cooler water can be applied to the jugular furrow along the neck where the jugular vein and carotid artery are superficial and free from large muscle groups, helping to increase heat exchange of these large vessels.

  VI.   During the cooling process it is important to monitor core body temperature. When body temperature drops to 103°–104°F (39.5°–40°C), stop active cooling measures, but continue to monitor core body temperature as it may continue to decline and warming procedures may be indicated.

  VII.   Because of the potential for severe tissue damage and the sequelae of tissue damage, it is imperative to obtain or transport the horse to definitive veterinary medical care as soon as possible. Recognize that a horse being transported in a trailer requires that he use muscles to stabilize himself, resulting in heat production. An enclosed trailer eliminates convection cooling and decreases evaporative cooling; therefore, be cognizant of transport time.

2.12.9. While definitive veterinary care may implement more aggressive cooling measures that are beyond the scope of first aid, such as cooled (≈65°–70°F/≈18.3°–22.8°C) IV fluids or cool water enemas, the benefit of the rapid response of applying cool water to the body surface should not be underestimated. It is worth repeating that while obtaining more definitive veterinary medical treatment is vital, implementing measures to lower core body temperature should NOT be delayed as a consequence.

2.13. Colic

2.13.1. *Colic* is a term that refers to acute paroxysmal abdominal pain.

  I.   Treatment for colic depends on its cause; some types of colic are amenable to resolution with supportive medical care, but others require surgical intervention. History, physical exam, and diagnostic tests are the basis for diagnosing colic and determining a medical versus surgical colic. Colic can be very dynamic, initially presenting as a medical colic and progressing to a surgical colic. This underscores the importance of assessment and reassessment of colic patients.

II.   Death from colic is the result of shock and cardiovascular collapse.

III.   Advancements in anesthesia, anesthetic agents, operating and recovery rooms, surgical instruments and techniques, and perioperative pharmacia continue to improve outcomes of surgical colic. The intraoperative and postoperative constant rate infusion of lidocaine in the management of ileus and ischemia-reperfusion injury is very encouraging.

2.13.2.   Clinical signs of colic include: wanting to lie down, wanting to roll, pawing, kicking at their belly, sweating, looking back at their flanks, tachypnea, tachycardia, prolonged capillary refill time, decreased or increased bowel sounds, or a change in the quality of bowel sounds (a tympanic "pebble in a culvert" sound versus normal "distant rumbling thunder"). Horses CANNOT vomit, so emesis will not be a sign of colic.

2.13.3.   First aid for colic is primarily to recognize that colic may exist and to obtain veterinary medical help as soon as possible.

I.   For many lay people, walking a colicky horse is a "standard treatment," although walking a horse for colic is controversial. Walking and the perfusion of muscles that it requires may tax an already compromised cardiovascular system, thereby worsening the level of shock. However, some horses are in so much pain that they will throw themselves down and thrash, violently injuring their head, eyes, legs, etc. In this case, keeping a horse walking may prevent this secondary trauma.

II.   If more definitive veterinary medical assessment and care will be delayed, administration of flunixin meglumine (Banamine) (1.1 mg/kg IV or PO [paste]) can provide analgesia and alleviate some of the systemic effects of endotoxins.

2.14. Tying-Up/Exercise-Related Myopathy/Sporadic Exertional Rhabdomyolysis

2.14.1.   There are a number of conditions, differing in etiology and pathogenesis, that fall under the umbrella complex of *exertional rhabdomyolysis*. Terms used to describe these various conditions include *tying-up, exercise-related myopathy, sporadic exertional rhabdomyolysis, Monday morning sickness, equine rhabdomyolysis syndrome,* and *azoturia,* among others. Within the literature, these terms are not used consistently or universally to describe these different pathologies.

I.   The condition discussed here is one seen with prolonged exercise/work, which places working horses at an increased risk for developing this exertional myopathy variously referred to as tying-up, exercise-related myopathy, or sporadic exertional rhabdomyolysis.

2.14.2.   The development of tying-up is related to muscle energy depletion (intramuscular glycogen and intramyocellular triglyceride as opposed to anaerobic metabolism from a lack of oxygen) and excessive sweating leading to electrolyte imbalances and dehydration.

I. Estimated fluid deficits from post exercise dehydration range from 5 to 50 liters (1.3–13.2 gal), and sodium (Na^+), chloride (Cl^-), and potassium (K^+) are the major electrolytes in the slightly hypertonic horse sweat. Profuse sweating, resulting in these large fluid losses and ion deficits, can lead to changes in skeletal muscle ion concentrations that increase the potential for muscular dysfunction and damage.

II. The electrolyte losses from sweating combined with electrolyte shifts from muscle damage result in serum electrolyte abnormalities including hyponatremia, hypochloremia, hyperkalemia, and hyperphosphatemia. A metabolic *alkalosis* is the most common acid-base disorder with sporadic exertional rhabdomyolysis because of the compensation for hypochloremia. It is important to recognize that hot humid conditions increase not only the risk of heat exhaustion but exertional myopathy as well.

2.14.3. Clinical signs of tying-up include muscle cramping, muscle fasciculation, a tucked-up appearance, sweating, stiff stilted gait, and reluctance to move. The largest muscle masses are often the most severely affected, and the large rump and leg muscles (gluteal, biceps femoris, and semitendonosus muscles) may be firm and painful to the touch.

I. It is important to note that a horse with *colic* may exhibit some of these same signs: a tucked-up appearance, sweating, reluctance to move, etc, but making a distinction is very important to prevent a horse with exertional myopathy from being mistaken for a horse with colic and either "therapeutically" walked or administered NSAIDs prior to fluid resuscitation.

A. Palpating and assessing the rump and leg muscles for hardness and pain that may be seen in tying-up but not with colic may help in distinguishing the two conditions.

2.14.4. First aid for these animals is primarily to recognize that this condition may exist and to obtain definitive veterinary medical help as soon as possible. These horses should **NOT** be moved, including walking or prolonged trailering, as this will worsen the condition.

I. A veterinarian may need to be transported to the horse to replace fluid and electrolyte losses, provide analgesia for muscle pain, and relieve anxiety.

II. Fluid resuscitation in these patients is paramount because the appropriate use of sedatives, analgesics, and NSAIDs can exacerbate perfusion problems in kidneys and damaged muscles.

A. Because of the risk of renal damage from hypoperfusion and rhabdomyolysis, urinary output should be closely monitored as aggressive IV fluid resuscitation requires appropriate renal function to manage the electrolyte and fluid load.

III. Fluid requirements can be calculated by adding estimated fluid deficits to the maintenance fluid volume.

A. Maintenance fluid requirements for adult horses are 2 ml/kg body weight/hr (48 ml/kg body weight/day or 1 L/hr/500-kg horse.)

B. Fluid deficit volume may be calculated by the formula:
% Dehydration × Body Weight (in kg). For example, a horse weighing 500 kg that is 6% dehydrated would have a fluid deficit of 30 L. This results in a total fluid replacement volume of 54 L over 24 hours (24 L maintenance + 30 L deficit

= 54 L). A 10- to 20-L bolus can be administered followed by a 24-hour calculated drip rate for the remaining volume.

1.   HR, pulse quality, MM/CRT, and skin turgor (assessed by lifting a pinch of skin on the neck or scapular region and noting how readily this tented skin returns to normal upon release) are used to estimate fluid deficits.

2.   HR 50–60, tacky MM, CRT 2–3 seconds, delayed recovery of tented skin: estimated dehydration 5–7%.

3.   HR >60, weak pulse, poor jugular distension, tacky MM, CRT >3 seconds, skin stays tented: estimated dehydration 8–10%.

C.   Because horses suffering from sporadic exertional rhabdomyolysis typically have a metabolic alkalosis and are hyponatremic, hypochloremic, and hyperkalemic, 0.9% NaCl is the initial crystalloid IV fluid of choice. Laboratory data should be obtained as soon as possible to detect additional electrolyte and metabolic abnormalities and also to monitor response to therapy.

APPENDIX A: FIRST AID CHEMICAL RESTRAINT AND NONSTEROIDAL ANTI-INFLAMMATORY DRUGS AND DOSAGES FOR WORKING HORSES

Chemical Restraint Drugs

Xylazine (100 mg/ml)

a) 0.5–1.1 mg/kg IV (CSU VTH Formulary, 2008)
b) For colic analgesia: 0.3–0.5 mg/kg IV (Plumb, 1999)
c) 1.1 mg/kg IV (package insert TranquiVed Injectable, Vedco, Inc.)
d) 2.2 mg/kg IM (package insert TranquiVed Injectable, Vedco, Inc.)

Xylazine + Butorphanol (Torbugesic) (10 mg/ml)

a) Xylazine 0.5 mg IV + butorphanol 0.02–0.03 mg/kg IV (Plumb, 2005)

Detomidine (Dormosedan) (10 mg/ml)

a) 20–40 micrograms (µg)/kg (0.02–0.04 mg/kg) IV or IM (package insert Dormosedan, Pfizer Inc. Pfizer Animal Health)

Detomidine + Butorphanol (Torbugesic) (10 mg/ml)

a) Detomidine 10–15 micrograms/kg (0.01–0.015 mg/kg) IV + butorphanol 20–30 micrograms/kg (0.02–0.03 mg/kg) IV. One can extend sedation/analgesic time if needed by repeating the same dose(s) of detomidine or butorphanol or both, IV. (Ko, 2002)

76

Acepromazine* (10 mg/ml)

a) 0.044–0.88 mg/kg IV (slowly) or IM (package insert Acepromazine Maleate Injection, Boehringer Ingleheim).
*Do NOT use in stallions (intact male horses). Do NOT use in hypovolemic animals.

Anti-inflammatory Drugs

Phenybutazone 20% (200 mg/ml, Oral Paste)

a) 1–2 grams IV or PO every 24 hours to every 12 hours per adult (≥450 kg [1000 lb]) horse. Injection should be made slowly and with care. Extravasation is extremely irritating to tissues. Limit IV administration to no more than 5 successive days of therapy and follow with oral forms if necessary (Plumb, 1999). Phenylbutazone is available in tablet form, but to avoid esophagitis the tablets should be pulverized and mixed with syrup, applesauce, grain, etc., which may not be practical in a first aid setting. Therefore, the oral paste is recommended.

Flunixin Meglumine (Banamine) (50 mg/ml, Oral Paste)

a) 1.1 mg/kg IV every 24 hours (package insert Banamine Injectable, Schering-Plough). Even though Banamine is labeled for IM administration as well, this route is not recommended due to local tissue reaction and sequelae.
b) For colic analgesia 1.1 mg/kg IV; dose may be repeated if signs of pain return (package insert Banamine Injectable, Schering-Plough).
c) 1.1 mg/kg PO every 24 hours (package insert Banamine Paste, Schering-Plough)

Suggested Reading

Barnett KC. *Equine Ophthalmology: An Atlas and Text*, ed 2. London, Elsevier Health Sciences, 2004.
Plumb DC. *Veterinary Drug Handbook*, ed 6. Ames, IA, Blackwell Publishing, 2008.
Rose RJ, Hodgson DR. *Manual of Equine Practice*, ed 2. Philadelphia, WB Saunders, 1999.
Stashak TS. *Adams' Lameness in Horses*, ed 5. Ames, IA, Blackwell Publishing, 2002.
Stashak TS. *Equine Wound Management*. Philadelphia, Lea & Febiger, 1991.

CHAPTER 3
VETERINARY TRIAGE

Wayne E. Wingfield, MS, DVM and Sally B. Palmer, DVM

In a disaster, triage must be conducted with the purpose of doing the greatest good for the largest number of patients. Rapid examination followed by classification of patients according to the urgency of their treatment needs is critical. Triage is an organized approach to multiple patients and ensures that the most critical animals are identified and normalized first. To that end, triage is based on two key points: (1) the medical needs of the patient and (2) the available medical resources (facilities, supplies, equipment, personnel, and time). Triage in local disasters requires knowledge of available facilities and capacities immediately adjacent to the disaster as well as knowing this same information for facilities located just outside of the disaster area. Without doubt, conventional triage is only the first step in a dynamic decision-making process.

3. Triage

3.1. Human Triage

3.1.1. *Triage* refers to the sorting of patients for treatment priority. Recognizing that there are different triage "protocols," the overall goal of any triage system is to provide the greatest good for the greatest number.

3.1.2. To that end, triage is based on two key points:
I. The medical needs of the patient.
II. The available medical resources—including facilities, supplies, equipment, personnel, and time.
  A. Depending on the situation, one or the other of these points will dictate the most appropriate treatment priority.

3.1.3. Triage in the field, or *prehospital triage,* is done to ensure priority transport of the most severely injured to the appropriate trauma level (I–IV) hospital.
I. *Multiple casualties*—When the number of patients and/or the severity of injuries does NOT exceed the capabilities of the available medical resources, those patients with the most severe injuries are treated first.

II. *Mass casualties*—When the number of patients and/or the severity of injuries DOES exceed the capabilities of the available medical resources, the patients with the greatest chance of survival requiring the least consumption of available medical resources are treated first.

3.1.4. In large-scale disasters, field triage is first accomplished and defines patients as they lay at the site.
  I.   Categories of field triage
      A.   Acute (red)
      B.   Nonacute (green)
  II.   From field triage, one then proceeds to "medical triage," and it is here that START and SAVE come into play.

3.1.5. One common protocol used in human triage is Simple Triage And Rapid Transport (START).
  I.   This system is based on primary observation of patients with regard to respiration, perfusion, and mental status (RPM) to assess patients in less than 60 seconds and assign an appropriate classification (Table 3.1).

Table 3.1. Triage categories used in human medicine.

Triage Color	Triage Category	RPM*
Red	Immediate (Emergent)	Altered
Yellow	Delayed (Urgent)	"Normal"
Green	Minor	Walking Wounded
Black	Unsalvageable (Dead, Dying)	Mortal wounds; will likely die despite medical attention or be found dead when initially assessed

*RPM = Respiration, pulse, and mental status.

3.1.6. Unlike first aid and basic life support, where the primary survey follows the ABCDs of trauma care and life-threatening conditions are identified and treated simultaneously, triage identifies those patients needing immediate care but does not administer that immediate care.
  I.   For example, when triaging, one may quickly attempt to clear an airway, but time is not spent to maintain an airway or to assist ventilation.

3.1.7. After START is completed, the transition phase begins, which is resource dependent:
  I.   Transport if possible.
  II.   Group like-categories of patients together.
  III.   Provide stabilizing care.
  IV.   Re-triage if the condition changes.

3.1.8. During incidents (most notably large-scale disasters) where transportation is significantly delayed or not available and facilities are overwhelmed or destroyed, the Secondary Assessment of Victim Endpoint (SAVE) method of triage may be used.

I. SAVE is based on the assumption that victims have been triaged based on START, there are limited medical and transport resources resulting in prolonged evacuation to definitive medical care, and patients may deteriorate because of these resource limitations.

II. The theory of SAVE can be represented by the following formula:

Benefit Expected × (Probability of Survival) = Value Resources Required

3.1.9. SAVE patients are categorized based on:
I. Those who will die regardless of care.
II. Those who will survive whether or not they receive care.
III. Those who will benefit from limited immediate (field) intervention.

3.1.10. SAVE begins with a reassessment of patients based on START triage. Immediate and delayed patients go to the treatment area, where they are treated based on severity and resources. Those patients who need limited resources with a high probability of surviving will probably be treated first. Minor and unsalvageable casualties proceed to observation areas (potentially in the same area depending on personnel resources) where they are periodically reassessed. Patients who do not respond to treatment are re-triaged, tagged, and sent to the observation area.

3.1.11. While different incidents will determine the triage method, the overall principle of assessing medical need and resource availability in order to provide the greatest good for the greatest number is the basic triage goal for humans.

3.2. Veterinary Triage

3.2.1. Assessing (1) the medical needs of the patient and (2) the medical resources available are still the basic principles of veterinary triage.
I. However, triage results and treatment decisions may be different because of the differences between human and veterinary medicine.

3.2.2. Factors responsible for these differences include:
I. The option of euthanasia.
II. Little tolerance for fair to poor outcomes of animal patients including long-term/permanent disabilities or intensive nursing care requirements.
III. Transport difficulties for large numbers of animals, or for certain species.
IV. Limited veterinary medical resources (facilities, equipment, supplies, and personnel, varying 24-hour emergency care capabilities).
V. Additional considerations that impact triage decisions within veterinary medicine include:
  A. Companion animals (dogs, cats, horses, pocket pets, birds, etc.) versus livestock animals (cattle, sheep, pigs, poultry, etc.).
  B. Small animals versus large animals.
  C. Presently, in veterinary medicine, there is no such designation of a Level I, II, III, or IV trauma clinic or hospital.

1. Most veterinary practices fall into two broad categories: general practice (of one or more species) or specialty practice (surgery, medicine, critical care, emergency, etc.).

2. Specialty practices tend to be limited to the larger metropolitan areas and academic institutions.

3. Many areas of the country are limited in their access to general practice care as well. Therefore, destination options may be limited, and triage will focus on identifying medical needs of the patient in light of available transport and medical resources, as well as the professional competency of the veterinarian.

D. Recognize that the treatment of animals is still dependent on the animal owner's disposable income; therefore, "medical resources" includes not only facilities, supplies, equipment, personnel, and time, but also money.

1. In a disaster, all animals will receive first aid care regardless of the owner's ability to pay.

3.2.3. Triage in veterinary medicine involves three systems
I. Field triage
II. Medical triage
III. Mobile veterinary unit triage

3.2.4. Field triage
I. Requires experienced veterinarians or rescuers.
II. Usually does not involve the individual examination of animals. More commonly, the animals are observed and decisions are made.
III. Designed to identify animals most likely to benefit from the available care under austere conditions.
IV. Divides animals into three categories (Table 3.2).
  A. Those that will likely die regardless of how much care they receive. Coded color = Black
  B. Those that will survive whether or not they receive care. Coded color = Green
  C. Those that will benefit significantly from austere interventions. Coded color = Red.

Table 3.2. Triage color codes used in veterinary field triage.

Triage Color	Triage Category	Explanation
Red	Immediate	Might benefit from austere interventions
Green	Minor	Walking wounded but likely to survive
Black	Dead, dying, or euthanatize	Dead, dying, or euthanatize

V. Advantages of the veterinary field triage system
  A. Focuses resources appropriately.
  B. Requires an experienced triage team.
  C. Tough decisions are made and adhered to.

D. After the disaster is over, the team will retrospectively examine decisions and dedicate themselves to an improved performance.

3.2.5. Medical triage

I.   Medical triage is done rapidly and involves examining individual animals.

II. One approach is to use the following four physiological criteria (RPPN):

A.   Respirations/minute

B.   Pulse rate/minute

C.   Pulse pressure

1.   Although subjective, pulse pressure has a linear relationship to stroke volume. Therefore, if the pulse pressure is decreased (as you might see in shock), the stroke volume is also likely decreased.

$$\text{Cardiac Output} = \text{Heart Rate} \times \text{Stroke Volume}$$

D.   Neurological status

III. Medical triage using RPPN (Table 3.3).

Table 3.3. Medical triage in veterinary patients using RPPN.

Category	Color	RPPN*
Immediate	**Red**	Abnormal RPP
Urgent	Yellow	Abnormal PPN
Minor	**Green**	"Normal RPPN"
Dead, Dying, or Euthanasia	**Black**	Mortal Wounds or <u>Severely</u> Abnormal Neurological

*RPPN = **R**espiration, **P**ulse rate, **P**ulse pressure, and **N**eurological status.

A.   In veterinary triage, it is important to recognize that limitations of treatment and injuries for certain species will affect the triage assessment.

1.   For example, a fractured femur in a dog may be tagged Yellow, but a fractured femur in a horse will be tagged Black.

IV. A relatively small number of animals can overwhelm the veterinary medical system, necessitating the implementation of the field triage system discussed earlier.

V.   The same basic triage principles apply to both veterinary and human patients. The theory can be represented by the following formula:

Benefit Expected × (Probability of Survival) = Value Resources Required

VI. Medical triage always begins with a reassessment of patients.

A.   Immediate and urgent patients go to the treatment area, where they are treated based on severity and resources. Those patients who need limited resources with a high probability of surviving will probably be treated first.

B.   Minor casualties go to an observation area where they are periodically reassessed.

C.   Patients that do not respond to treatment are re-tagged and sent to the observation area or euthanatized.

D.   One critical difference in veterinary triage is that the category of patients that will die regardless of how much care they receive and those that will suffer for the lack of care will be euthanatized.

    1.   Therefore, it is very important to properly identify those animals that will survive whether or not they receive care and those that will benefit significantly from available interventions.

    2.   Of note, while euthanatizing an injured animal is done for humane reasons, these decisions need to be well documented and supported.

        a.   It is not uncommon for some animals (horses especially) to be insured, and the insurance company must authorize the euthanasia when possible. When contacting the insurance company is not feasible, documentation and witnesses are very important.

VII.   Flow chart for medical triage using RPPN (Figure 3.1).

Medical Triage Using RPPN

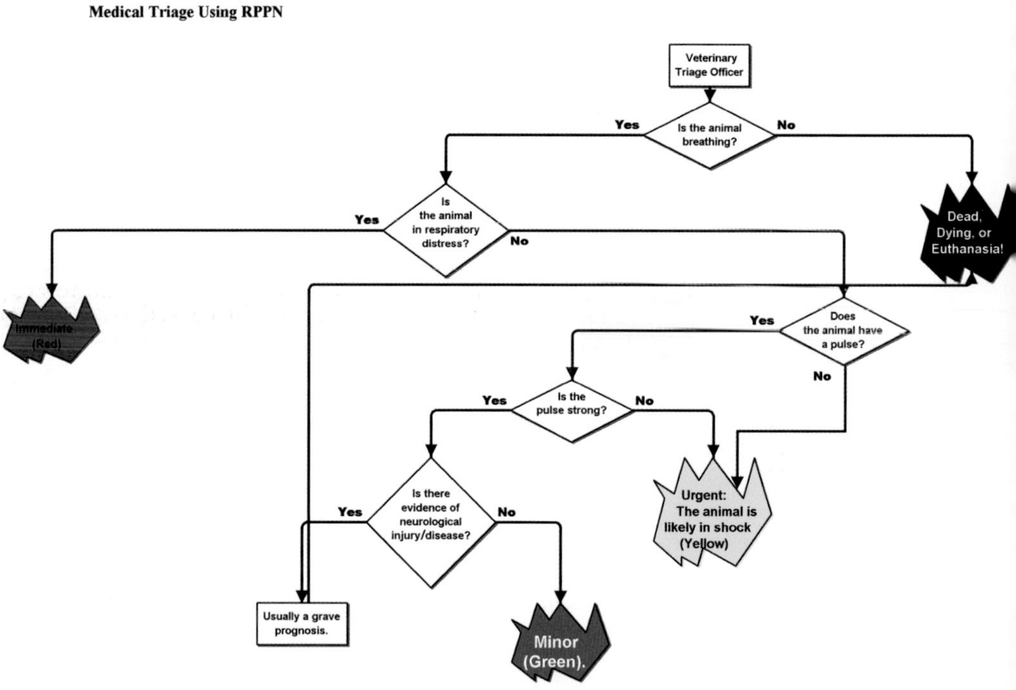

Figure 3.1   Flow chart to provide guidance in learning medical triage.

VIII.   All animals must be identified and a variety of methods can be used.

A.   Ribbons of the appropriate triage color may be attached to the animal. These will have no information regarding the patient.

B.   An alternative would be to attach a triage tag to the animal (Fig. 3.2). This tag uses an image of a dog, but this should not deter its use on other veterinary species. The idea is to identify wounds, fractures, burns, etc. by marking an approximate location on the triage tag image.

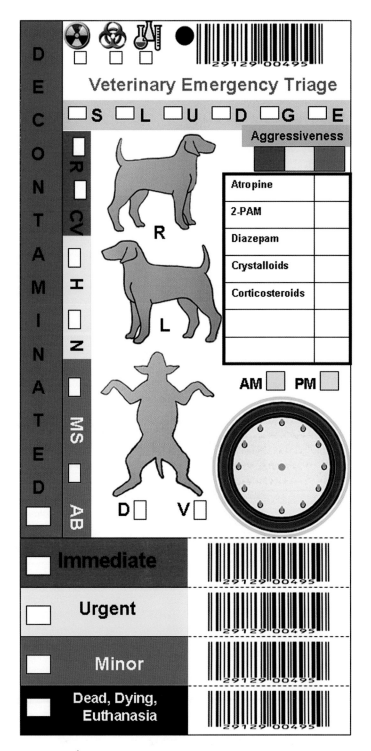

Figure 3.2 Proposed veterinary triage tag.

85

    1. It is also important that the behavioral disposition of the animal be identified to make other responders aware of potential aggressiveness.

3.2.6. Mobile veterinary unit triage

I. Triage in a mobile veterinary unit utilizes a physiological systems approach entitled Veterinary Systems Triage and Rapid Treatment (V-START)
    A. Physiological systems priorities in V-START
        1. Respiratory
        2. Cardiovascular
        3. Hemorrhage
        4. Neurological
        5. Musculoskeletal
        6. Abdominal injuries
II. Categories and coding (Table 3.4)

Table 3.4. Triage coding for mobile veterinary unit triage. Notice the blue category has been added to indicate whether an animal has been decontaminated.

Group	Color	Types of Injuries
Immediate	Red	Critical: May survive if life-saving measures are administered.
Urgent	Yellow	Likely to survive if care is given within hours.
Minor	Green	Minor injuries: Care may be delayed while other patients receive treatment.
All Groups	Blue	Animal has been decontaminated.
Dead, Dying, or Euthanasia	Black	Dead or severely injured and not expected to survive.

III. Guidelines in coding using V-START (Table 3.5)
    A. Working dogs and horses
    B. Similar to the human START protocol, a rapid assessment, based on the ABCDEs of emergency care, is done to appropriately categorize and tag patients based on their medical needs.
        1. A—Airway
        2. B—Breathing
        3. C—Circulation
        4. D—Disability (neurological and musculoskeletal)
        5. E—Environmental (hypothermia/hyperthermia)
IV. Flow charts and table to assist in the use of V-START during mobile veterinary unit triage (Figs. 3.3–3.5).

Table 3.5. Triage categories using V-START.

Triage Color	Category	Physiological System Involvement
Red	Immediate	Respiratory, Cardiovascular, (Hypothermia, Hyperthermia)
Yellow	Urgent	Cardiovascular, Musculoskeletal, Neurological, Abdominal Injuries
Green	Minor	Musculoskeletal, Neurological, Abdominal Injuries
Black	Dead, Dying, or Euthanasia	Dead or dying when initially assessed. Mortal wounds not compatible with "Quality of Life" issues. Euthanasia.

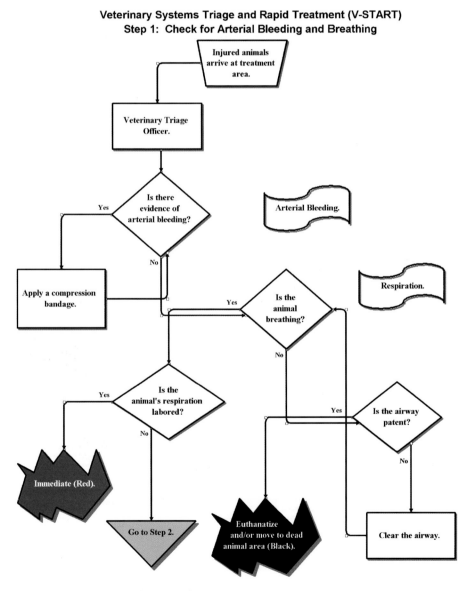

Veterinary Systems Triage and Rapid Treatment (V-START)
Step 1: Check for Arterial Bleeding and Breathing

Figure 3.3 Step 1 guides you in learning V-START.

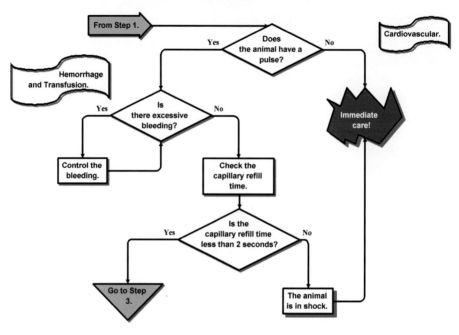

Figure 3.4 Step 2 guides you in learning V-START.

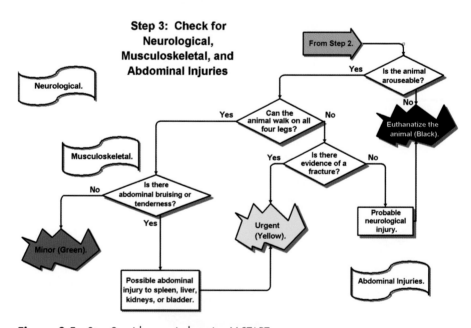

Figure 3.5 Step 3 guides you in learning V-START.

3.3. Additional Veterinary Triage Support

3.3.1. Livestock

I.   Triage of injured food animals (cattle, sheep, pigs, poultry, etc.) is based on three factors:

  A.   Economic concerns

  B.   Public health concerns

  C.   Humane concerns

II.   Unless there is an economic benefit to treating an injured food animal, treatment will not be given and the animal will be euthanatized. If the disaster involves a zoonotic disease, it is likely the entire population in the affected area will be euthanatized.

III.   As a guideline, triage of livestock will use the field and medical methods consecutively.

  A.   Without benefit of chutes or alleyways, a hands-on V-START assessment is not practical and observation of animals may suffice for initial triage.

  B.   If corrals or pens are available, animals may be sorted into triage groups rather than individually "tagged."

  C.   "Tagging" livestock, especially cattle, buffalo, etc., is problematic.

   1.   Different colored grease crayons may be used, but they have limitations.

   2.   Neck ribbons may work for sheep and goats.

   3.   Spray paints may have some application depending on species, weather, etc.

  D.   While field and medical triage identifies those animals classified as Immediate and Urgent, these animals will frequently be reassessed as Black during the mobile veterinary unit triage (V-START) categorization—based on the lack of resources.

   1.   Most surviving animals will be tagged as minor and are categorized as "those who will survive whether or not they receive care."

   2.   Very few animals will be in the category of "those benefiting from intervention," primarily because of the economics of administering medical treatment.

  E.   Another consideration in the triage and treatment of livestock is whether or not an animal will be imminently slaughtered for food (human or animal) products. Many medications have regulated drug withdrawal periods for animals going to slaughter, so judicious use and intervention with drugs must be considered if treatment is attempted.

3.4. Summary

3.4.1.   Both human and veterinary medicine use triage to sort and prioritize treatment of patients.

3.4.2.   Both require an understanding of the medical needs of the patient, and the available medical resources.

I. While the medical decision making process is similar in human and veterinary triage, the triage results and treatment decisions may differ because of the differences between human and veterinary medicine.

3.4.3. Recognizing these similarities and differences is important in order to optimize the triage goal of doing the greatest good for the greatest number.

Suggested Reading

Bozeman WP. Mass casualty incident triage. Ann Emerg Med 2003;41:582–583.

Buono CJ, Lyon J, Huang J, et al. Comparison of mass casualty incident triage acuity status accuracy by traditional paper method, electronic tag, and provider PDA algorithm. Ann Emerg Med 2007;50:S12–S13.

Ducharme J, Tanabe P, Todd K, et al. A comparison of triage systems and their impact on initial pain management: A multicenter study. Ann Emerg Med 2006;48:61.

Garner A, Lee A, Harrison K, Schultz CH. Comparative analysis of multiple-casualty incident triage algorithms. Ann Emerg Med 2001;38:541–548.

Hirshberg A, Holcomb JB, Mattox KL. Hospital trauma care in multiple-casualty incidents: A critical view. Ann Emerg Med 2001;37:647–652.

Iserson KV, Moskop JC. Triage in medicine, part I: Concept, history, and types. Ann Emerg Med 2007;49:275–281.

Meredith W, Rutledge R, Hansen AR, et al. Field triage of trauma patients based upon the ability to follow commands: A study in 29,573 injured patients. J Trauma 1995;38:129–135.

Moskop JC, Iserson KV. Triage in medicine, part II: Underlying values and principles. Ann Emerg Med 2007;49:282–287.

Pesik N, Keim ME, Iserson KV. Terrorism and the ethics of emergency medical care. Ann Emerg Med 2001;37:642–646.

Richards ME, Nufer KE. Simple triage and rapid treatment: Does it predict transportation and referral needs in patients evaluated by disaster medical assistance teams? Ann Emerg Med 2004;44:S33–S34.

Ross SE, Leipold C, Terregino C, O'Malley KF. Efficacy of the motor component of the Glasgow Coma Scale in trauma triage. J Trauma 1998;45:42–44.

Torres HC, Moreno-Walton L, Radeos M. The reliability of triage classification as a predictor of severity in major trauma. Ann Emerg Med 2007;50:S106–S107.

CHAPTER 4
BOMB BLASTS AND EXPLOSIVES

Wayne E. Wingfield, MS, DVM

Explosive devices have become the destructive agents of choice for many terrorists, primarily because the materials used to construct them are so easily accessible. During the 1990s, a number of bombing incidents diminished Americans' sense of security. In February 1993, the World Trade Center bombing in New York City killed 6 people and injured more than 1000. In April 1995, a truck bomb exploded at the Murrah Federal Building in Oklahoma City, killing 168 people and injuring more than 750. In June 1996, the bombing of Khobar Towers in Dhahran, Saudi Arabia, killed 19 U.S. airmen. A year later, a bomb attack at Olympic Centennial Park in Atlanta was intended to harm not only bystanders but also the law enforcement officers who went to the scene after receiving a telephone call announcing the pending explosion. Similarly, in 1997, also in Atlanta, a secondary device was aimed at firefighters, emergency medical services (EMS) personnel, and police officers called to bombings at a health care clinic and a nightclub. Finally, the use of aircraft to attack the World Trade Center and the Pentagon resulted in nearly 3000 human deaths on September 11, 2001. The use of roadside and suicide bombers in Iraq has accounted for most injuries and deaths in this conflict. Undoubtedly, these tactics will one day make their way to our homeland, and we need to be prepared to identify and respond to these devices.

4. Bomb Blasts and Explosives

4.1. Explosives are Categorized as High-order Explosives (HE) or Low-order Explosives (LE)

4.1.1. HE produces a defining supersonic overpressurization shock wave.
  I. Examples of HE include TNT, C-4, Semtex, nitroglycerin, dynamite, and ammonium nitrate fuel oil (ANFO).

4.1.2. LE creates a subsonic explosion and lack HE's overpressurization wave.
  I. Examples of LE include pipe bombs, gunpowder, and most pure petroleum-based bombs such as Molotov cocktails or aircraft improvised as guided missiles.

4.1.3. Explosive and incendiary (fire) bombs are further characterized based on their source.

   I. *Manufactured* implies standard military-issued, mass produced, and quality-tested weapons.

     A. Manufactured (military) explosive weapons are exclusively HE based.

   II. *Improvised* describes weapons produced in small quantities or use of a device outside its intended purpose, such as converting a commercial aircraft into a guided missile.

4.1.4. Terrorists will use whatever is available—illegally obtained manufactured weapons or improvised explosive devices (also known as IEDs) that may be composed of HE, LE, or both.

4.2. Three Basic Types of Explosions

4.2.1. *Mechanical:* Involves a buildup of pressure inside a container, often due to overheating. Once the internal pressure exceeds the structural capacity of the container, the container fails.

4.2.2. *Chemical:* Caused by an almost instantaneous conversion of a solid or liquid explosive compound into gases that have a much greater volume than the substance from which they were generated. All manufactured explosives (except nuclear) are chemical explosives.

4.2.3. *Nuclear:* May be induced by either fission (the splitting of nuclei of atoms) or fusion (the joining of the nuclei of atoms under great force).

4.3. Mechanisms of Blast Injury

4.3.1. Disaster response personnel (including veterinarians) must understand the pathophysiology of injuries associated with explosions and must be prepared to assess and treat the injured animals.

4.3.2. The early presentation of victims can be deceiving, because the initial manifestations of significant injury can be subtle.

4.3.3. The four basic mechanisms of blast injury are termed *primary, secondary, tertiary,* and *quaternary* (Table 4.1). "Blast wave" (primary) refers to the intense overpressurization impulse created by a detonated HE. Blast injuries are characterized by anatomical and physiological changes from the direct or reflective overpressurization force impacting the body's surface. The HE "blast wave" (overpressure component) should be distinguished from "blast wind" (forced superheated airflow). The latter may be encountered with both HE and LE.

   I. Explosions cause injury through four principal mechanisms.

     A. Primary blast injury, secondary injury, and tertiary injury. Primary blast injury is caused by the effect of the blast wave or pressure wave on the body.

Table 4.1. Mechanisms of Blast Injury.

Category	Characteristics	Body Part Affected	Types of Injuries
Primary	Unique to HE, results from the impact of the overpressurization wave with body surfaces	Gas-filled structures are most susceptible—lungs, gastrointestinal tract, and middle ear	Blast lung (pulmonary barotrauma) TM rupture and middle ear damage Abdominal hemorrhage and perforation Globe (eye) rupture Concussion (TBI without physical signs of head injury)
Secondary	Results from flying debris and bomb fragments	Any body part may be affected	Penetrating ballistic (fragmentation) or blunt injuries Eye penetration (can be occult)
Tertiary	Results from individuals being thrown by the blast wind	Any body part may be affected	Fracture and traumatic amputation Closed and open brain injury
Quaternary	All explosion-related injuries, illnesses, or diseases not due to primary, secondary, or tertiary mechanisms Includes exacerbation or complications of existing conditions	Any body part may be affected	Burns (flash, partial, and full thickness) Crush injuries Closed and open brain injury Asthma, COPD, or other breathing problems from dust, smoke, or toxic fumes Angina Hyperglycemia Hypertension

After *Explosions and Blast Injuries: A Primer for Clinicians.* Atlanta, Centers for Disease Control and Prevention (CDC), May 9, 2003.

B.   Secondary injury is the result of debris propelled by the blast wind of the explosion. These flying projectiles can produce both penetrating and blunt trauma.

C.   Tertiary injuries are caused by the displacement of the body by the blast winds into environmental objects. Regardless of the mechanism of explosion-related injury, the basic principles of trauma care still apply.

D.   Quaternary injuries are all explosion-related injuries, illnesses, or diseases not due to primary, secondary, or tertiary mechanisms and include exacerbation of complications of existing conditions.

4.3.4.   Blast waves are produced by the detonation of munitions, the firing of large-caliber guns, and any type of explosion. These waves can be powerful enough to injure exposed animals.

4.3.5. The organs most vulnerable to this type of injury are the gas-filled organs, namely, the ear, the lungs, and the gastrointestinal tract.

    I. An important concept that defines injury patterns is the medium in which the blast occurs. An underwater blast wave has particular lethality because water is incompressible compared with air. Therefore, a wave resulting from a blast occurring underwater travels farther and faster than a wave from a similar explosion on land. Hence, blast injuries in water occur at greater distances from the detonation point and are often more severe.

        A. Another characteristic of blast waves is that they are indeed waves, traveling in a sinusoidal pattern. The injury patterns they produce are caused not only by the medium in which they travel but also by the position of the victim's body in relation to the wave and any reflective/deflecting objects in the environment. For example, as a blast wave strikes a wall, it is reflected, subsequently magnifying the wave's energy. An animal standing in front of a wall reflecting a blast wave can be subjected to devastating forces. Similarly, the use of body armor on both humans and animals may provide a false sense of security. Body armor does protect from shrapnel, but significant underlying blunt trauma may result from exposure to a wave blast coming from an explosion. (The advantages of body armor far outweigh this risk.) As the wave strikes the body of someone wearing armor, the energy is reflected against the inside of the body protection, producing injuries far greater than if no armor was worn at all.

        B. Therefore, a person or animal wearing body armor cannot be presumed to have been protected from explosion-related injury. Explosions in confined spaces have a similar effect. Injuries are magnified by the effect of reflective surfaces within a closed room.

4.3.6. *Primary blast injury:* Primary blast injury is caused by the direct effect of a blast wave created by an explosion. When an explosion occurs, gases expand suddenly and spherically from the center of the explosion. Because of the compressibility of air, this expansion of gases compresses the surrounding air, creating a high-pressure front. This blast wave travels outward at supersonic speeds of more than 900 mph. Primary blast injury is the direct result of this dense wave striking the body. Bystanders feel the explosion as a sudden thump in their chest, which is the arrival of the pressure/blast wave (Fig. 4.1). Under some circumstances, this force is magnified several thousand times, causing significant injury.

    I. *Primary blast injury* has three primary mechanisms.

        A. The first is *spalling*, which occurs when the shock wave (blast wave) transfers from a dense medium (liquid) such as water to a less-dense medium (gas) such as air. In an underwater explosion, for example, the shock wave travels in front of the detonation, reaches the surface, and reflects off the less-dense air. This scenario is comparable to the effect of striking the outside of a rusty bucket with a hammer. The transfer of energy displaces rust from the inside of the bucket, even though the hammer did not strike it directly. During naval battles, depth charges are released into the water. It appears as if there are two explosions for each depth charge. The first is the *spalling* effect. It causes injury by the transfer of reflected blast wave energy through a body's' dense substrates (liver, muscle) into the less-dense material of the gastrointestinal tract and lungs. An upward explosion of water follows because of expanding gases caused by the detonation.

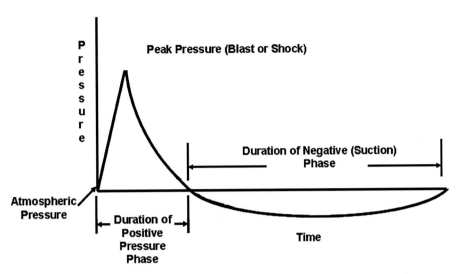

Figure 4.1. Blast injuries. Idealized graph of a blast pressure wave over time. (After Bowen TE, Bellamy RF, editors. *Emergency War Surgery.* Washington, DC, U.S. Government Printing Office, 1988.)

Table 4.2. Selected Pressure Effects of Explosions.*

Pressure (PSI)	Effect
5	Possible tympanic membrane rupture
15	50% incidence of tympanic membrane rupture
30	Possible lung injury
40	Concrete shatters
75	50% incidence of lung injury
100	Possible fatal injuries
200	Death more likely than not

*Adapted from Kizer KW. Dysbarism. In Tintinalli JE, Kelen GD, Stapyczynski JS, editors. *Emergency Medicine: A Comprehensive Study Guide*, ed 5. New York, McGraw-Hill, 2000, p 1276.

    B. The second mechanism of injury is the implosion of gas-filled spaces as the high pressure in the surrounding fluid or solid compresses them.
    C. Third, primary injuries are related to differences in tissue density, which affects rates of acceleration and deceleration. These differences result in shearing and tearing forces.
       1. The organs most vulnerable to primary blast injury are those containing air (Table 4.2).
          a. The body is able to respond to pressure change well if the change in pressure is slow. The ear uses the Eustachian tube to equilibrate the pressures of the middle ear. Diving to the bottom of a pool induces a similar effect of pressure changes. The atmospheric pressure increases toward the bottom of the pool, squeezing the middle ear. A diver can open the Eustachian tubes by holding his or her nose and blowing (performing a

Valsalva maneuver), which relieves the pressure on the middle ear. Diving-induced increases in pressure are minimal (1 to 2 atmospheres above normal), yet they can cause profound discomfort to the middle ear if equalization does not occur. Similar venting is used by the lungs through the respiratory tree and by the gastrointestinal tract through expulsion of gases. Each of these mechanisms allows the body to equilibrate with the ambient atmospheric pressure. An explosion that produces a pressure wave 1000 times the magnitude of the example above, traveling at supersonic speed, will impose tremendous damage when it strikes any body in its path. Hollow organs are disrupted by the rapid increase in atmospheric pressure. As the pressure wave strikes the body, it compresses the air-filled organs and collapses them. Gas-filled organs are like balloons filled with air. If they are squeezed by applying hard pressure rapidly (as during the impact of a pressure wave), they will burst. The resulting force causes shearing of vascular beds, pulmonary contusions, pneumothorax, and gastrointestinal hemorrhage. In fact, the force of a pressure wave can be significant enough to force air into blood vessels, resulting in air emboli (Fig. 4.2).

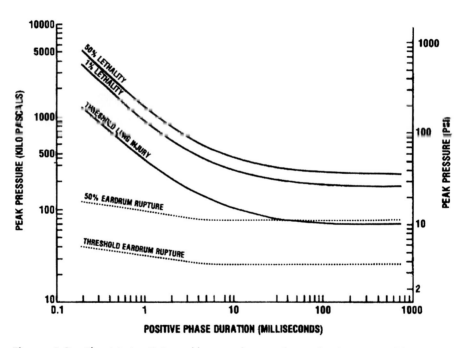

Figure 4.2. Blast injuries. Estimated human tolerances for single, sharp, rising blast waves. (After Bowen TE, Bellamy RF, editors. *Emergency War Surgery.* Washington, DC, U.S. Government Printing Office, 1988.)

II.   *Secondary blast injuries:* Secondary blast injuries (penetrating or blunt) result from debris acting as projectiles as the blast wave propels them. Since the blast wave travels at supersonic speeds, there is little chance that people in its path will be able to dodge the wavefront or the debris it carries. Therefore, scene safety is vitally important. Since the energy of the blast wave dissipates with distance, it is important for responders and victims to move (or be moved) a safe distance away. This distance depends on the degree of threat.

III.   *Tertiary blast injuries:* Tertiary injuries are the result of animals and humans being thrown by the blast wave and associated wind. The victim becomes a projectile. Injuries in this category vary depending on what the victim hits in the environment. This category also includes "miscellaneous effects": burns from fire or radiation, crush injury associated with structural collapse, as well as smoke and carbon monoxide inhalation (which has particular importance if an explosion occurred in a closed space).

IV.   *Quaternary blast injuries:* Quaternary injuries are all explosion-related injuries, illnesses, or diseases not due to primary, secondary, or tertiary mechanisms and include exacerbation of complications of existing conditions.

4.3.7.   Assessment of the working animal following blast injury (Table 4.3).

Table 4.3.   Overview of Explosive-related Injuries.

System	Injury or Condition
Auditory	TM rupture, ossicular disruption, cochlear damage, foreign body
Eye, orbit, face	Perforated globe, foreign body, air embolism, fractures
Respiratory	Blast lung, hemothorax, pneumothorax, pulmonary contusion and hemorrhage, AV fistulas (source of air embolism), airway epithelial damage, aspiration pneumonitis, sepsis
Digestive	Bowel perforation, hemorrhage, ruptured liver or spleen, sepsis, mesenteric ischemia from air embolism
Circulatory	Cardiac contusion, myocardial infarction from air embolism, shock, vasovagal hypotension, peripheral vascular injury, air embolism–induced injury
CNS injury	Concussion, closed and open brain injury, stroke, spinal cord injury, air embolism–induced injury
Renal injury	Renal contusion, laceration, acute renal failure due to rhabdomyolysis, hypotension, and hypovolemia
Extremity injury	Traumatic amputation, fractures, crush injuries, compartment syndrome, burns, cuts, lacerations, acute arterial occlusion, air embolism–induced injury

Note: Up to 10% of all blast survivors have significant eye injuries. These injuries involve perforations from high-velocity projectiles, can occur with minimal initial discomfort, and present for care for days, weeks, or months after the event. Symptoms include eye pain or irritation, foreign body sensation, altered vision, periorbital swelling or contusions. Findings can include decreased visual acuity, hyphema, globe perforation, subconjunctival hemorrhage, foreign body, or lid lacerations. Liberal referral for ophthalmologic screening is encouraged. (After *Explosions and Blast Injuries: A Primer for Clinicians.* Atlanta, Centers for Disease Control and Prevention [CDC], May 9, 2003.)

I.   The approach to the casualty with explosion-induced injury is the same as for any trauma victim, i.e., initiation of life support measures. Attention should be directed to the common life-threatening manifestations of thoracic and abdominal injuries. Pulmonary manifestations include hemorrhage, barotrauma, and arterial air embolism; abdominal manifestations include hemorrhage and hollow organ rupture. Therapy is directed at the specific manifestations as well as avoiding iatrogenic injury.

II.   Signs and symptoms

A.   The initial assessment begins with the early recognition of potential injuries. Affected animals may appear disoriented and confused, and they may have difficulty hearing because of eardrum rupture. The organ most sensitive to pressure change is the ear. The ear is designed with the specific purpose of collecting and amplifying pressure signals. Acoustic energy is converted to mechanical energy by displacement of the tympanic membrane (eardrum) into the middle ear. If the rise of energy is too rapid, the eardrum cannot accommodate the rapid pressure change and therefore ruptures (Figs. 4.3 and 4.4). The threshold of tympanic rupture is approximately 5 pounds per square inch (PSI). Fifty percent of people exposed to pressures above 15 PSI over atmospheric pressure will have eardrum rupture (Table 4.2). Therefore, not all animals exposed to a blast will present with ruptured eardrums, but those who do will require special attention because further underlying injury may exist. Isolated eardrum perforation in survivors of explosions does not appear to be a marker of concealed pulmonary blast injury or of poor prognosis. Thus, if an animal presents with isolated eardrum rupture, a thoracic film should be obtained and the patient should be admitted for 24 hours to rule out pulmonary injury. In a mass casualty event, persons who have sustained isolated eardrum perforation from explosions may be discharged from the emergency hospital after chest radiography and a brief observation period.

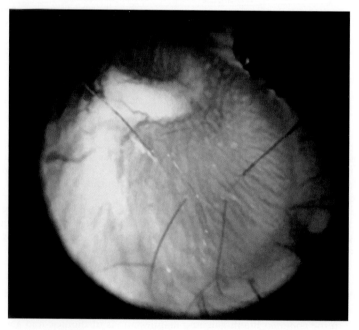

Figure 4.3. Normal tympanic membrane in the external ear of the dog.

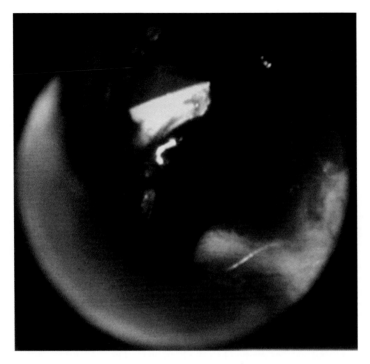

Figure 4.4. Ruptured tympanic membrane in the ear of a dog.

B.   A careful examination may reveal ruptured tympanic membranes (eardrums) or hypopharyngeal petechial hemorrhages. These early findings should alert the rescuer to the fact that the victim sustained a significant exposure to a blast wave. Hence, underlying injuries to the pulmonary and gastrointestinal tract should be suspected and a thorough clinical examination should be performed.

C.   *Pulmonary:* Disorientation and confusion may be the result of head injury. If these symptoms coincide with tympanic membrane rupture, air embolism may be present. In addition, medical personnel should observe victims for shortness of breath, chest tightness, and hemoptysis (bloody cough). Each of these complaints is related to blunt trauma of the chest caused by the blast wave. Pulmonary contusions are delayed in their development and may not be evident for several hours. "Blast lung" may not be present for 48 hours. Hence, it is important to obtain a thoracic film on all animals suspected of blast wave exposure, along with observation for at least 24 hours. There are no laboratory studies that offer any diagnostic help. An arterial blood gas measurement may be helpful in the diagnosis if hypoxia is present.

D.   *Gastrointestinal:* Gastrointestinal injuries are much more difficult to identify, so clinical suspicion must be entertained. Early signs of gastrointestinal injury include decreased bowel sounds, abdominal tenderness, and rectal bleeding. Early radiographs of the abdomen may reveal free air under the diaphragm or air in the lumen of the intestine. These findings indicate significant abdominal injury. Their emergence may be delayed for several days.

4.3.8. Treatment

I.   Regardless of the mechanism of explosion-related injury, the basic principles of trauma care still apply. As with any trauma patient, attention to life support measures should be implemented. A thorough history and examination can yield diagnostic clues of underlying injuries. Tympanic membrane rupture and hypopharyngeal hemorrhages require only conservative management. Neither of these carries any increase in morbidity. However, because they can be indicators of exposure to a significant pressure wave, further evaluation is required.

II.   The most important aspect of care is airway management. Respiratory distress requires the use of supplemental oxygen. Progressive deterioration of a patient's respiratory status may be an indicator of pulmonary barotrauma, pneumothorax, or air emboli. The caregiver should also consider whether there has been exposure to a toxic gas (carbon monoxide). Pneumothorax and air emboli require prompt diagnosis, as they can be lethal in minutes if untreated. Treatment for pneumothorax consists of supplemental oxygen and needle thoracostomy if tension occurs.

4.3.9. Summary of findings in animals affected by explosives or bomb blasts.

I.   Blast injuries are not confined to the battlefield. They should be considered for any human/working animal exposed to an explosive force.

II.   Clinical signs of blast-related abdominal injuries can be initially silent until signs of acute abdomen or sepsis are advanced.

III   Standard penetrating and blunt trauma to any body surface is the most common injury seen among survivors. Primary blast lung and blast abdomen are associated with a high mortality rate. "Blast lung" is the most common fatal injury among initial survivors.

IV.   Blast lung presents soon after exposure. It can be confirmed by thoracic radiography. Prophylactic chest tubes (thoracostomy) are recommended prior to general anesthesia and/or air transport.

V.   Auditory system injuries and concussions are easily overlooked. The symptoms of mild TBI and post traumatic stress disorder can be identical.

VI.   Isolated TM rupture is not a marker of morbidity; however, traumatic amputation of any limb is a marker for multisystem injuries.

VII.   Air embolism is common and can present as stroke, myocardial infarction, acute abdomen, blindness, deafness, spinal cord injury, or claudication. Hyperbaric oxygen therapy may be effective in some cases.

VIII.   Compartment syndrome, rhabdomyolysis, and acute renal failure are associated with structural collapse, prolonged extrication, severe burns, and some poisonings.

IX.   Consider the possibility of exposure to inhaled toxins and poisonings (e.g., CO, CN) in both industrial and criminal explosions.

X.   Wounds can be grossly contaminated. Consider delayed primary closure and assess tetanus status. Ensure close follow-up of wounds, head injuries, eye, ear, and stress-related complaints.

XI.   Communications and instructions to the animal handler may need to be written because of tinnitus and sudden, temporary, or permanent deafness.

Selected Reading

Auf der Heide E. *Disaster Response: Principles of Preparation and Coordination.* Accessed August 12, 2008, from http://orgmail2.coe-dmha.org/dr/index.htm.

Centers for Disease Control and Prevention. Mass casualty event preparedness and response. Accessed August 12, 2008, from www.bt.cdc.gov/masscasualties.

Hill JF. Blast injury with particular reference to recent terrorists bombing incidents. Ann R Coll Surg Engl 1979;61:411.

Hogan D, et al. Emergency department impact of the Oklahoma City terrorist bombing. Ann Emerg Med 1999;34:160–167.

Katz E, et al. Primary blast injury after a bomb explosion in a civilian bus. Ann Surg 1989;209:484–488.

Landesman LY, Malilay J, Bissell RA, Becker SM, Roberts L, Ascher MS. Roles and responsibilities of public health in disaster preparedness and response. In: Novick LF, Leibovici D, et al, editors. Blast injuries: Bus versus open-air bombings—a comparative study of injuries in survivors of open-air versus confined-space explosions. J Trauma 1996;41:1030–1035.

Mallonee S, et al. Physical injuries and fatalities resulting from the Oklahoma City bombing. JAMA 1996;276:382–387.

Mays GP, editors. *Public Health Administration: Principles for Population-Based Management.* Gaithersburg, MD, Aspen Publishers, 2001.

Phillips YY. Primary blast injuries. Ann Emerg Med 1986;15:1446–1450.

Quenemoen LE, Davis YM, Malilay J, Sinks T, Noji EK, Klitzman S. The World Trade Center bombing: Injury prevention strategies for high-rise building fires. Disasters 1996;20:125–132.

Stein M, Hirshberg A. Trauma care in the new millinium: Medical consequences of terrorism, the conventional weapon threat. Surg Clin N Am 1999;79.

Wightman JM, Gladish SL. Explosions and blast injuries. Ann Emerg Med 2001;37:664–678.

CHAPTER 5
WORKING ANIMAL PREPARATION FOR WEAPONS OF MASS DESTRUCTION THREATS

Wayne E. Wingfield, MS, DVM

Disaster response teams risk being exposed to potential chemical toxins, radiation, explosives, and biological agents. These teams are often accompanied by working dogs (search-and-rescue, bomb-sniffing, cadaver, illicit drugs, guard dogs, etc.). Additionally, handicapped individuals in the private sector are often accompanied by service animals (guide dogs for the blind, hearing dogs for the deaf, etc.). Also encountered in a disaster will be horses used by mounted police and mini-ponies used as guide animals for the blind. In this document, the term *working animal* (WA) refers to both dogs and horses. The term *working dog* (WD) refers to all dogs present at a disaster for the purpose of assisting in recovery efforts. The purpose of this section is not to provide a complete review of the chemical, explosive, radiological, and biological (CERB) warfare threat but to address several key concerns for WAs.

WAs are potentially at the highest risk of becoming contaminated during the course of their duties. It is important to remember the WA's risk often differs from that of the human handler. The human handler is wearing clothes that can easily be removed, thus eliminating a substantial amount of contamination. The WA is covered in hair (fur) that collects hazardous particles and obviously cannot remove his/her "coat." The WA's contaminated hair coat thus becomes a means to spread the contaminant to other animals, including humans! Additionally, especially with dogs, the animal cleans him/herself with its tongue, thereby ingesting the contaminant.

5. Principles of Working Animal Operation Following Chemical (C), Explosive (Blast) Injury (E), Radiological (R), and Biological (B) Threat

As part of the disaster response team, WAs may have to operate in areas subject to CERB threats. Operation in these areas requires that we recognize we cannot completely protect WAs during an attack. While personnel have personal protection equipment (PPE), functional protective apparatus for WAs does not currently exist and, even if it did, the WA could not function normally while so protected. This means that the only sure way to protect the WA from these threats is to remove it from the area; however, removing the WA may not be operationally possible due to mission requirements or limitations of evacuation assets. Under these circumstances, the best that can be done is to place the WA in as protected a location as possible and return to duty or complete evacuation when the threat has passed. The principles of threat detection, surveillance and decontamination, and victim treatment are the same as for other disaster response teams and very similar to planning for placement and protection of medical and food storage facilities, but there are some special concerns.

5.1. WA Handler

The WA will arrive with an assistant, the handler, who will assist with the care of the animal, have the responsibility to restrain and muzzle the dog, if necessary, and will provide information on health history, immediate chief complaint, or injury. These handlers can also assist with follow-up and re-evaluation following treatment.

5.1.1. Importantly, the role of the medical assistance team is to assist the WA handler in health maintenance issues and to care for the animal with minor to moderate injuries/illness. If further treatment is necessary, the team can help arrange definitive veterinary care.

5.2. Welfare of Human Personnel

Disaster response personnel must always keep the welfare of human personnel foremost in the decision process of how to manage WAs in the CERB threat environment. Personnel safety must not be jeopardized in efforts to protect or treat WAs. All personnel involved in a disaster must remain in approved PPE. Treatment of WAs with clinical signs of illness due to chemical agents may not be possible without endangering WA handlers or veterinary personnel. In this scenario use of expedient euthanasia may be appropriate.

5.3. Chemical and Biological Agent Exposure May Occur by Three Primary Routes

5.3.1. *Inhalation/absorption through mucous membranes:* Inhaled gases, vapors, and aerosols may be absorbed by any part of the respiratory tract including mucosa of the nasal passages, mouth, airways, and lungs. Due to permeability and surface area along with the direct and systemic effects, especially of chemical agents, this is the route most likely to cause severe intoxication. There is currently no equipment designed to protect WAs from this route of exposure. Protective shelters are under investigation but until available the only means to protect from this route is evacuation or expedient shelter.

5.3.2. *Absorption through the skin:* Liquid droplets and solid particles that come in contact with skin may be directly absorbed and have both direct and systemic effects. Due to the protective effect of the thick coat and the lower density of sweat glands in canine skin, we expect that WDs are inherently less sensitive to cutaneous toxicity from chemical agents. All nonhaired portions of the skin, the dense eccrine sweat gland areas of the foot pads and nose, and damaged or inflamed skin will likely promote absorption of chemical agents. In the horse, sweat glands are prominent over the body despite the dense hair coat, and absorption of chemical weapons is likely in this species. WAs can only be protected from cutaneous absorption by preventing contact with the agent using shelters or evacuation. There is no protective garment for WAs. Protection of skin integrity (maintaining healthy skin) and use of skin protectants should help reduce risk of cutaneous absorption.

5.3.3. *Ingestion:* Ingestion of agents may occur due to feeding of contaminated food or water or the WD licking a contaminated surface including its own skin and hair. Ingested agents will have direct effects on the gastrointestinal tract and absorption may result in systemic toxicity. The most important prevention is to prevent the WA from being exposed to contaminated food, water, and environments.

5.4. Working Animal Preparation for Chemical and Biological Threats

Most of these preparations will be the responsibility of the WA master, handler, or owner and not the disaster response team. However, it is important that the disaster response team be familiar with areas of concern so they can help prepare the WA during pre-deployment training.

5.4.1. *Location and preparation of kennels/stalls/pens:* WA primary holding areas should be located upwind from prime threat areas and on high ground so that any CERB agent blows away from and settles below them (Fig. 5.1).

The location concerns must be balanced against the operational requirements of the mission and with terrain and threat analysis. The ability to protect the field holding area from overhead is ideal, and at high threat levels, movement of off-duty WAs to an indoor area (see 5.5) may be appropriate.

5.4.2. *Storage of WA food:* Unlike most initial disaster response personnel food rations, the WA diet is not distributed in resistant or easily decontaminated containers. Therefore, any WA rations exposed to attack must be presumed to be contaminated unless proven otherwise. (Do not forget the disaster response team can help inspect the WA food if presence/ absence of contamination is not clear.) In the event of attack, adequate food must be available to support the WA pending delivery of new food or evacuation. A 1-week per WA supply of food should be stored in a location where it is protected from contamination in case of attack, e.g., tightly sealed plastic storage cans inside a tightly sealed freezer/refrigerator, or in a nearby common protective shelter or a filtered and shielded vehicle.

5.4.3. *Storage and availability of WA equipment:* WA muzzles, leads, halters, and leashes are usually made of plastic, leather, and cloth, which will be difficult to decontaminate after attack and thus will present a risk to the

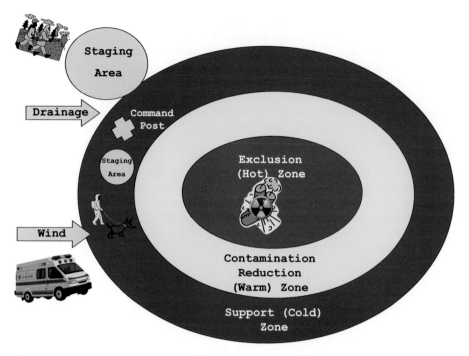

Figure 5.1. Hot, contamination, and support zones in a disaster area. Staging areas are upwind and uphill from the hot zone.

WA and associated personnel. Extra equipment should be available for each WA and stored in a protected location (as with food, discussed earlier) for use after an attack.

5.5. Identification of Supplemental Collective Protection in Case of Attack

The delivery route for most CERB threats is via airborne, missile, or artillery delivered aerosol or gas. The different agents have variable ability to drift, penetrate structures or ventilation systems, and absorb into skin, clothing, and equipment. In general, we can expect the agents to settle to the ground in patterns predicted by local wind patterns. Some agents are persistent while others will disseminate or decay almost immediately. If the main animal holding facility is not protected against chemical threat, additional locations should be identified so WAs can be placed in protected transport kennels/ trailers during and immediately after attack. Keep in mind that in many operational environments the temperature in tightly sealed protective structures will rapidly increase. Heat injury may be a concern and water must be available to the WAs. Possible locations will include the following:

5.5.1. *Common protective shelters and vehicles:* Chemical resistant and air-filtered overpressure shelters and vehicles are in the military inventory, but most personal protection is based on use of individual PPE gear followed by decontamination. Space in common shelters is generally limited to functions that must be completed by teams (e.g., medical care), and space for additional personnel will be limited. Allocation of space for WAs may not be possible due to prioritization for personnel and concern about continued function, which may be impeded by WAs (e.g., noise, sanitation issues).

5.5.2.   Shelter in the interior of a fixed facility, preferably above ground level, with exterior openings (doors, vents, windows) sealed with plastic and tape. Noise, heat, sanitation, and maintaining WAs and personnel hydration will rapidly become concerns in such a shelter.

5.5.3.   Tents with all flaps down will provide limited protection from gross contamination as liquid/droplet agents disseminate and settle to the ground, but little protection will be provided against vapor or gas. Noise, heat, and hydration will be rapidly developing problems.

5.6. Individual Protection of the WA

The first choice for protection of the WA should be shelter in a CERB-protected facility during and after an attack, but it is possible that the WA may be in an exposed area during an attack or that movement of WAs is essential prior to area decontamination. In these situations, field expedient shelters and protection may be used to reduce direct contact of liquid and droplet agents, and foot protection for WDs may be needed to prevent contact if the WA must be moved out of a contaminated area.

5.6.1.   *Shelter options:* The development of a modified "patient chemical wrap" for protection of the WA in its transport kennel/trailer is being evaluated for the future. NOTE: Unfortunately, until this equipment becomes available, there is no standard protection for WAs in a CERB environment. The best that can be done is to cover the WA to prevent CERB agent from settling directly on exposed skin and hair and to reduce the concentration of agent that may be inhaled. Tents, tarps, plastic sheets, and extra PPE garments may all be used. The ideal situation is to place the WA in its transport kennel/trailer and drape a cover over it until the holding area and animal can be moved out of the contaminated area. Care must be taken to observe the WA for hyperthermia that may occur while covered. If a vehicle is available, the WA may be placed in the vehicle, but as there will be no air exchange, the WA may be subject to rapid heat injury.

5.6.2.   *Decontamination considerations:* There are several views regarding the decontamination of a WA following a biological exposure.
  I. Familiarization training
     A. The effectiveness of decontamination efforts will largely depend on the cooperativeness of the WA. The WA's first reaction to humans in protective gear will vary. If the animal has no familiarization and is introduced to persons dressed as aliens who spray him with soap and water and get soap in his eyes, he will likely be less than cooperative. Conversely, if the animal is introduced to these "alien-dressed" humans, watches them dress into PPE, and then goes through decon slowly and gently, the WA will likely have improved

success in forthcoming decon sessions. The handler should thus train regularly while wearing PPE and protective mask. Obviously the presence of the mask will often impede obeying commands given by the handler. In all cases, avoid spraying the WA in the face and ears. This will only frighten the animal and make things much worse.

B. HAZMAT personnel safety

    1. Always have a muzzle available for WDs. This reduces the likelihood of being bitten by providing a physical barrier from the rescuer and prevents the WD from attempting to clean itself with its tongue. Thus, the muzzle will reduce the ingestion of the hazardous substance and the decontamination solutions.

    2. Utilize a rigid capture noose or chain lead and collar/halter to maintain control of the WA at all times. This prevents the WA from running free and potentially spreading contaminants to "clean" areas and individuals.

C. Decontamination procedure

    1. If at all possible, protect the animal's eyes and ears from further contamination and from decontamination solutions.

        a. Moist towelettes (Wet Ones) are used to decontaminate the facial area, including the nose and nares, area around the eyes, and the exterior of the mouth and lips.

    2. If possible, have the handler maintain the WA or stand by for assistance whenever possible.

    3. Maintain control of the animal's feet. The WD's nails (claws!) can easily shred PPE. In the case of the horse, hooves should be considered lethal weapons!

    4. Be alert! Decontamination may seem routine to the rescuer but this is a highly stressful event for the WA. The resulting fear and anxiety of the animal provide a danger to any personnel in the vicinity.

    5. The WA should be thoroughly rinsed, starting directly behind the ears and working down the back of the neck and then rinsing from the top of the back downward until all four paws/hooves have been rinsed.

        a. Sterile water or saline is used to flush the eyes and an ophthalmic ointment should be applied to the eyes at this time. It will help wash out contaminants and prevent further damage by these agents. The ointment will also soothe pain and inflammation from the contaminants.

    6. The WA should then be washed and scrubbed with soap and water. The scrubbing starts directly behind the ears and proceeds down the back of the neck. This is followed by scrubbing the top of the back and moving downward until the legs and paws/hooves have been scrubbed individually.

    7. The head and face are carefully cleaned using moist towelettes, gauze pads, and clean, warm water.

    8. The WA exits the wash point and is monitored for further contamination.

    9. If contamination is found, the washing process is repeated.

    10. If the WA is found to be free of contaminants, it should be dried with towels, and a heated blower if tolerated. Drying of the animal is important in preventing hypothermia.

    11. The WA exits the decontamination line and is seen by a veterinarian for a follow-up examination and further treatment, if necessary.

12. If the WA's equipment is successfully decontaminated, it may be returned to work. Replacement collars/halters and leads should be available.
   D. Decontamination of WA gear and equipment
   1. In most cases, it may be more realistic to dispose of the contaminated equipment rather than to put it through decontamination.
      a. Leather (leashes, collars, muzzles, halters, saddles, etc.)
         • Soak the leather in water heated to approximately 126°F for 4–6 hours, and then air dry without heat.
         • Monitor for contamination and repeat or dispose of if necessary.
      b. Nylon and canvas (leashes, halters, muzzles, safety vests, foot booties, etc.)
         • Boil in water for 1 hour. Soap can be added to improve efficiency.
         • Remove from water, rinse thoroughly, and air dry.
         • Monitor the equipment for residual contamination and repeat or dispose of if necessary.
      c. Metal (leashes, collars, bits, bridles, etc.)
         • Wash thoroughly with a soap and water solution or apply a 5% bleach solution and let stand for 30 minutes. Rinse thoroughly.
         • Monitor for residual contamination and repeat or dispose of if necessary.
II. Decontamination station layout
   A. WAs are considered responders and are thus processed through the technical decontamination station.
   1. In the ideal world, a separate decontamination station for WAs, away from human personnel, is desired.
   B. Components of a decontamination station for WAs (Fig. 5.2)
   1. *Equipment drop:* area where equipment (leashes, muzzles, leashes, leads, halters, bridles, saddles, blankets, etc.) can be dropped and decontaminated.
   2. *Primary decon:* water supply, long-handled soft bristle brushes, soap, and multiple hoses.
      a. Water-proof tarps or tubs to help collect and control contaminants. This is true in standard decontamination operations and the incident does not include mass casualties. In all situations, animal (and human!) decontamination should not be delayed to allow for runoff containment. With mass casualties, runoff containment may not be feasible because of the volume of water used. The Environmental Protection Agency (EPA) says that during a true mass casualty incident, runoff is of secondary concern; the primary concern is decontamination of the victims. This policy can be found on the EPA website (http://yosemite.epa.gov/oswer/ceppoweb.nsf/vwResourcesByFilename/onepage.pdf/$File/onepage.pdf). The EPA will not pursue hazardous waste violations against first responders who are not able to contain runoff during mass casualty decontamination operations. Remember to contact local authorities and water treatment plants if the runoff cannot be contained.
   3. *Secondary decon:* Water supply, long-handled soft bristle brushes, soap, and multiple hoses.

4. *Drying station:* Dry animals with towels, paper towels, blow dryers, etc.

5. *Veterinary evaluation:* Exit point to the cold zone where veterinary medical personnel may attend to illnesses or injuries of the animal(s) and monitor for hypothermia and hyperthermia.

6. *Recovery and rehab:* Animals (and humans!) need periodic rest times in order to prepare to return to mission.

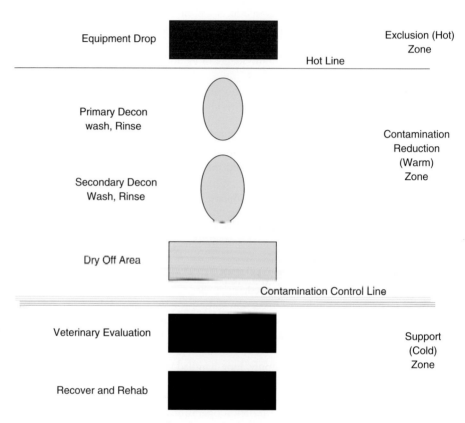

Figure 5.2. Decontamination line for working dogs and horses.

III. Decontamination solutions

A. *Liquid soap and water:* When comparing risks to benefits, soap and water is the best all-around choice as a decontamination solution. The liquid soap can be spread liberally over the animal and worked under the hair coat using a soft bristle brush or gloved fingers. Work the soap through the hair using an S-pattern beginning at the neck, working down the back, and ending up on ventral abdomen and legs. The soap is then rinsed off with copious volumes of warm water. Do not overlook using a swimming pool for dogs or a body of water (lake, ocean, etc.) as possible means of providing decontamination to WAs.

1. The types of soaps recommended are either baby shampoo (to reduce effects on the eyes), good old-fashioned "green soap," or *liquid* dishwasher detergent. (Do not use powdered dishwasher soap!)

B. *Hypochlorite/bleach solution:* Diluted bleach solutions have been recommended in the past for decontamination of WAs. The effect this agent has on the WA varies from animal to animal and will depend on the concentration of the solution. In order to minimize effects on the WA, the dilution is often to a level that the desired decontamination effect is lost. To counter this loss of effectiveness, greater contact time is required. This in turn leads to more adverse health effects on the animal. These effects are on the skin and through inhalation.

C. *Betadine:* Diluted Betadine was also promoted as the best solution when decontaminating the WA exposed to a biological agent. As with hypochlorite solutions, the dilution to make the solution effective is likely ineffective on the biological agent.

D. *Chlorhexidine solution:* In order to get the full effect from chlorhexidine solution, it would have to be left on the WA for several minutes. Time is often a luxury when dealing with decontamination.

5.6.3. *Skin Exposure Reduction Paste Against Chemical Warfare Agents (SERPACWA).* SERPACWA is a barrier cream for use by the military to protect against the effects of chemical agents. New military doctrine (Interim, 8 January 2003) authorizes individual working members to carry six packets, equivalent to 2 days' protection, to be started when directed by the responsible field commander. SERPACWA will NOT protect the respiratory tract and mucous membranes, so protecting the WD from exposure by evacuation or shelter are always recommended. If the WD must be moved through a lightly contaminated area and cannot be carried in a protected crate, then the use of SERPACWA may reduce the risk of cutaneous absorption of nerve agent and skin injury by vesicants.

I. The effectiveness of SERPACWA is dependent on the thickness and integrity of the SERPACWA layer and the length of time between application and agent exposure. A properly applied intact SERPACWA layer protects the skin from chemical agent for 4 hours after exposure.

II. *Application of SERPACWA to WDs:* SERPACWA should be applied (rubbed over skin and worked in) to all nonhaired portions of the abdomen, groin, and axillae (armpits). It should NOT be applied on or around the eyes. It is estimated that one or two packages will be needed per WD per initial application. Reapplication should not be required as use is only appropriate during evacuation through a lightly contaminated area.

A. *Foot protection by SERPACWA:* WDs should not be required to walk through a contaminated area. If there is no other option, foot protection (see later) other than SERPACWA is needed. Application of SERPACWA to the feet is likely to collect dirt and debris, thus increasing risk of injury to the foot. This may compromise the integrity of the SERPACWA coating, reducing its effectiveness and increasing the risk of agent absorption through the damaged skin.

III. *WD decontamination and cleaning with SERPACWA:* SERPACWA will increase the effectiveness of decontamination because it is easier to remove the chemical agent from the SERPACWA layer than from the skin itself. SERPACWA can be removed from the skin by rubbing or washing with soap and water.

5.6.4. *Foot protection:* WDs should not be walked through a contaminated area without some form of foot protection.

Ideally the WD should be carried through a contaminated area in its transport kennel. Field expedient foot covers should only be used if there is no alternative. Available appropriate materials may include the following: The resistant and easily decontaminated outer bag from an MRE, extra chemical protective gloves, Mylar specimen bags (we recommend at least two bags per foot as they tear easily), or patches from damaged PPE not in use by personnel. Nonabsorbent tarp, tent, or plastic sheets are also options. These items should be placed over the foot to form a "sock" and secured with duct tape. They should be removed and the feet decontaminated as soon as possible.

Suggested Reading

American Veterinary Medical Association (AVMA). *AVMA Emergency Preparedness and Response Guide.* American Veterinary Medical Association, 1931 N Meacham Road Suite 100, Schaumburg, IL 46204-2760, 1995.

Currance P. Decontamination procedures. In Currance P, editor. *Medical Response to Weapons of Mass Destruction,* St. Louis, Mosby-JEMS, 2005; 165–182.

Thorman DC, Poisoned animal management, part 1. NAPINet Rep 1989;2-3.

Mershon MM, Tennyson AV. Chemical hazards and chemical warfare. JAVMA 1987;190:734–745.

Osweiler GD, et al. *Clinical and Diagnostic Veterinary Toxicology.* Dubuque, IA, Kendall/Hunt Publishing, 1985.

Soric S, Belanger MP, Wittnich C. A method for decontamination of animals involved in floodwater disasters. J Am Vet Med Assoc 2008;232:364–370.

CHAPTER 6
CHEMICAL INJURY TO WORKING ANIMALS

Wayne E. Wingfield, MS, DVM

The basic nature of the chemical agent threat to working animals (WAs) is the same as for human personnel. There are five basic types of chemical warfare agents: nerve, blister (vesicant), blood, pulmonary, and riot control agents. Nerve (acetylcholinesterase inhibitor) agents and vesicants (mustards) are thought to be major threats. Blood (cyanides) and pulmonary toxicants (phosgenes) are less likely threats. WAs are most likely to encounter riot control agents in the United States. Treatment of a WA casualty due to chemical attack is similar to other canine or equine intoxication and to treatment of human casualties. The WA's hair coat may provide limited protection against skin exposure, thereby slightly limiting the effects of chemical injury. Additionally, inhalation exposure may be more severe in working dogs (WDs) than in humans as the dog must pant to cool itself.

6. Chemical Injury to Working Animals:

6.1. Introduction to Chemical Agents

A toxic chemical agent is any chemical that, through its chemical action on life processes, can cause death, temporary incapacitation, or permanent harm to humans or animals.

6.2. Classification

6.2.1. *Chemical warfare (CW) agents:* These agents include nerve, blister, blood, pulmonary, and incapacitating agents. Their physiological actions are as follows:

  I. *Nerve agents:* Nerve agents inhibit cholinesterase (ChE) enzymes (Figs. 6.1 and 6.2). This inhibition permits acetylcholine (ACh), which transmits many nerve impulses, to collect at its various sites of action. The body's muscles and glands become overstimulated due to excessive amounts of ACh. At sufficient doses, this can lead to an inability of the body to sustain breathing.

  II. *Blister agents (vesicants):* Blister agents are noted for producing reddening and blistering of the skin, but the eyes and respiratory tract are more sensitive than

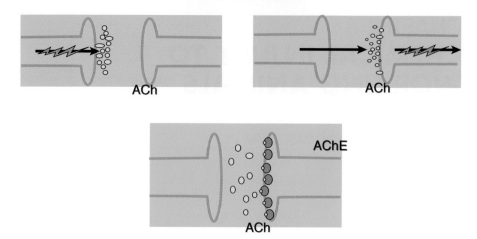

Figure 6.1. Acetylcholine (ACh) is normally released and acts as the primary chemical neurotransmitter of the parasympathetic nervous system. It rapidly moves across the postsynaptic gap and stimulates nerve function. Acetylcholinesterase (AChE) is then released, thus blocking any additional effects of ACh.

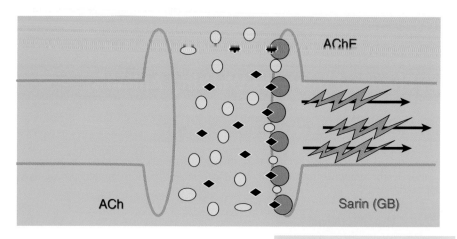

Body's muscles and glands are overstimulated due to excessive amounts of ACh.

Figure 6.2. Nerve agents (♦) (i.e., Sarin [GB]) directly affect the enzyme acetylcholine (ACh), resulting in excessive acetylcholinesterase (AChE). The AChE cannot hydrolyze the ACh, and it accumulates and continues to stimulate the affected organ or muscle.

the skin. Eye exposure results in reddening of the eyes and temporary blindness or permanent effects. Inhaled mustard damages mucous membranes and the respiratory tract.

III.   *Blood agents:* The blood transports these agents to all body tissues. Hydrogen cyanide (AC) and cyanogen chloride (CK) are cellular poisons, and they disrupt the oxidative processes used by the cells. Arsine (abbreviated "WA") is different. It causes hemolysis of the red blood cells. The central nervous system (CNS) is especially vulnerable to lack of oxygen regardless of the etiology, and respiratory and cardiovascular collapse resulting from AC and CK poisoning. In the case of arsine poisoning, the cause of death is myocardial failure.

IV.   *Choking agents (pulmonary):* Pulmonary agents cause damage to the lungs, irritation to the eyes and the respiratory tract, and pulmonary edema ("dry-land drowning").

V.   *Riot control agents:* The riot control agents are chemicals that rapidly produce sensory irritation or disabling physical effects that disappear within a short time following termination of exposure.

6.3. Nerve Agents (Tabun/GA, Sarin/GB, Soman/GD, Cyclosarin/GF, V-Agent/VX)

6.3.1.   *Action:* Nerve agents act via the same mechanism of action as organophosphate insecticides. Both are acetylcholinesterase inhibitors that increase the persistence of ACh neurotransmitters in the neuromuscular (nicotinic) junctions of the somatic nervous system and within the autonomic ganglia (nicotinic) of the sympathetic and parasympathetic nervous systems (PNS) and neuroeffector sites of the PNS.

6.3.2.   Identification and description (Table 6.1)

Table 6.1.   Identification and Description of Nerve Agents.

Agent	UN No.	Class	ERG Guide	Vapor Pressure (mm Hg)	Vapor Density (Air = 1)
Tabun (GA)	2810	6.1	153	0.07 at 68°F/20°C	5.63
Sarin (GB)	2810	6.1	153	2.1 at 68°F/20°C	4.86
Cyclosarin (GF)	2810	6.1	153	0.044 at 77°F/25°C	6.2
Soman (GD)	2810	6.1	153	0.4 at 77°F/25°C	6.33
V Agent (VX)	2810	6.1	153	0.0007 at 68°F/20°C	9.2

6.3.3.   The commonly used mnemonic "DUMBELS" is helpful for recognizing the *muscarinic* (eyes, airways, gastrointestinal, skin, and cardiac sites). This mnemonic is as follows: **D:** diarrhea; **U:** urination; **M:** miosis (pupil constriction); **B**: bradycardia, bronchorrhea, bronchospasm; **E**: emesis; **L**: lacrimation; and **S**: salivation. There is also a mnemonic using the days of the week to help recognize *nicotinic* (skeletal muscle) signs: **M**: mydriasis (pupil dilation); **T**: tachycardia; **W**: weakness; **tH**: hypertension; **F**: fasciculations (muscle twitching).

6.3.4. *Treatment:* Nerve agent antidotes Atropine and 2-PAM chloride are of limited effectiveness with GD. 2-PAM chloride must be given within 2 minutes of exposure. WAs that suffer chemical injury by inhalation will likely require emergent respiratory support and immediate pharmacological therapy, and need intensive care if they survive the attack. Attempts to treat and decontaminate WAs with severe respiratory distress due to chemical agent inhalation may be inappropriate due to a poor prognosis and risk of injury to the handler and veterinary personnel. Expedient euthanasia is appropriate, when possible.

6.3.5. *Decontamination:* If the WA's skin/coat was exposed to liquid agent, decontamination is necessary as the agent may absorb to the fur and then through the skin. Vapor agent does not typically adhere to human skin but may absorb to a WA's hair coat so decontamination may still be needed after vapor agent exposure. In other ways, decontamination of the exposed WA is similar to decontamination of human casualties.

I.   Remove collar(s), muzzles, halters, leads, and other gear that may be contaminated. These items can initially be decontaminated by soaking in 5.0% sodium hypochlorite (commercial bleach is 5%–6% sodium hypochlorite) or 5% sodium carbonate and then must be thoroughly rinsed prior to reuse. NOTE: Plastic and leather items may absorb agent, which then "off-gasses" even after soaking in decontamination solutions. These items should be checked by qualified chemical defense personnel and certified as decontaminated.

II.   *Definitive decontamination:* In general, the most expedient way to decontaminate the WA will be to place a veterinary working decontamination substation within the central decon station used by personnel, or simply to decontaminate the WA with the handler using conventional decontamination techniques.

III.   Options for definitive decontamination include:

A.   *Physical removal and hydrolysis:* Washing the WA with soap and warm water, or copious water alone, will physically remove the agent and promote hydrolytic deactivation. This is the easiest and fastest method and least likely to cause additional harm to the WA. It may also aid in treatment of possible heat injury induced or developing secondary to closed confinement in protective structures. Large quantities of water must be available and runoff water must be considered contaminated. Soap, other than tearless baby shampoo, must not be used around the eyes.

B.   Adjunctive decontamination procedures previously reported:

1.   *Oxidation and hydrolysis using active chlorine solutions:* Sodium or calcium hypochlorite 0.5% solution (dilute bleach) was the standard decontamination solution for human skin in decontamination stations and was STRONGLY preferred for WA decontamination over 5.0% sodium carbonate solution. The WD should be soaked with decontamination solution for 2–5 minutes and then must be rinsed well with water to prevent skin irritation or

burns. Irritation to the skin due to chemical decontamination may increase skin permeability and agent absorption, thus increasing risk of toxicity from chemical agents. This risk of skin irritation must be considered when planning chemical decontamination versus just washing with soap and water or copious rinsing with water alone.

2. *Oxidation and hydrolysis using sodium carbonate solution:* If other decontamination methods are not available, 5% sodium carbonate solutions may be used to decontaminate grossly contaminated areas of the WA but this solution is VERY alkaline and must be rinsed off VERY well to avoid skin burns. Sodium carbonate MUST NOT be used if VX agent exposure is present as it DOES NOT work against VX and toxic metabolites will form. It should not be used around the eyes. It should not be used as a full body soak or dip solution. Increased agent absorption due to skin irritation is a great concern if the solution is applied too liberally or is not rinsed off promptly and completely.

3. *Eye and head decontamination:* The use of copious water irrigation is the safest method of decontaminating the eyes and periocular face. This may be supplemented with the use of tearless baby shampoo. No other decontamination solutions should be used around the eyes. Use of eye lubricants or ointment to protect the eyes from irritation by decontamination solutions (specifically 5% sodium carbonate) is NOT currently recommended. If application is to be done, use care as it may actually promote eye injury since personnel will be in PPE and the WA may not cooperate with medication application. Ointment may also hinder decontamination efforts and may absorb and concentrate some agents, actually increasing ocular trauma and toxicity.

6.3.6. *Emergent pharmacological therapy:* Medical treatment of the WA with nerve agent exposure is similar to treatment for organophosphate insecticide intoxication. Treatment should be based on clinical signs and history of exposure. Recurrent treatment may be needed for severe casualties or if complete decontamination is not possible. Mark I autoinjectors may be used by WA handlers for initial intramuscular (IM) injection in the large paraspinal muscles in the lumbar region or in the large muscles of the caudal thigh. After the initial doses, listed below, redosing based on clinical signs and intervals used for human postexposure treatment is appropriate. Veterinary personnel should provide appropriate retreatment using conventional doses and the intravenous (IV) routes as soon as possible.

I. Atropine

    A. *Action:* Atropine is the prototype antimuscarinic agent and competitively inhibits ACh activity at parasympathetic neuroeffector junctions, controlling parasympathetic signs including miosis, salivation, lacrimation, digestive signs, and respiratory distress. Atropine should only be administered if clinical signs are present or if gross and confirmed contamination or inhalation of nerve agent has just (within minutes) occurred.

    B. Dosage

        1. *Working dogs:* The recommended dose for WD organophosphate toxicity is 0.22 mg/kg with ¼ IV and the remainder SQ or IM.

        2. *Working horses:* In the horse, the dosage of atropine is 0.22–1 mg/kg (the average-sized horse is 1000 to 1200 lb [≈455–545 kg]).

    a. Because colic is a significant complication in the horse following atropine administration, a guideline for administering atropine would be to START with a dosage of 0.22 mg/kg either IV to effect or $\frac{1}{4}$ given IV and the remainder given IM. This dosage should allow a redosing of at least 4 times and still it would be under the 1 mg/kg dosage, thus reducing the likelihood of colic.

    b. Obviously, with a full-blown exposure, one might have to commit to using a full 1 mg/kg dosage and repeat every 1.5–2 hours with the atropine being given IM as needed.

  C. Formulations

    1. The AtroPen auto injector may be issued individually or in the Mark I kit. The AtroPen contains 2 mg of atropine. In order to provide the 0.22 mg/kg dosage, it would require one Mark I for each 9.09 kg (20 lb).

      a. WD Aid: The WD with signs or confirmed nerve agent exposure should receive an initial dose of 1 AtroPen autoinjectors IM for each 20 lb of body weight. Additional doses of atropine may be given every 10–20 minutes if signs continue or go away and then return. Premeasured doses of atropine may be dispensed to handlers in high-risk areas as an alternative to autoinjector use.

      b. If the average-sized horse needs 455–545 mg of atropine ($\approx$250 AtroPen Injectors/average-sized horse!), then using the autoinjectors is not reasonable. The horse receiving atropine sulfate should be administered $\frac{1}{4}$ of the dose IV and the remainder given IM.

    2. A veterinary injectable atropine is available for use.

      a. Available as 0.5 mg/ml (30 and 100 ml vials), 2 mg/ml (100-ml vials), and 15 mg/ml (100-ml vials).

D. *Veterinary working aid:* Continued atropine therapy via IV route at appropriate dose is the most likely required retreatment of a severely exposed WA. Atropine therapy should be continued as directed until clinical improvement is noted. As previously noted, miosis due to ocular contamination may persist despite adequate systemic therapy. If other signs have resolved, continued atropine redosing is not warranted just because miosis persists. In the horse, large doses of atropine will likely result in intestinal colic and their use must be carefully monitored.

E. *Signs of atropine toxicity:* Excessive administration of atropine may result in toxicity. The effects of atropine toxicity in WAs are expected to be similar to those in humans with atropinization, but it may be difficult to evaluate some toxic effects in WAs. Signs of atropine toxicity include decreased salivation, dry mouth and mucous membranes, difficulty swallowing, tachycardia, and hyperthermia, difficulty urinating, and altered or dull mentation. Decreased salivation will further contribute to hyperthermia due to decreased evaporative cooling during panting (WD). These signs may be difficult to appreciate in WAs that are often tachycardic and hyperthermic due to stress/excitement during work and veterinary care. More severe atropinization causes disorientation, hallucinations, depression, or restlessness. In WAs, this may manifest as inappropriate aggression or poor response to commands. In the horse, signs of abdominal pain, kicking at the abdomen, and other signs of colic can be expected. The handler may be the most able to assess these changes in an individual WA.

II. 2-PAM (pralidoxime) chloride

A. *Action:* 2-PAM acts to reactivate acetylcholinesterase to aid in control of muscarinic signs and address nicotinic signs (muscle fasciculation and tremors) of nerve agent. Its efficacy decreases with time after exposure as the agent acetylcholinesterase bonds age, making the enzyme resistant to reactivation.

B. Dosage

1. *Working animals:* The recommended dose for WA organophosphate toxicity is 20 mg/kg IM or slowly IV. In horses, the dosage may require 35 mg/kg.

C. *Formulations:* The ComboPen autoinjector contains 600 mg of 2-PAM chloride, therefore:

1. *WA aid:* Each Mark I autoinjector will treat an animal weighing 30 kg (66 lb). Again, the horse is too large to conveniently use the autoinjectors.

2. Pralidoxime chloride is available as a 1-gram cake in containers of six, 20-ml vials without diluents, or syringes.

D. *Veterinary working aid:* Redosing of the WD with conventional SC or IM injections every 8–12 hours for 2–3 days after intoxication may be necessary.

E. *Signs of 2-PAM chloride toxicity:* 2-PAM chloride is safe and free of significant adverse affects at recommended normal doses. At high doses, it will cause anticholinesterase effects including ataxia, vomiting, hyperventilation, muscle rigidity, tachycardia, seizures, and respiratory arrest. The acute LD_{50} for 2-PAM Chloride in the dog is 190 mg/kg.

III. Valium (Diazepam)

A. *Action:* Diazepam is the prototypic benzodiazepine used in animals with seizure disorders and as a sedative and preanesthetic.

B. *Dosage:* An initial dosage for diazepam is calculated at 0.25–5 mg/kg IV. Most commonly, diazepam is administered at the veterinary anticonvulsant dose of 10–50 mg as needed for acute seizure in serial doses of 10 mg IV.

C. Formulation

1. Diazepam injection 5 mg/ml in 2-ml ampules and syringes and 1-, 2-, and 10-ml vials.

2. The convulsant antidote nerve agent (CANA) Valium autoinjector contains 10 mg of diazepam for use in WAs with nerve agent induced seizures; therefore:

a. *WA aid:* If an exposed WA is seizuring, the handler may give up to 3 CANA autoinjectors at 5- to 10-minute intervals, as needed to control WA seizures. If CANA treatment is necessary, additional atropine should also be administered. Premeasured doses of diazepam may be dispensed to WA handlers in high-risk areas as an alternative to Mark I use, but dispensed medication must be accounted for and use/disposal/destruction monitored as a controlled drug.

D. *Veterinary working aid:* Preliminary information from overseas research indicates that intramuscular diazepam may not successfully control nerve agent–induced seizures. Veterinary personnel should be prepared to give additional diazepam IV. If this cannot be achieved, diazepam per rectum at double the IV dose has been used to treat seizures. *Do not forget to remove the needle from the syringe before administering diazepam per rectum!*

IV. *Activated charcoal:* Oral contamination through grooming/licking and biliary excretion and reabsorption through the GI tract have been reported after cutaneous organophosphate toxicity. Based on this observation, treatment with activated charcoal per os or by orogastric tube is appropriate after an exposed affected WD is stabilized with initial treatments. This is particularly warranted if signs of toxicity recur after thorough decontamination.

6.3.7. *Prophylactic treatment:* Prophylactic treatment in WAs has not been evaluated as to its effect on performance and reliability. If the threat warrants pretreatment of personnel, evacuation of WAs to a lower-risk area or shelter is appropriate. If this is impossible due to mission requirements or evacuation concerns, preplanning for expedient shelter and treatment should be initiated. The sections that follow are not intended to advocate pretreatment of WAs but are provided for information purposes only.

I.   WA handlers may use pyridostigmine pretreatment when authorized by senior commanders in high-threat areas of operation. Pyridostigmine at 5–30 mg/dog has been used as a treatment of myasthenia gravis in dogs. Side effects are related to cholinergic effect and include GI signs (vomiting, diarrhea, nausea), salivation, miosis, and lacrimation, increased airway secretions and respiratory distress, etc. This mimics signs of nerve agent. A WD can be administered one pyridostigmine tablet (30 mg) every 8 hours at the discretion of the responsible veterinarian.

II.   Transdermal sustained-release scopolamine and physostigmine have been investigated as nerve agent pretreatment using beagle dogs as a test model. Efficacy was reported, but operational feasibility and potential effect on WA performance have not been examined. Anticholinergic adverse effects of scopolamine mimic those of atropine toxicity. These may include dry mucus membranes, altered vision and mydriasis, tachycardia and hypertension, vomiting and constipation, sedation, and ataxia.

6.3.8. Triage (Table 6.2)

Table 6.2. Triage Guidelines for Nerve Agents.

Triage Category	Clinical Signs
Immediate	Unconscious, seizuring, or postictal; breathing difficulty or apneic with immediate therapy available (MARK I, Valium, ventilation).
Delayed	Working animal recovering from exposure and has already received treatment.
Minor	Neither apparent signs nor symptoms noted following exposure.
Dead/Dying	Apneic, no pulse, or no heart sounds.

6.3.9. *Aftercare:* The most important aspects of treating the WA for nerve agent exposure—decontamination and stabilization—have been discussed. The treated WA may well have partial respiratory obstructions due to exudates and fluid accumulation. There may also be residual effects of therapeutic medications. The ABC (airway, breathing, and circulation) principles apply in these cases. Supportive care, symptomatic management of residual effects and injuries, and watchful waiting should allow most effects of nerve agent intoxication to dissipate in WAs with sublethal exposures. However, dull mentation, mild dyspnea, altered vision, and muscle weakness have been reported to persist for hours to days in people with nerve agent and organophosphate toxicity. This may manifest as altered behavior and performance in WAs. Past exposure to nerve agent may be a consideration in evaluating WA fitness for duty even after apparent recovery from relatively mild intoxication.

6.4. Blister Agents (Vesicants)

6.4.1. *Actions:* Vesicants are chemical agents, including sulfur mustards (H/HD/HT) and Lewisite (L), that cause development of vesicles or blisters on contaminated skin and membranes. In addition, phosgene oxime (CX), which is not a true vesicant, causes urticaria, wheals, and pruritus. The agents cause local and systemic effects, but the mechanism of action is unclear. In addition to their primary action, mustards have some cholinergic toxicity. Sulfur mustard is unique in that its freezing point is ≈57°F, so in cooler temperatures, it will be in a very thick, viscous form that will not volatilize. After contact with skin or mucous membranes, the agents are rapidly broken down into reactive compounds that are absorbed and bind to the contaminated tissue. Intact agent is not persistent on skin or mucous membranes for more than a few moments but may persist on contaminated hair, clothing, and equipment and in the environment. These contaminated surfaces may serve as fomites for recontamination of the exposed patient or other personnel.

I.   The susceptibility of dogs to mustard agents is similar to, or slightly less than, the susceptibility of humans, but the presence of the thick fur coat may partially protect the skin from agent contact. The initial effects of mustard agents may not be apparent for hours after exposure. Lewisite causes pain and erythema within seconds, while phosgene exposure causes instantaneous pain. Mustards are the best studied and most significant military threat. Unless otherwise specified, comments in the following sections relate primarily to mustard agents.

6.4.2. *Clinical signs:* Signs of vesicant injury to animals are not well described. Exposure to mustard gas in an open environment caused the following observations:

I.   In humans, the severity and scope of clinical signs depend on the degree (concentration and time dependent), route of exposure, and variation in individual susceptibility. Cutaneous effects include erythema, pain, pruritus, blister formation and bursting, skin necrosis, and secondary infections. Severity of skin lesions are graded as first-, second-, and third-degree burns. Ophthalmic exposure causes tearing, itching, burning, blepharospasm, and photophobia. More severe exposure may cause corneal damage. Mild inhalation of mustard gas causes nasal discharge, sneezing, epistasis, and coughing. Severe inhalation may cause respiratory distress due to airway obstruction by exudates or vesicular membranes and progresses to secondary infection and sepsis. Initial GI signs, including nausea and vomiting, may be caused by the unpleasant smell or by cholinergic activity. Persistent or late-onset GI signs are likely due to irritation of GI mucosa.

6.4.3. Treatment

I. *Sulfur mustard (HD/H/HT):* There is no antidote for sulfur mustard. Clinical effects of exposure to mustard do not occur for hours after contact. Mustard is an oily liquid with color ranging from light yellow to brown. The odor is unreliable, but when detectable, it is that of a slight sulfur, garlic, onion, or mustard. Below an environmental temperature of 100°F, mustard is a liquid, but above 100°F, it is a vapor, making it an inhalation hazard. Because of this, the WA exposed to mustard requires immediate and thorough decontamination using soap and warm water. Exposed skin will have a sunburned appearance, with blisters forming later. Observation of potentially exposed WA for at least 8 hours is advised.

II. *Lewisite (L):* Unlike mustard, Lewisite causes pain on contact. Lewisite is an oily, colorless liquid with the scent of geraniums. It is more volatile than mustard, and the exact mechanism of tissue damage is unclear. Within 5 minutes of exposure, the skin will develop a grayish cast, a result of epithelial necrosis. Blister formation occurs in 12–18 hours. WAs exposed to Lewisite requires immediate decontamination.

III. *Phosgene oxime (CX):* Phosgene oxime is classified as a vesicant, although it causes erythema, urticaria, or wheals instead of fluid-filled blisters on the skin. The vapor is extremely irritating. Both the liquid and vapor cause almost immediate tissue damage on contact. Below 95°F, phosgene oxime is a solid but the vapor pressure is high enough to produce symptoms. Contact with phosgene oxime results in a sudden rash, with exposed skin appearing pale and blanched with rings of erythema forming within 20 minutes of contact. Skin may have wheal-like lesions of pale up to 30 minutes after exposure. Immediate decontamination is required.

6.4.4. *Decontamination:* The only effective means to prevent or reduce damage from vesicants is vigorous, early (within seconds!) decontamination. Copious volumes of water should be applied to the WA to reduce itching and burning. Eyes should be flushed for several minutes using water or normal (0.9% sodium chloride) saline.

6.4.5. *Triage:* Triage of WA following vesicant contact is given in Table 6.3.

Table 6.3. Triage Guidelines for Exposure to Vesicants.

Triage Category	Clinical Signs
Immediate	Moderate to severe respiratory signs and symptoms.
Delayed	Skin lesions up to 50% of the body surface area (BSA), mild to moderate respiratory signs.
Minor	Skin lesions less than 5% BSA, and not in vital areas of the respiratory or oral tract.
Dead/Dying	Severe respiratory effects develop within 4–6 hours after contact. Lesions over 50% of the BSA and limited resources.

6.4.6. Pharmacological therapy

I.   British–anti-Lewisite (BAL; Dimercaprol) is the antidote for Lewisite, and a decreased mortality of exposed dogs is reported when given within 100 minutes of contact. This antidote will also alleviate some systemic effects. BAL is often not immediately available, and thus a heavy metal–chelating agent such as edetate calcium disodium (CaEDTA) may be suitable. For the WD, dilute to a 1% solution (10 mg/ml) with either normal saline or 5% dextrose in water (D_5W), and give 27.5 mg/kg SQ every 6 hours for 5 days and then give 5 days' rest; repeat if necessary. Alternately, may give 50 mg/kg SQ every 12 hours for 5 days if every 6 hours is too inconvenient. In horses, if severely affected, give CaEDTA at 75 mg/kg IV slowly in D_5W or saline daily for 4–5 days (may divide daily dose into 2–3 administrations per day). Stop therapy for 2 days and repeat for another 4–5 days.

II.   Topical ophthalmic analgesics such as proparacaine may be useful. Proparacaine is a rapid-acting topical anesthetic useful for relief of corneal pain. Proparacaine primarily anesthetizes the cornea, with limited penetration into conjunctiva. Anesthesia is of short duration (5–10 minutes). The usual dose is 1–2 drops, and you may repeat 1-drop doses every 5–10 minutes for 5–7 doses. Prolonged use may retard wound healing and cause corneal epithelial ulcers. Because the blink reflex may be suppressed, the eye should be protected from external injury during use. Repeated use may lead to rapid development of tolerance.

III.   As with thermal burns, IV analgesics may also be helpful.

IV.   Parenteral administration of crystalloid fluids is important when the WA has received a significant exposure and is showing signs of vesicant injury.

6.4.7.   *Aftercare*: Wound care, analgesics, and maintaining fluid balance and nutrition are the hallmarks of aftercare for vesicant contact.

6.5. Blood Agents

6.5.1.   Cyanide (AC/CK)

I.   *Actions*: Cyanide is often referred to as a "blood agent" because it will turn venous blood bright or cherry red. It is a highly lethal agent causing death within minutes of exposure. Under temperate conditions, cyanide evaporates quickly to form a poisonous gas or vapor. Two forms of cyanide that are likely weapons include hydrogen cyanide (AC), which is lighter than air and quickly dissipates, and cyanogen chloride (CK), which is heavier than air and accumulates in low spots. Most munitions contain the liquid cyanide and these rapidly vaporize upon detonation. Cyanide appears to be the least toxic of the "lethal" chemical agents. The mechanism of action of the cyanides is to inhibit the cytochrome oxidase enzymes present in all cells. These enzymes utilize oxygen and produce cellular energy. When these enzymes are inhibited, the cell cannot produce needed energy and soon dies. Before death, the cell switches to anaerobic metabolism resulting in a significant systemic acidosis.

II.   *Clinical signs*: Central nervous system cells, because of their high metabolic rates, are most sensitive to the lack of oxygen, and thus most signs and symptoms are related to this system's involvement. The clinical signs of inhalation of cyanide vapor are fast and few. One may see an initial rapid and deep breathing (about 5 breaths) during the first 15 seconds of inhalation. The skin is usually

flushed and very pink. The WA quickly loses consciousness, and seizures begin
within 30 seconds. After 3–5 minutes, breathing stops, and after 5–8 minutes, there
is cardiac arrest.

  A. Inhalation of lesser amounts of cyanide, or ingestion of a solution of cyanide
  salts, causes an anxious appearance in the WA. The animal becomes agitated, is
  unsteady on its legs, begins to salivate excessively, and finally shows muscle
  twitching. This is followed by unconsciousness and cardiopulmonary arrest.
  Antidotes can be very effective in these animals.
  B. In contrast to what is seen in a seizuring nerve agent WA victim, a seizuring
  cyanide victim has normal-sized pupils, normal amounts of secretions, and few
  or no muscular fasciculations.

III. *Treatment:* The WA exposed to cyanide, but showing no clinical signs of
toxicity, will not likely require treatment.

  A. Oxygen does appear to be useful as the sole treatment in mild to moderate
  exposure to cyanide.

IV. Pharmacological therapy

  A. Medical interventions approved in the United States
    1. Medical professionals in the United States currently have access to an
    antidote called the Cyanide Antidote Kit (also called the Taylor, Lilly, or
    Pasadena Kit). This kit contains three different medicines—amyl nitrite,
    sodium nitrite, and sodium thiosulfate—to be used in a specific sequence: the
    amyl nitrite is administered as an inhalant, followed by the sodium nitrite and
    sodium thiosulfate, which are given IV.
      a. The nitrites are given to convert hemoglobin in the red blood cell to
      methemoglobin, which attracts the cyanide away from the cytochrome
      oxidase and allows the cell to continue the process of aerobic metabolism.
      Thiosulfate is given to facilitate detoxification of cyanide by the body's own
      cyanide clearance system.
      b. Because the amyl nitrate is administered via inhalation, it seems unlikely
      this will be useful in the working animal.

  B. Medical interventions in other parts of the world
    1. In countries throughout the world, other antidotes have been developed
    and are currently used by emergency medical personnel in various situations.
    2. Hydroxocobalamin, a precursor of vitamin B_{12}, has been used safely and
    effectively in France (with the trade name Cyanokit, made by Merck Sant S.
    A.S.) since 1996 to treat smoke inhalation victims with cyanide exposure,
    including as an empiric therapy, and in cases of suspected cyanide poisoning.
    While not currently available in the United States, it is being investigated for
    possible use in the United States. The mechanism of action of
    hydroxocobalamin is fairly straightforward. The hydroxocobalamin attaches to
    the cyanide directly, creating cyanocobalamin, a natural form of vitamin B_{12},
    which is excreted in the urine. The advantage of this approach is that
    methemoglobin is not produced and the oxygen-carrying capacity of the
    victim's blood is not lowered. Therefore, it is suitable for use in smoke
    inhalation victims as well as other causes of cyanide poisoning. The most
    common side effect of hydroxocobalamin in humans is temporary pink
    discoloration of the skin, urine, and mucous membranes.
    3. Dicobalt ededate is used in the United Kingdom to treat cyanide poisoning.
    Cobalt compounds fixate to the cyanide ion. One 300-mg ampule is

administered IV at a regular rate over 1 minute followed by 50 ml glucose IV infusion. The most common side effects include vomiting, hypotension or hypertension, and tachycardia. Dicobalt edetate can be extremely toxic in the *absence* of cyanide ions and can only be given when the presence of severe cyanide poisoning is detected.

   4.   4-Dimethylaminophenol (DMAP) is used in Germany as an antidote for severe cyanide poisoning in patients that are in a deep coma and that have dilated nonreactive pupils and deteriorating cardiorespiratory function. DMAP converts part of the hemoglobin of the blood from ferrous hemoglobin to ferric; this creates a pool of binding potential that can divert cyanide from the cytochromes it poisons. Patients are given an IV dose of 3.25 mg/kg body weight. There are differences in individual susceptibility, which may result in an unacceptably high level of methemoglobin after normal therapeutic doses. Adverse side effects include hemolysis, mild headache, dizziness, hyperventilation, cyanosis, and discoloration of the urine.

C.   Additional information regarding treatment of cyanide toxicity.

   1.   Three antidotes for cyanide poisoning have been widely recommended: Ferrous sulfate dissolved in aqueous citric acid and aqueous sodium carbonate given orally, amyl nitrate by inhalation, and IV dicobalt edentate (Kelocyanor).

   2.   The oral solutions are only of value in reducing the absorption of swallowed cyanide, whereas most WAs will be exposed by inhalation or skin contact. These oral solutions also have a very limited shelf life. Recent reviews have questioned the effectiveness of the oral solutions and have also pointed out the likelihood of iron toxicity. Thus, currently the use of these solutions is not recommended.

   3.   Amyl nitrate, given by inhalation, has a long history of use in cyanide poisoning, although there is little scientific evidence that is of significant benefit. It has a limited shelf life and can be quite difficult to obtain as it is manufactured only in small quantities. Again, it is unlikely amyl nitrate will be of benefit in treating the WA exposed to cyanide.

   4.   Kelocyanor, given by IV injection, has been proven of use when administered to seriously ill human victims of confirmed cyanide poisoning. It is itself toxic, however, and can kill if used wrongly. Kelocyanor should only be used when the diagnosis is certain and the patient is seriously ill. Otherwise, prompt IV administration of cyanide antidote drugs is required. These antidotes can be effective so long as the animal has a pulse. Oxygen must be administered via face mask, needle tracheostomy, or endotracheal tube.

D.   *Conclusions:* It is unlikely that antidotes will be of value in treating cyanide toxicity. There is a great deal of anecdotal evidence of the value of oxygen in treating human victims of mild to moderate cyanide toxicity.

   1.   *For cyanide toxicity in large animals:* First give sodium nitrite at a dose of 16 mg/kg IV followed with a 20% solution of sodium thiosulfate given at a dose of 30–40 mg/kg IV. If symptoms reoccur, then repeat the treatment, using sodium thiosulfate only. Be aware that sodium nitrate may result in significant hypotension and thus be prepared for the animal to fall to the ground. This is most important when dealing with the full-sized horse. This approach has been noted to be effective, especially in cattle.

V.   *Decontamination:* Decontamination is usually unnecessary unless the hair coat is wet from exposure to cyanide. If this is the case, thoroughly rinse the WA

with copious volumes of water. Immediately irrigate the eyes with water for at least 10 minutes.
VI.   Triage (Table 6.4)

Table 6.4. Triage guidelines for Exposure to Cyanide.

Triage Category	Clinical Signs
Immediate	Apneic, but pulses are present. Move immediately to fresh air. Immediate antidote therapy is required!
Delayed	Recovering from the effects of therapy.
Minor	Mild effects, not life-threatening.
Dead/Dying	Cardiopulmonary arrest.

VII.   *Aftercare:* Pulse oximetry will be of no use in cyanide toxicity as the problem does not result from a lack of oxygen, but from the inability of the animal's body to use the available oxygen. Severe metabolic acidosis resulting from cyanide exposure requires correcting this acidosis with parenteral crystalloids and possible use of sodium bicarbonate. An empirical dosage of sodium bicarbonate would be 0.25 mEq/kg given slowly IV. One should not place the sodium bicarbonate in crystalloid solutions containing calcium or magnesium (i.e., Ringer's lactate or Normosol-R) as these may result in precipitation of calcium or magnesium carbonate crystals.

6.6. Choking (Pulmonary) Agents

Pulmonary edema results when animals are exposed to compounds categorized as pulmonary agents. There are three primary pulmonary agents to which the WA may be exposed during a disaster: phosgene (CG), chlorine (Cl), and ammonia (anhydrous). Of all the terrorism agents, these should be considered the most dangerous. They are chemicals that are easily obtained, usually require little in the manufacturing process to be used as a weapon, and are all on the FBI's top 10 list of agents most likely to be used as a weapon of mass destruction. Being pulmonary agents, one expects them to immobilize the WA through inhalation of the chemical, causing severe lung damage, and eventually, death.

6.6.1.   Specific pulmonary agents
I.   Phosgene is a liquid that evaporates very quickly and enters the body through the airways. It causes pulmonary edema by damaging the thin membrane (alveolar-capillary membrane) between the pulmonary capillaries and the alveoli. When inhaled, phosgene travels to the bronchioles where it breaks down the alveolar-capillary membrane. Plasma from the blood then leaks into the disrupted membrane and finally into the alveoli, filling these with fluid (i.e., pulmonary edema). The pulmonary edema quickly results in hypoxia and difficulty in breathing for the WA. Inhalation of phosgene can result in varying degrees of pulmonary edema, usually after a symptom-free period that varies with the amount inhaled. Phosgene is a liquid, with rapid vaporization after an explosion. It has a characteristic white cloud, and an odor of sweet, newly mown hay.

II. Chlorine is a greenish-yellow gas or amber liquid (under pressure) with a pungent odor. It exists as a gas at room temperature, with inhalation being the most lethal route of exposure. Skin and eye exposure are also quite harmful to the WA. Chlorine is heavier than air when the temperature is <32°F. Chlorine can be quite hazardous as noted in Table 6.5:

Table 6.5. Effects of Various Chlorine Concentrations on Animals.

Concentration of Chlorine	Symptoms
5–8 ppm	Pharyngeal and eye irritation
34–51 ppm	Lethal in 1–1.5 hours
430 ppm	Lethal in 30 minutes
1000 ppm	Lethal after a few breaths

III. Ammonia is a colorless gas with a very distinct pungent odor. It is typically found, transported, and stored in a liquefied form. It has widespread use as an industrial chemical and is commonly employed in agriculture. Additionally, it is often found in meth labs. Anhydrous ammonia has a high affinity for water and will rapidly penetrate deeply into tissues. Ammonia is lighter than air at 68°F. When released from a container, anhydrous ammonia will have an expansion ratio of 850:1.

6.6.2. *Clinical signs:* Initially, WAs exhibit transient irritation to the eyes, nose, and throat immediately after exposure to the pulmonary agents. This is manifested by watery eyes, pawing at their eyes (dogs), and then coughing and respiratory distress ensue. Time to effect often depends upon the dose inhaled but may be anytime between 2 and 24 hours. The greater the exposure and the shorter the time to onset of signs, the greater is the pulmonary damage. With pulmonary injury and resultant edema, the WA will show signs of hyperpnea, exercise intolerance, cough, and, finally, the production of a clear to slightly blood-tinged sputum when pulmonary edema becomes severe.

6.6.3. *Treatment:* Realistically, the WA with severe respiratory distress will have minimal likelihood of survival. Appropriate management would include high-flow oxygen following either tracheostomy or anesthesic-induced anesthesia. Because airway reflexes are depressed, continuous positive airway pressure (CPAP) or positive-end expiratory pressure (PEEP) ventilation is required. Administration of diuretics (i.e., furosemide) is of minimal value because the pulmonary edema is not of cardiac origin (the pulmonary edema results from damage to the alveolar-pulmonary membrane). Addition of diuretics to an animal on CPAP/PEEP should be carefully monitored as the combination of the two might result in cardiovascular collapse due to severe hypotension. Aerosolized alpha$_2$-agonist (albuterol) may help with acute bronchospasm, but this will only be possible in the WA when the animal is already on a ventilator.

I. Of special note in the horse, there are reports of people receiving dimethylsulfoxide (DMSO) and oxygen administration, resulting in the incapacitation of rescuers. It was theorized that when paramedics drew a blood sample from a person on DMSO and exogenous oxygen, the sudden temperature change caused the DMSO to chemically convert to dimethyl sulfate, a known chemical warfare agent. **Just a small whiff of this chemical from the patient's drawn blood was enough to incapacitate ER staff within seconds!** Since DMSO is commonly used in the horse, caution must be applied to avoid a catastrophe.

6.6.4. *Decontamination:* Large volumes of water are used for decontamination of the WA.

6.6.5. Triage of animals exposed to pulmonary agents (Table 6.6).

Table 6.6. Triage Guidelines of Animals Exposed to Pulmonary Agents.

Triage Category	Clinical Signs
Immediate	Severe respiratory distress with pulmonary edema.
Delayed	Respiratory distress without signs of pulmonary edema. This animal must be closely monitored for progression of signs.
Minor	Asymptomatic following a known exposure.
Dead/Dying	Pulmonary edema, cyanosis, and hypotension. Onset of pulmonary edema occurring within 4–6 hours of exposure will probably not do well even with optimal care.

6.6.6. *Supportive care:* Supportive management of the airway and management of liquid burns are recommended for the WA with minimal symptoms. With severe symptoms, euthanasia should be considered.

6.6.7. *Aftercare:* Oxygen and supportive airway management are used for the WA following survival of exposure to pulmonary agents.

6.7. Riot control agents (RCA) (tear-producing compounds)

The RCAs are chemicals that rapidly produce sensory irritation or disabling physical effects that disappear within a short time following termination of exposure. The standard tear-producing agents are o-chlorobenzylidene (CS), other agents in the same family (CS1, CS2, CSX), and dibenz(**b,f**)-1:4-oxazepine (CR). Generally, they produce a rapid onset of effects (seconds to several minutes) and they have a relatively brief duration of effects (15–30 minutes) once the victim has escaped the contaminated atmosphere and has removed the contamination from clothing or hair coat. Because tear compounds produce only transient casualties, they are widely used for training, riot control, and situations where long-term incapacitation is unacceptable. When released indoors, they may cause serious illness or death. It is not uncommon for WAs to become exposed to RCAs. Many of these agents will cause temporary discomfort but seldom have long-term or fatal effects. Tests have been conducted by various credible organizations and it has been determined that working WDs can most often continue with their operations even after being exposed to these chemicals. If the environment requires the handler to wear a protective mask, one should avoid taking a WA into that environment.

6.7.1. *Clinical signs:* Clinical signs include an initial burning feeling or irritation to the eyes that progresses to pain accompanied by blepharospasm and lacrimation. The mucous membranes of the mouth have a sensation of discomfort or burning, with excess salivation. Rhinorrhea is accompanied by pain inside the nose. When inhaled, these compounds cause a burning sensation or a feeling of tightness in the chest, with coughing, sneezing, and increased secretions. On unprotected skin, especially if the air is warm and moist, these agents cause tingling or burning.

6.7.2. Specific agents

I. o-*Chlorobenzylidene malononitrile (CS):* In 1959, CS was adopted for combat training and riot control purposes. CS produces an intense burning and irritation of the eyes, with mild to severe conjunctivitis. It also produces a burning sensation in the nose and mucous membranes of the respiratory tract, followed by draining of the nasal sinuses. The chest feels constricted, with a sensation of choking and being unable to breathe. CS is also a primary skin irritant and can produce erythema, edema, and vesication. CS exists as a family of four forms: CS, CS1, CS2, and CSX. Different forms of CS have different persistence characteristics because of their formulation, dissemination, and rate of hydrolysis. CS has been found to persist in snow for as long as 30 days but its persistency in soil varies, depending on the condition of the soil.

II. *Dibenz(b,f)–1 : 4-oxazepine (CR):* In 1974, CR was approved for use in riot control situations. CR is more potent and less toxic than CS. CR is not used in its pure form but is dissolved in a solution of 80 parts of propylene glycol and 20 parts of water to form a 0.1% CR solution. The severity of symptoms increases with the CR solution concentration and in any environment of high temperature and humidity. CR does not degrade in water, and it is quite persistent in the environment. Under suitable conditions, CR can persist on certain surfaces (especially porous) for up to 60 days.

III. *Capsaicin (OC) (pepper spray):* Capsaicin, also called oleoresin capsicum, is derived from cayenne peppers. OC stimulates sensory nerve endings, causing reflex changes in blood pressure and respiration. It causes pain, edema, and erythema of the tissues with which it makes contact. It also produces bronchoconstriction and edema of the airway mucosa. Contact with the eyes is extremely painful. OC is a powerful irritant and lacrimator. Although it may not have been the cause of death, it has been associated with deaths in humans.

IV. *Chloroacetophenone (tear gas or mace) (CN):* Inhalation of CN causes a burning sensation, cough, sore throat, nausea, and shortness of breath. Exposure to skin causes redness and pain. Eye exposure causes redness, pain, and blurred vision. CN can cause pulmonary edema. High concentrations can cause blisters to form, and CN is a potent skin sensitizer. The indiscriminate use of large amounts of CN in confined spaces has caused injuries requiring medical attention or even death.

V. *Smokes and obscurants:* Smoke is an aerosol that owes its ability to conceal or obscure to its composition of many small particles suspended in the air. These particles scatter or absorb the light, thus reducing visibility. When the density or amount of smoke material between the observer and the object to be screened exceeds a certain minimum threshold value, the object cannot be seen. Many types and combinations of smokes are used, but the three basic types of screening smokes are hexachloroethane (HC) smoke, phosphorus smoke, and fog oil smoke. White phosphorus (WP) and HC are hygroscopic; they absorb water vapor from the atmosphere. This increases their diameters and makes them more efficient at reflecting light rays. Fog oils are nonhygroscopic and depend upon vaporization techniques to produce extremely small-diameter droplets to scatter light rays. Most smokes are not hazardous in concentrations that are useful for obscuring purposes. However, any smoke can be hazardous to health if the concentration is sufficient or if the exposure is long enough. The protective mask gives the respiratory tract and the eyes adequate protection against all smokes.

6.7.3. *Treatment:* Specific treatment is generally not required since the signs and symptoms subside on their own once animals have been moved to fresh air. The eyes should be rinsed with either sterile water or saline. A topical ophthalmic ointment can then be applied to soothe and reduce inflammation caused by the exposure.

6.7.4. *Decontamination:* No form of hypochlorite should be used in an attempt to decontaminate RCAs. Bleach reacts with riot control agents to form a strong irritant. Do not decontaminate riot control agents with any form of bleach.

I.   Move the animal to fresh air; brush or vacuum powders from the hair coat.

II. Flush the skin with plain water, soap and water, or a weak solution of sodium bicarbonate (baking soda). Water and soap may cause a temporary worsening of the burning sensation, but it will not cause additional damage.

Suggested Reading/Resources

Agent Characteristics

Centers for Disease Control Emergency Preparedness and Response website and associated agent fact sheets for sulfur mustard and nerve agents: http://www.bt.cdc.gov/agent/.

Chemical Stockpile Emergency Planning and Preparedness Program. Website. http://www.cma.army.mil/csepp.aspx. CSEPP Reentry & Restoration Guidance & IPT Monitoring Plan.

Cyanide Poisoning Treatment Coalition (CPTC). Website. http://www.cyanidepoisoning.org/.

Department of the Army. *USAMRICD'S Medical Management of Chemical Casualties Handbook,* ed 4. Aberdeen Proving Ground, MD, U.S. Army Medical Research Institute for Chemical Defense, February 2001.

Department of the Army. *U.S. Army Textbook of Military Medicine (TMM): part 1: Medical Aspects of Chemical and Biological Warfare.* Washington, DC, Office of the Surgeon General, Department of the Army, 1997.

Department of the Army/Department of Defense, 2005. *Field Manual (FM) 3–11.9, Potential Military Chemical/ Biological Compounds, Multiservice Tactics Techniques and Procedures,* January 2005. http://chppm-www.apgea.army.mil/chemicalagent/.

Department of the Army (ECBC). *US Army Material Safety Data Sheets (MSDS) for GB, HD, and VX.* Aberdeen Proving Ground, MD, Edgewood Chemical and Biological Center, December 2004. http://chppm-www.apgea.army.mil/chemicalagent/.

Department of the Army Office of the Surgeon General. Memorandum, Subject: Nerve Agent Percutaneous Exposure Criteria and Airborne Exposure Levels (AELs) for GD. GF in Use of Interim DA Guidance on Implementation of the New AELs, 29 June 2004.

Headquarters, Department of the Army. Memorandum Subject: Implementation Guidance Policy for New Airborne Exposure Limits for GB, GA, GD, GF, VX, H, HD, and HT; signed by Mr. R. J. Fatz, Deputy Assistant Secretary of the Army (Environment, Safety and Occupational Health); OASA (I&E), June 2004. http://chppm-www.apgea.army.mil/chemicalagent/.

Kingery AF, Allen HE. The environmental fate of organophosphate nerve agents: A review. Toxicol Environ Chem 1995;47:155–184.

Munro NB, et al. The sources, fate, and toxicity of chemical warfare agent degradation products. Environ Health Perspect 1999;107(12):933–974. http://chppm-www.apgea.army.mil/chemicalagent/.

National Research Council-COT. *Volume 3, Acute Exposure Guidelines for Selected Airborne Chemicals.* Washington, DC, National Academies Press, 2003. www.nap.edu.

OSHA Guidance. http://www.osha.gov/SLTC/emergencypreparedness/guides/blister.html; http://www.osha.gov/SLTC/emergencypreparedness/guides/nerve.html.

Talmage SS, et al., The fate of chemical warfare agents in the environment. In Maynard R, et al, editors. *Chemical Warfare Agents: Toxicology and Treatment.* New York, John Wiley and Sons, 2006.

U.S. Army Center for Health Promotion and Preventive Medicine (USACHPPM). *USACHPPM CHPPM Technical Guide 244: The Medical NBC Battlebook.* August 2000. http://chppm-www.apgea.army.mil/.

U.S. Army Center for Health Promotion and Preventive Medicine (USACHPPM). The Army Chemical Agent Safety Program; Safety; 28 February 1997. http://chppm-www.apgea.army.mil/chemicalagent/.

U.S. Army Chemical Materials Agency. Chemical Stockpile Disposal Project (CSDP). http://www.cma.army.mil/csdp.aspx.

Watson AP, et al. Cholinesterase inhibitors as chemical warfare agents: Community planning guidelines. In Gupta R, editor. *Toxicology of Organophosphate and Carbamate Compounds.* New York, Elsevier/Academic Press, December 2005.

Williams JM, Rowland B, Jeffery MT, et al. Degradation kinetics of VX on concrete by secondary ion mass spectrometry. Langmuir 2005;21:2386–2390.

Release Scenarios Health Effects (Signs and Symptoms) and Personnel Safety

Centers for Disease Control and Prevention. DHHS CDC interim recommendations for airborne exposure limits for chemical warfare agents H and HD (sulfur mustard). Fed Reg 2004;69:24164–24168. http://chppm-www.apgea.army.mil/chemicalagent/.

Centers for Disease Control and Prevention, Notice; Department of Health and Human Services (DHHS) Centers for Disease Control and Prevention (CDC); Final recommendations for protecting human health from potential adverse effects of exposure to agents GA (Tabun), GB (Sarin), and VX. Fed Reg 2003;68:58348–58351. http://chppm-www.apgea.army.mil/chemicalagent/.

Chemical Stockpile Emergency Preparedness Program, US Army and US Federal Emergency Management Agency (FEMA). Policy Paper #20 (revised), Subject: Adoption of acute exposure guidelines levels (AEGLs); February, 2003. http://chppm-www.apgea.army.mil/chemicalagent/.

Department of the Army Office of the Surgeon General. Memorandum subject: Nerve agent percutaneous exposure criteria and airborne exposure levels (AELs) for GD.GF in use of interim DA guidance on implementation of the new AELs, June 2004. http://chppm-www.apgea.army.mil/chemicalagent/.

Department of the Army (ECBC). *US Army Material Safety Data Sheets (MSDS) for GB, HD, and VX.* Aberdeen Proving Ground, MD, Edgewood Chemical and Biological Center, December 2004. http://chppm-www.apgea.army.mil/chemicalagent/.

DuPont. *Permeation Guide for DuPont™ Tychem® Protective Fabrics.* June 2004. 1-800-931-3456. http://www2.dupont.com/Personal_Protection/en_US/assets/downloads/tychem/permguide82004.pdf.

Environmental Protection Agency. http://www.epa.gov/oppt/aegl/pubs/tsd45.pdf.

Environmental Protection Agency. (TOPOFF 3) Email (sent April 26, 2006, Mark Mjoness, EPA) and associated attachments and follow on teleconference: SUBJECT Inter-Agency Technical Expert Panel–EOC Event Room 1–Additional Meeting Documents (establishes the clearance levels used for HD event–concurrence by EPA, OSHA, and CDC/HHS).

Headquarters, Department of the Army. Memorandum subject: Implementation guidance policy for new airborne exposure limits for GB. GA, GD, GF, VX, H, HD, and H; signed by MF Hayambhill I, Pulfa, Taylor, Assistant Secretary of the Army (Environment, Safety and Occupational Health); OASA (I&E), June 18, 2004. http://chppm-www.apgea.army.mil/chemicalagent/.

Interagency Mass Personnel Decontamination Guidance: TSWG. *Best Practices and Guidelines for CBR Mass Personnel Decontamination.* 2004. Contact: cbrncsubgroup@TSWG.gov.

National Research Council-COT. *Volume 3, Acute Exposure Guidelines for Selected Airborne Chemicals.* Washington, DC, National Academies Press, 2003. www.nap.edu.

Talmage SS, et al. Chemical warfare agent degradation and decontamination. Curr Org Chem 2006.

Watson AP, et al. Cholinesterase inhibitors as chemical warfare agents: Community planning guidelines. In Gupta, editor. *Toxicology of Organophosphate and Carbamate Compounds.* New York, Elsevier/Academic Press, 2006, pp 47–68.

Watson AP, et al. Development and application of acute exposure guidelines levels for chemical warfare nerve and sulfur mustard agents. J Toxicol Environ Health B 2006;9:173–263.

Soil

Environmental Protection Agency. (TOPOFF 3) Email (sent April 26, 2006, Mark Mjoness, EPA) and associated attachments and follow on teleconference: SUBJECT Inter-Agency Technical Expert Panel–EOC Event Room 1–Additional Meeting

Documents (establishes the clearance levels used for HD event–concurrence by
   EPA, OSHA, and CDC/HHS).
Headquarters Department of the Army, Office of the Assistant Secretary for
   Installations, Logistics, and Environment. Memorandum, SUBJ: Derivation of
   Health-Based Environmental Screening Levels (HBESLs) for Chemical Warfare
   Agents, May 28, 1999.
U.S. Army Center for Health Promotion and Preventive Medicine (USACHPPM /
   ORNL, 1999. USACHPPM Technical Report: Health-Based Environmental
   Screening Levels for Chemical Warfare Agents, March 1999. http://chppm-www.
   apgea.army.mil/chemicalagent/ NOTE: values selected were those based on EPA
   Region IX PRGs and EPA Region III RBCs.

Water

Environmental Protection Agency. (TOPOFF 3) Email (sent April 26, 2006, Mark
   Mjoness, EPA) and associated attachments and follow on teleconference: SUBJECT
   Inter-Agency Technical Expert Panel–EOC Event Room 1–Additional Meeting
   Documents (establishes the clearance levels used for HD event–concurrence by
   EPA, OSHA, and CDC/HHS).
Headquarters, Department of the Army. TB Med 577; Field Sanitation, Control and
   Surveillance of Field Water Supplies. 2005. http://chppm-www.apgea.army.mil/
   chemicalagent/.
Headquarters Department of the Army, Office of the Assistant Secretary for
   Installations, Logistics, and Environment, Memorandum, SUBJ: Derivation of
   Health-Based Environmental Screening Levels (HBESLs) for Chemical Warfare
   Agents, May 28, 1999. http://chppm-www.apgea.army.mil/chemicalagent/.

Hazardous Waste Criteria

U.S. Army. Proposed Utah Chemical Agent Rule (UCAR), May 1999 (Volume 1,
   Section XI). Development of health-based waste management concentration levels.
U.S. Army Center for Health Promotion and Preventive Medicine (USACHPPM).
   Information Paper, Management criteria for chemical warfare agent (CWA)-
   contaminated waste and media. October 10, 2000, as well as USACHPPM
   technical paper, Chemical warfare agent health-based waste control limits,
   September 2000. http://chppm-www.apgea.army.mil/chemicalagent/.

Toxicity Values (e.g., Reference Doses)

National Research Council—COT. *Review of the U.S. Army's Health Risk
   Assessments for Oral Exposure to Six Chemical-Warfare Agents.* Washington, DC,
   National Research Council, National Academies Press, 1999. www.nap.edu.
Opresko DM, et al. Chemical warfare agents: Estimating oral reference doses. *Rev
   Environ Contamin Toxicol* 1998;156:1–183. http://chppm-www.apgea.army.mil/
   chemicalagent/.
Watson AP, Munro NB. *Reentry Planning: The Technical Basis for Offsite Recovery
   Following Warfare Agent Contamination.* ORNL-6628. Oak Ridge National
   Laboratory, Oak Ridge, TN, 1990.

(Civilian) Effect Levels: Air Effect Levels: Media Other Than Air

Opresko DM, et al. Chemical warfare agents: Current status of oral reference doses.
   Rev Environ Contamin Toxicol 2001;172:65–85. http://chppm-www.apgea.army.
   mil/chemicalagent/.

Watson A, Opresko D, Hauschild V. *Evaluation of Chemical Warfare Agent Percutaneous Vapor Toxicity: Derivation of Toxicity Guidelines for Assessing Chemical Protective Ensembles.* ORNL/TM-2003/180. Oak Ridge, TN, Oak Ridge National Laboratory, 2003. http://www.osti.gov/bridge; http://chppm-www.apgea.army.mil/chemicalagent/.

Breakdown Product Toxicity

Bausum HT. Toxicological and related data for VX, suggested breakdown products and additives; suggested RfD and RfC values. Prepared by the U.S. Army Center for Health Promotion and Preventive Medicine, Aberdeen Proving Ground, MD, for the Newport (IN) Chemical Agent Disposal Facility, in HBESL document, Appendix F, 1998.

Bausum HT, Reddy G, Leach GJ. Suggested interim estimates of the reference dose (RfD) and reference concentration (RfC) for certain key breakdown products of chemical agents. Report to the U.S. Army Center for Health Promotion and Preventive Medicine (USACHPPM Chemical Standards Working Group, December 10, 1998.

National Research Council—Institute of Medicine. Chemical and Biological Terrorism: Research and Development to Improve Civilian Medical Response. Washington, DC, National Academies Press, 1999.

Field Detection Tool Manufacturers

AP2Ce: Proengin Inc., 405 NE 8th Street, Fort Lauderdale, FL 33304; www.proengin.com; (Tel) 954-760-9990; (Fax) 954-760-9955; contactusa@proengin.com.

APD2000: Smiths Detection–Danbury, 21 Commerce Drive, Danbury, CT 06810, www.sensir.com; (Tel) 203-207-9700, toll free: 888-473-6747; (Fax) 203-207-9780; danbury@smithsdetection.com; For technical problems or questions during normal business hours, email support.danbury@smithsdetection.com.

Black RM, Clarke RJ, Cooper DB, et al. Application of headspace analysis, solvent extraction, thermal desorption and gas chromatography-mass spectrometry to the analysis of chemical warfare samples containing sulfur mustard and related compounds. J Chromatogr 1993;637:71–80.

CSEPP Planning Guidance, Appendix M, Planning Guidelines for Recovery Phase Activities for the Chemical Stockpile Emergency. http://chppm-www.apgea.army.mil/.

Draeger tubes: Draeger Safety, Inc., 101 Technology Drive, Pittsburgh, PA 15275-1057; www.draeger.com; (Tel) 412-787-8383; (Fax) 412-787-2207.

LLNL, T. M. Carlsen et al. *Sampling Requirements for Chemical and Biological Agent Decontamination Efficacy Verification.* UCRLAR-143245; US Department of Energy, Lawrence Livermore National Laboratory, March 29, 2001.

M256 and M272 kits: (manufacturer) Truetech Inc., Riverhead, NY 11901; (Tel) 631-727-8600; (vendor) Safeware Inc. (Tel) 1-800-359-4617, M8 and M9 papers: (manufacturer) Truetech Inc., Riverhead, NY 11901; (Tel) 631-727-8600; (vendor) Safeware Inc. (Tel) 1-800-359-4617, Preparedness Program, May 1997.

Talmage SS, et al. Chemical warfare agent degradation and decontamination. Curr Org Chem 2006.

Trace Atmospheric Gas Analyzer (TAGA), EPA Environmental Response Team (Tel) 732-321-6660.

U.S. Army, 1998. CSEPP Reentry and Restoration Guidance and IPT Monitoring
Plan. http://chppm-www.apgea.army.mil/chemicalagent/.

U.S. Army Center for Health Promotion and Preventive Medicine (USACHPPM).
Health-Based Environmental Screening Levels for Chemical Warfare
Agents. Technical report prepared by U.S. Army Center for Health
Promotion and Oak Ridge National Laboratories, March 1999.
http://chppm-www.apgea.army.mil/chemicalagent/.

U.S. Army Center for Health Promotion and Preventive Medicine (USACHPPM).
USACHPPM CHPPM Technical Guide 244: The Medical NBC Battlebook, August
2000.

Vogt BM, Sorensen JH. How clean is safe? Improving the Effectiveness of
Decontamination of Structures and People Following Chemical and Biological
Incidents. ORNL/TM-2002/178. Oak Ridge National Laboratory, Oak Ridge, TN,
2002. http://www.osti.gov/bridge.

Watson AP, Munro NB. Reentry Planning: The Technical Basis for Offsite Recovery
Following Warfare Agent Contamination. ORNL-6628. Oak Ridge, TN, Oak
Ridge National Laboratory, 1990. Website. www.safewareinc.com.

Decon—Agent Degradation by Control of pH, Temperature, Photolysis

Kingery AF, Allen HE. The environmental fate of organophosphate nerve agents: A
review. Toxicol Environ Chem 1995;47:155–184.

Williams JM, Rowland B, Jeffery MT, et al. Degradation kinetics of VX on concrete
by secondary ion mass spectrometry. Langmuir 2005;21:2386–2390.

Animal/Livestock Decon and Treatment

American Veterinary Medical Association (AVMA). *AVMA Emergency Preparedness
and Response Guide*, 1995. American Veterinary Medical Association, 1931 N.
Meacham Rd. Suite 100, Schaumburg, IL 46204–2760.

Dorman DC. Poisoned animal management, part I. NAPINet Rep 1989;2:3.

Mershon MM, Tennyson AV. Chemical hazards and chemical warfare. JAVMA
1987;190:734–745.

Osweiler GD, et al. *Clinical and Diagnostic Veterinary Toxicology*. Dubuque, IA,
Kendall/Hunt, 1985.

Field Detection, Sampling for Confirmatory Results Decontamination/Cleanup: Planning and Methods

AR 385-61: The Army Chemical Agent Safety Program; Safety; 28 February 1997.
http://chppm-www.apgea.army.mil/chemicalagent/.

Chemical Stockpile Emergency Preparedness Program, US Army and US
Federal Emergency Management Agency (FEMA) Policy Paper #20 (Rev),
Subject: Adoption of Acute Exposure Guidelines Levels (AEGLs); February
2003.

Department of Health and Human Services/Centers for Disease Control and
Prevention. *Review of the U.S. Army Proposal for Off-site Treatment and Disposal
of Caustic VX Hydrolysate From the Newport Chemical Agent Disposal Facility*.
Atlanta, GA, U.S. Dept. of Health and Human Services, Centers for Disease
Control and Prevention, April 2005.

Department of the Army. *U.S. Army Textbook of Military Medicine (TMM): Part 1: Medical Aspects of Chemical and Biological Warfare.* Washington, DC, Office of the Surgeon General, Department of the Army, 1997; use of "M9 tape" and "M256A1 ticket" in certifying decon.

Headquarters, Department of the Army. Guidelines for decontamination and disposal of tools, supplies, equipment, and facilities, memorandum subject: Implementation guidance policy for new airborne exposure limits for GB. GA, GD, GF, VX, H, HD, and HT; signed by Mr. Raymond J. Fatz, Deputy Assistant Secretary of the Army (Environment, Safety and Occupational Health); OASA (I&E), June 18, 2004. http://chppm-www.apgea.army.mil/chemicalagent/.

Headquarters, Department of the Army. Memorandum subject: Implementation guidance policy for new airborne exposure limits for GB. GA, GD, GF, VX, H, HD, and HT; signed by Mr. Raymond J. Fatz, Deputy Assistant Secretary of the Army (Environment, Safety and Occupational Health); OASA (I&E), June 18, 2004. http://chppm-www.apgea.army.mil/chemicalagent/.

Heath SE. *The Development of the Veterinary Service and Animal Care Annex to the Indiana State Emergency Operations Plan.* Proceedings of the Indiana Veterinary Medical Association Disaster Preparedness Committee (1993–1995). Indianapolis, IN, State Emergency Management Agency, Indiana Government Center South, 1995.

NATO. *NATO Handbook for Sampling and Identification of Biological and Chemical Agents. Vol 1, Procedures and Techniques.* AEP-10, 2000, Vol 1 (Edition 5). NATO/PFP Unclassified.

Talmage SS, et al. Chemical warfare agent degradation and decontamination. Curr Org Chem 2006

Talmage SS, et al., The fate of chemical warfare agents in the environment. In Maynard R, et al., editors. *Chemical Warfare Agents: Toxicology and Treatment.* New York, John Wiley and Sons, 2006.

U.S. Army—Proposed Utah Chemical Agent Rule (UCAR), May 1999 (Volume 1, Section XI), Development of Health-Based Waste Management Concentration Levels.

U.S. Army Center for Health Promotion and Preventive Medicine (USACHPPM). Information paper, Management Criteria for Chemical Warfare Agent (CWA)-Contaminated Waste and Media, 10 October 2000, as well as USACHPPM Technical paper, Chemical Warfare Agent Health-Based Waste Control Limits, dated September 2000. http://chppm-www.apgea.army.mil/chemicalagent/.

U.S. Army Center for Health Promotion and Preventive Medicine (USACHPPM). Health-Based Environmental Screening Levels for Chemical Warfare Agents. Technical report prepared by U.S. Army Center for Health Promotion and Oak Ridge National Laboratories, March 1999. http://chppm-www.apgea.army.mil/chemicalagent/.

Watson AP, et al. Cholinesterase inhibitors as chemical warfare agents: Community planning guidelines. In Gupta R, editor. *Toxicology of Organophosphate and Carbamate Compounds.* New York, Elsevier/Academic Press, December 2005.

Watson AP, et al. Development and application of acute exposure guidelines levels for chemical warfare nerve and sulfur mustard agents. J Toxicol Environ Health B 2006;9:173–263.

CHAPTER 7
RADIOLOGICAL EVENTS

Jerry J. Upp, DVM, EMT

Radiation elicits the most fear as a weapon of mass destruction. This is likely due to the thought of a nuclear holocaust. The potential use of radioactive materials by terrorists includes sources from medical diagnostics, oncological therapy, and production of energy. Many of these agents can result in significant mortality, but more likely, the fear factor perpetuated by news media will result in more casualties than those of the actual device. Nevertheless, working animals and their handlers are likely to be exposed to radiation, and a basic understanding of the types, injuries, and treatment will be useful.

7. Radiological Events

7.1. Basic Terminology

7.1.1. Radiological events caused by terrorism are a real threat in today's society. Working animals (WAs) may be grossly contaminated before the first responders even know that a release of radiation has occurred.

7.1.2. Radiation is colorless and odorless, which may lead to improper detection of a serious event. The goal here is not to make nuclear scientists out of the reader but to give the first responder some basic knowledge of what may be encountered and how we can use this knowledge to help the WA and the handlers.

7.1.3. When dealing with radiation, the major problems that can be encountered are alpha particles, beta particles, gamma rays, x-rays, and neutron radiation. The most likely in a terrorist attack are the alphas, betas, and gammas (Fig. 7.1). The main modes of contamination are absorption, ingestion, inhalation, and injection.

    I.   Alpha particles are given off from the breakdown of many radioactive isotopes. They are the heaviest and most highly charged particles. Because of this, they are the least penetrating of the three. Even dead layers of skin will stop their penetration into the body. The major modes of contamination from alpha particles are from inhalation and ingestion. WAs have hair that

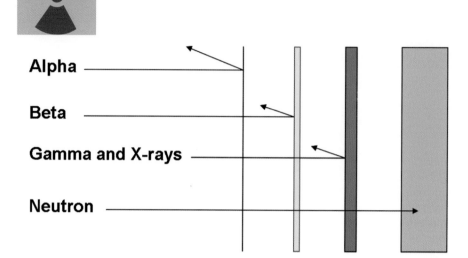

Paper Plastic Lead   Concrete

Figure 7.1. Radiation symbols must use the conventional radiation caution colors: magenta or purple on yellow background. The most common types of radiation include alpha particles, beta particles, gamma and x-rays, and neutrons. Alpha particles are heavy and doubly charged which cause them to lose their energy very quickly in matter. They can be shielded by a sheet of paper or the surface layer of our skin. Alpha particles are only considered hazardous if an alpha emitting material is ingested or inhaled. Beta particles are much smaller and have only one charge, which cause them to interact more slowly with material. They are effectively shielded by thin layers of metal or plastic and are again only considered hazardous if a beta emitter is ingested or inhaled. Gamma emitters are associated with alpha and beta decay. X-Rays are produced either when electrons change orbits within an atom, or electrons from an external source are deflected around the nucleus of an atom. Both are forms of high-energy electromagnetic radiation which interact lightly with matter. X-rays and gamma rays are best shielded by thick layers of lead or other dense material and are hazardous to people when they are external to the body. Neutrons are neutral particles with approximately the same mass as a proton. Because they are neutral, they react only weakly with material. They are an external hazard best shielded by thick layers of concrete.

will also prevent any penetration, but due to their constant cleaning, grooming, and sniffing, ingestion and inhalation avenues are a concern. Most alpha particles are very slow in leaving the body once they have entered.

II. Beta particles are smaller than alpha and can travel slightly farther distances; therefore, they penetrate more than do alpha particles. They can travel slightly deeper into the skin and can be responsible for burns in the skin called *beta burns* and damage to the lens of the eye. When dealing with the WA, this may be more likely in the lesser-haired regions of the head, feet, ventral abdomen, and pinna of the ears. Once again, ingestion and inhalation are the more dangerous avenues for contamination. The particles can also enter through abrasions, lacerations, or penetrations. If WAs do not have breathing protection, inhalation and ingestion from grooming and breathing contaminated air are concerns.

III.   Gamma rays travel as waves. They are the most penetrating of the three types. They can travel the farthest, and shielding is needed to prevent damage to internal organs and tissues. They travel through the patient, so external contamination is not a concern but the internal damage is a concern.

7.1.4.   An important concept to remember when dealing with radiation is the concept of *time*, *distance*, and *shielding*. The less time the WA, handler, and responder are exposed, the better. The farther distance and the more shielding that are used, the better the chance of survival. There is a rule called the *seven/ten rule*. This states that for every 7-fold increase in time (in hours) after a radiological release, there is a 10-fold decrease in radiation. For example, if the initial dose rate is 1000 rad/hr, after 7 hours, this dose rate is down to 100 rad/hr. After 49 hours (approximately 2 days), this rate is down to 10 rad/hr. If you multiply 49 hours by 7, you get ≈2 weeks, and the dose rate is down to 1 rad/hr. This is important when dealing with search and rescue dogs, especially when using cadaver-locating dogs. If corpses are being searched for by these dogs, there is no reason to search immediately. Increasing the time from release will decrease the radiation that the WA and handler will encounter.

7.2.   Possible Methods of Radioactive Release

7.2.1.   *Nuclear weapons* are a possibility when dealing with terrorism but not a probability. The chance that terrorist organizations have the components to make a nuclear bomb is still rather small. The WA would probably not be used initially after a blast due to the large amount of radiation that would be present. A nuclear blast is due to a fission reaction, which is much more deadly than some of the more likely scenarios. The one area that is a possibility is in the area of suitcase bombs. These are smaller nuclear devices that can still cause nuclear explosions. Russia may have constructed many of these in the past, and due to that country's lack of security, some suitcase bombs have ended up missing. Some say as many as 84 of these bombs were unaccounted for in 1997. A suitcase bomb can have the equivalent of a 1-kiloton bomb.

7.2.2.   A *dirty bomb, or RDD (radiological dispersal device)*, is a much more likely scenario when dealing with terrorism. A dirty bomb is composed of conventional explosives and has radioactive material added. Depending on the type of radiation used, the conventional explosives will probably be the most deadly component. The public perception of a dirty bomb and their misconceptions about the "radiation" involved may lead to more terror and panic. This is a reason that a dirty bomb has been called a "weapon of mass disruption." The actual radiation dispersal from a dirty bomb may not be great depending on the isotope used. The radioactive agents can either be high-level radiation or low-level radiation. High-level radiation involves actual fission byproducts from a nuclear facility or blast, making it harder for a terrorist to obtain. Low-level radiation is much more likely and includes industrial and medical radiation or waste. These would be much easier to obtain. WAs could have been exposed to radiation after a blast that was considered conventional, when in reality it was a dirty bomb.

7.2.3. *Dispersal of radiation without explosives* is the last scenario. This could occur if a radioactive substance is left in the open and contaminates people or animals in the vicinity.

7.3. Possible radioactive agents: There are many possible radioactive substances that may be encountered. The following are some of the more common, and one should be familiar with some of their basic characteristics.

7.3.1. *Americium (Am):* Americium is not a naturally occurring substance. Instead, it is a manmade metal produced from plutonium. The isotope has uses in industry and medicine and is called americium-241 or Am-241. The most common place that Am-241 is found is in household smoke detectors. Am-241 is an alpha emitter with some weak gamma waves. Our main concern with this in our WA is with ingestion or inhalation. Once Am-241 is in the body, it concentrates in the bone, liver, and muscles. If Am-241 is inhaled, it will be retained in the lung tissue. It has a half-life (t½) of 432 years; therefore, it is very slow to clear. Lung and bone cancers are a concern with Am-241. It is excreted in the urine and feces, so monitoring the waste of the WA will need to be done safely.

7.3.2. *Cesium (Cs)* is a naturally occurring element found in rock and granite. The radioactive form of cesium is cesium-137, or Cs-137. It is formed by the fission of uranium and is used commercially to calibrate radiation detection equipment, used medically as a cancer treatment, and used in industry to detect flow rates of some liquids. When Cs-137 decays, it gives off beta particles and gamma rays. It is one of the more serious gamma ray emitters. Because of the beta particles emitted, the WAs and the handlers will have to be monitored for beta burns and for internal organ and tissue damage due to the gamma rays. Cs-137 was one of the major isotopes found in the 1986 Chernobyl nuclear plant accident. Through ingestion or inhalation, Cs tends to localize in muscle. It may also concentrate in milk. The t½ of Cs-137 is around 30 years, and most of the elimination from the body is via the kidneys. A small amount will pass in the feces. In animal testing, it was noted that behavioral changes occurred at higher doses. This could make handling these animals fairly dangerous, and the emergency responders and handlers should watch for these behavioral changes.

7.3.3. *Cobalt (Co)* occurs naturally in many metals and has been used as a blue coloring in glass and pottery. Radioactive cobalt, or Co-60, is used medically as a cancer therapy and is used commercially in plastic manufacturing and food sterilization. Co-60 is another isotope that gives off beta particles and is a strong gamma wave emitter. Observing for beta burns and organ damage will be a necessity. Inhalation causes extensive lung damage and ingestion leads to concentration in the kidneys, heart, liver, bone, and blood. High doses of Co-60 have also shown behavioral changes in animals so care needs to be taken when decontaminating and treating these animals. The t½ of Co-60 is 5.27 years and, if ingested in a large amount, is found in the feces. Longer-term elimination is through the kidneys.

7.3.4. *Iodine (I):* The radioactive form of iodine is I-131. It is formed from uranium and plutonium, and its biggest use is in medicine. Iodine is taken up in the thyroid gland of humans and animals. I-131 is used in the treatment of thyroid disorders and tumors. Too much I-131 has adverse effects on the thyroid gland and actually causes tumors and/or complete damage of the gland. I-131 gives off beta particles and gamma rays; therefore, burns and organ damage are a possibility if the dose is high enough. From an external source, it can also damage the eyes. One of the few treatments for radioactive exposure works against I-131 if instituted early. It is potassium iodide (KI), which will compete with the I-131 for thyroid uptake. Many emergency preparedness kits have potassium iodide included even though the only radiation that it works against is I-131. It must be given prior to exposure or immediately after to have any effect. The t½ of I-131 is rather short, being only around 8 days. I-131 will concentrate to some extent in milk; therefore, any dairy operations close to a release will have to be monitored closely. Vegetative plants will also take up the iodine and may then be consumed by the animals.

7.3.5. *Plutonium (Pu):* Plutonium is listed here due to its familiarity with the public but is probably farther down the list as a possibility in a dirty bomb. Plutonium is used almost exclusively in nuclear facilities and would be fairly hard to obtain for a terrorist. It is produced by a fission reaction and is a byproduct in weapon production and in nuclear power plants. The isotope of concern is plutonium-239 (Pu-239) and has a t½ of 24,000 years. Plutonium is an alpha emitter, which means the main mode of contamination is through inhalation. Unlike most of the other alpha emitters, ingestion is a concern but not a major one. It is not absorbed well from the gastrointestinal tract. It passes out of the feces rather quickly. Once inhaled, it can cause major problems in the lungs, and once in the bloodstream it concentrates in the kidneys, liver, spleen, and especially in bone. Once the Pu-239 breaks down, it will form other isotopes that give off beta particles and gamma rays. Any WAs that have had plutonium exposure must be handled with the idea that beta particles and gamma waves may be given off, even though the initial particle is an alpha. Pu-239 is excreted by the kidneys so it will be present in urine. Due to the long t½, the radioactivity will be present and shed from the tissues for a long period of time.

7.3.6. *Strontium (Sr):* Strontium-90 is the most radioactive isotope of strontium. It is actually a waste product from fission reactions. A medical isotope of strontium is Sr-89, which is used as pain relief in certain bone cancers. Sr-90 gives off heat when decaying and is also used as a power source in space vehicles. It is a beta emitter; therefore, WAs and handlers need to be monitored for burns. The t½ of Sr-90 is 29 years and always gives off Yttrium during decay. Strontium behaves in the body much like calcium and accumulates in bone and teeth, thereby increasing the likelihood of bone cancers. Sr-90 is excreted in the urine for long periods and in the feces for the first few days.

7.3.7. *Uranium (U):* Uranium has three major isotopes of concern: U-234, U-235, and U-238. U-235 is the enriched or concentrated form. The t½ of all three is extremely long. The t½ of U-234 is 244,000 years, U-235 is 710 million years, and U-238 is 4.5 billion years. U-234 and U-235 are the more radioactive isotopes and are formed through enrichment of U-238. U-235 is the most talked about isotope, when dealing with nuclear reactors and power sources. Uranium is also is used in armor-piercing shells due to its extremely hard structure. It is 65% more dense than lead. Once again, emergency responders will probably not be confronted with a uranium release due to the difficulty in obtaining enriched uranium. Uranium is an alpha emitter, as is Thorium, which is a byproduct; therefore, ingestion and inhalation are the major concerns. Ingestion causes bone, liver, and kidney damage, whereas inhalation can cause lung cancers. Uranium is also considered a toxic chemical, meaning that acute kidney failure can occur well before any cancers will form.

7.4. Radioactivity Detection Devices

7.4.1. Many devices are on the market, with the most common being the Geiger-Mueller counter. Most emergency medical services (EMS)/hazmat responders have this available. Some Geiger-Mueller counters are not very specific for alpha and some beta radiations. Special "pancake" detectors are used to give a more accurate reading. Personnel can and should use dosimeters. These can be direct reading dosimeters, self-reading dosimeters, film badge dosimeters, or, more uncommonly, thermoluminescent dosimeters. Whichever dosimeter is used, it should be evaluated after each exposure or shift done by the responder. It would be a good idea to have a dosimeter attached to the WA in addition to the handler. The readings may be more accurate in the WA due to their possibly closer proximity to the radiation in search-and-rescue operations.

7.5. Acute and Chronic Medical Problems Due to Radiation

The problems seen from radiation exposure in the WA will correlate closely with human signs and symptoms. The following effects deal with human exposure but are extrapolated to the animal population.

7.5.1. Acute radiation syndrome (ARS) (Table 7.1).

Table 7.1. Triage of Animals Based on Radiation Dosage.

Injury Without Radiation	Injury With Radiation		
	<150 rad	150–450 rad	450–1000 rad
Dead, dying, euthanasia	Dead, dying, euthanasia		
Immediate	Immediate		Euthanasia
Urgent	Urgent	Variable	Euthanasia
Minor	Minor	Follow ARS management guidelines	Euthanasia
Absent	Ambulatory monitoring	Ambulatory monitoring with routine care. Hospitalization as needed in mass casualty setting but indicated in non–mass casualty setting	Euthanasia

I. The following need to occur:

   A. The radiation dose must be high, usually exceeding 70 rad. Milder symptoms can occur at doses of 30 rad.

   B. The source is usually external and not deposited in the body. The opposite can occur but only rarely.

   C. The radiation must be penetrating, meaning gamma rays and, more unlikely, x-rays and neutrons. For the WA in an emergency setting, gamma rays would be the most likely.

   D. A large portion or area of the body will need to receive the dose. Localized exposures rarely cause ARS.

   E. The dose is usually delivered over a short period of time.

II. ARSs are as follows:

   A. The *hematopoetic syndrome* usually occurs with a dose between 70 and 1000 rad, but milder signs occur at as low as 30 rad. The survival rate decreases with increases in radiation, and the usual cause of death is bone marrow suppression.

   B. The *gastrointestinal syndrome* is the next in progression. The signs of the bone marrow suppression occur in addition to irreversible damage to the gastrointestinal tract. The usual dose range is between 1000 and 10,000 rad. Survival in this syndrome is unlikely in humans or animals. If this type of dose were to occur to any WA, euthanasia would probably be opted for. Death usually occurs within 2 weeks.

   C. The *central nervous syndrome* is the last syndrome. This requires a dose greater than 5000 rad and is always fatal. Death in humans usually occurs within 3 days.

III. *Four stages of ARS:* It is assumed that the WA will go through similar stages. Depending on the extent, the syndrome, and the treatment capabilities, humane euthanasia may be the most viable option.

A. *Prodromal stage* consists of nausea, vomiting, and occasional diarrhea. If the vomiting occurs less than 4 hours after exposure, the prognosis is much poorer than after 4 hours.

B. *Latent stage* is the next stage. In this stage, the patient will feel more normal and look better clinically. This can last from hours to weeks.

C. *Illness stage* is the third stage. This is where the signs can become more severe and the patient feels much worse. The signs can last up to several months.

D. *Recovery* or *death stage* is last. This will occur from weeks up to 2 years.

IV. Average amounts of acute radiation and their mortalities are as follows:

A. <200 rad—Can be lethal to small numbers.

B. 350 rad—5% die within one month without treatment.

C. 450 rad—Half of those exposed will die without treatment.

D. 650 rad—Most die even with treatment.

E. >1000 rad—Central nervous system death within 3 days. No survival.

V. A *cutaneous syndrome* does occur with exposure to the skin. Beta radiation is most often implicated, but x-rays and gamma rays can also damage the skin. Localized inflammation, erythema, and hair follicle damage can occur. The lesser-haired areas in the WA are more likely to sustain this damage. Pay particular attention to the face, muzzle, eyes, ventral abdomen, feet, and pinna of the ears. Most of these lesions will heal but may lack hair follicles or the affected areas may become necrotic.

VI. Chronic exposures and their sequelae are less well understood. A chronic radiation syndrome has been described in Russia involving humans. This would be unlikely in our WA due to not being in the radioactive zone for long periods of time. Cataract formation and tumor formation are the two most likely problems. Behavioral changes, gastrointestrinal changes, leukopenias, and anemias can occur.

7.5.2. Management of working animals in a radiological emergency.

I. The first thing that should be done by the responders is in the area of *personal protection*. Setting up *upwind and uphill* is crucial. A mask with a full face and HEPA filter or fit-tested respirators should be used as a minimum for respiratory protection. Disposable polyethylene suits with foot protection and multilayer rubber gloves should also be used. These guidelines may be altered slightly depending on other possible hazards such as chemicals or fire. The protection listed is effective for alpha and beta particles but not gamma waves. It is imperative to obtain information about the type of release that is being responded to and the isotopes involved. Remember time/distance/shielding. Also remember the 7/10 rule. Some controversy exists when dealing with radiation exposure and injuries. One school of thought says to treat the wounded and then decontaminate. The other school of thought says to decontaminate and then treat. For our purposes, we will be decontaminating our service animals and then treating. Due to the possibility of cross-contamination and the safety of the handlers and responders, we cannot afford to treat first and then decontaminate.

II. *Decontamination*

A. Radiological contamination of the WA will most likely occur as a result of radioactive dust particles on the hair coat. The removal of these contaminants is very important in avoiding inhalation or ingestion after the fact.

The primary goals in regards to radiological decontamination are the removal of the contaminants and to screen the WA prior to leaving the decontamination containment (warm zone). Radiation levels should be within an acceptable range based upon the standards established by standard operating procedures, OSHA, and the Federal Emergency Management Agency (FEMA).

    1.   Keep in mind that alpha radiation can easily be masked by water. Be sure to thoroughly clean and rinse the WA prior to release.

B.   We will set up very similar decontamination stations for the WA as has been done with human patients. Remove and bag any contaminated collars, leashes, and muzzles while in the exclusion zone (hot zone). Most of these animals are well trained and will be able to be sent through decontamination tents, especially if their handlers are with them. The handlers can be decontaminated at the same time. An exception to this type of decontamination will be in the area of the equine patients. These animals may have to be run through portable stalls and manually decontaminated. Mild tranquilization may be needed due to the horses spooking when they see the Level A/B/C suits. Most of the particulate radiation will be in the hair coats; therefore, complete bathing and rinsing will need to be done in an expedient but thorough manner. The thicker hair coat will require more cycles and time than our human counterparts, and monitoring will have to be done before calling them clean. Have clean leashes, collars, and muzzles available. Be sure to prepare for repeat decontamination if needed. Remember that these animals will want to lick their hair, especially when wet, so open-ended fairly loose muzzles should be applied. A fairly loose muzzle will be desirable in a nonfractious patient in case vomiting was to occur from exposure. The muzzles will also help eliminate any possible danger to the personnel in case of any possible behavioral changes in a normally nonfractious animal. Mild sedation may be a benefit for the safety of the handler, the emergency personnel, and the animal. Washing with soap and water will suffice since soap emulsifies and dissolves the contamination. Dry decontamination is also a possibility. Vacuuming the hair coat with HEPA-filtered vacuums can be done prior to wet decontamination if vacuums are available. Do not use vacuums if not filtered. The hair can be shaved and bagged but time restraints will prohibit this technique. Eye flushing should occur to remove any particles from the conjunctiva. Flush medial to lateral and use saline or water. Ointments are not recommended due to the possibility of trapping any unflushed contamination. Decontaminate any wounds first and cover when decontaminating the uninjured areas. If abrasions are present, gentle washing will suffice. If punctures or lacerations are present, sedation may be needed for debridement. If radioactive pieces are inside any wounds, remove and place in lead containers or remove from the direct vicinity of the decontamination station. If any questions arise that more expert help is needed, call Radiation Emergency Assistance Center/Training Site (REAC/TS) at 865-576-3131 or 865-576-1005.

III.   *Treatment options:* The medical treatments of the WA will be dependent on availability of medications. Unfortunately, in a mass casualty situation, the availability of these drugs will probably be funneled to the human victims and supportive care will be our method of therapy. Never forget the ABCs when dealing with trauma. A savable contaminated patient needs to have life-threatening injuries addressed after decontamination but before any other supportive care to combat the effects of radiation. Fluids will be used in these patients due to possible shock and dehydration from their search-and-rescue work. The fluids will also enhance urinary output and quicker removal of internal contamination. After the initial emergency care consider the following:

A. *Potassium iodide* can be used if exposed to radioactive iodine (I-131). This is one of the medications that may be in short supply due to human use. KI does nothing for any isotope other than I-131. It competitively binds to thyroid tissue so the I-131 cannot bind to the thyroid. It must be used immediately after exposure or prior to any exposure to be effective. It may have some effects up to 3–4 hours post exposure but probably has minimal effects after that time. Remember, it is only salvaging the thyroid and other problems from I-131 need to be addressed from the beta and gamma effects. The human adult dose is a 130-mg tablet and will probably be used at this level for the larger dogs. A one-time dose is usually sufficient, and allergic reactions are a possibility.

B. *Prussian Blue* is another drug that can theoretically be used but once again may be in short supply. It is used in Cesium and Thallium exposures. It must be taken under the guidelines of REAC/TS. It is used for internal contamination from either ingestion or inhalation. It will help speed up the removal of Cesium or Thallium from the body. It traps the Cesium in the intestine and cuts down on the biological t½. It is a rather safe drug, and human dosages are 500-mg capsules given 3–4 times per day up to 180 days.

C. *Calcium or zinc diethylenetriamine (Ca-DTPA or Zn-DTPA)* is a chelating agent that is being used experimentally for Plutonium and Americium contamination. Other agents that may be treated are Yttrium, Curium, and Californium. Its lack of availability will limit its use in WAs. Ca-EDTA has also been used experimentally and may be more readily available to the veterinarian responders.

D. *Aluminum phosphate or barium sulfate* can be readily obtained to help in the elimination of Strontium.

E. *Emetics* can be used if ingestion is a possibility. Hydrogen peroxide at 2 ml/kg (not to exceed 45 ml/dose) can be used. Apomorphine at 0.04 mg/kg SQ, IV, or in the conjunctival sulcus can be used if available.

F. *Gastric lavage* can be done if ingestion is known. It will need to be done within 1–2 hours post ingestion and will probably have to be done under anesthesia.

G. *Activated charcoal* may have some benefits if ingestion has occurred. A dose of 1–3 g/kg may help bind some of the isotopes and expedite removal.

H. *High-fiber materials* may also be of some benefit. Oral Metamucil, canned pumpkin, or high-fiber foods such as Hill's R/D or W/D may be effective.

I. *Docusate sodium (DSS) enemas* can be used to help with colon evacuation. Most of the isotopes will pass in the feces, so this will help decrease the exposure time.

7.5.3. Remember that **personal protective equipment should be used when treating these animals.** Urine and feces should be monitored if possible and strict quarantines should be practiced. Expedient treatments should occur due to the time exposure of the veterinarian or technician. Feces and urine should be collected and disposed of following recommended guidelines depending upon the isotope involved. Nasal swabs can be done to help determine inhalation exposure, although a negative swab does not rule out inhalation contamination.

7.5.4. Dead or euthanatized animals

I. Minimal exposure possibilities exist if protective clothing and masks are used. External contamination should still be decontaminated as normal. Even though it has not been shown on the human side that autopsies of deceased patients carry a great risk to the coroner, necropsies of these animals are not recommended by the author. Large lead-lined boxes are not needed for burial, but care should be taken to bury in nonporous soil away from any water supplies. In the event of a mass casualty event, the EPA will set up guidelines for the burial of humans and the animal caretakers should follow the same protocols. Gamma rays do not cause a person or animal to become radioactive; therefore handling these bodies is not a major concern if only gamma rays were present.

Suggested Websites

http://www.acr.org/dyna/?doc=departments/educ/disaster_prep/disaster_planning.html
http://www.afrri.usuhs.mil/
http://www.atsdr.cdc.gov
http://www.bt.cdc.gov/radiation
http://www.epa.gov
http://www.nrc.gov
http://www.ocrwm.doe.gov
http://www.orau.gov/reacts/guidesitemap.htm

CHAPTER 8
BIOLOGICAL AGENTS AS WEAPONS OF MASS DESTRUCTION

Sherrie L. Nash, MS, DVM

Biological warfare can be defined as the use of microorganisms or toxins derived from living organisms to induce death or disease in humans, animals, or plants. Animal disease agents have long been used as biological warfare agents. As far back as the 14th century, armies catapulted plague-infected corpses over their enemy's city walls. In 1984, members of a cult in Oregon spread *Salmonella* over salad bars of four restaurants, causing illness in 700 people, all to influence an election. Most recently, anthrax was used as a terrorist agent, killing 5 people and causing illness in 22 in the United States.

Covert biological attack will not produce immediate casualties. Animals may serve as sentinels in the event of a bioterrorism incident and veterinarians may diagnose the disease first. Economic targets such as livestock, crops, tourism, and transportation are likely to become terrorist choices. Even small outbreaks of exotic disease in livestock or crops could remove the United States from the large world market of agricultural products, which we have enjoyed for so long. On the other hand, working animals (WAs) exposed to biological agents provide the potential for that WA to serve as a vector and spread contamination to other areas and humans.

Most of the bacteria, viruses, rickettsiae, and toxins involve agents that are zoonotic (Fig. 8.1). Each of the zoonotic agents is addressed here. Additionally, other species have been added to the discussion since it is possible a biological attack may be seen first in domestic and/or wild animals. One will quickly note that there are species differences in susceptibility to the various agents and there are certainly differences in presentations in regard to signs seen in humans. For example, dogs are naturally resistant to anthrax. All natural anthrax reports in dogs have been from the ingestion of contaminated meat and resulted in gastrointestinal disease. Prognosis was excellent when these dogs were treated with penicillin drugs. Experimental inhalant anthrax infections in dogs (at dosages 125 times what would make a human ill!) were very mild and manifested solely as mild or transient fever. The exposed dogs were not clinically sick. There are no reports of dogs developing the cutaneous form of anthrax. In general, dogs as a species, are resistant to infection with agents of significant biowarfare interest. Therefore, bioterrorism diseases are likely to be selected for efficacy against human personnel and not companion animals.

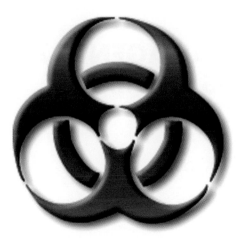

Figure 8.1. Biohazard placard indicating the presence of biological agents, some of which may be zoonotic.

8. Biological Agents as Weapons of Mass Destruction

8.1. Bacteria

Bacteria are single-celled, microscopic organisms. Bacteria may be beneficial to animals and humans, such as when they make up the normal flora of the intestinal tract. They may also cause disease in some animals, many animals, and/or humans. Many of the bacteria that infect animals will also infect humans are therefore zoonotic.

8.1.1. Anthrax (woolsorter's disease, malignant pustule, charbon, malignant carbuncle, splenic fever, Siberian ulcer, Milzbrand)
   I.   Centers for Disease Control and Prevention (CDC) category A; OIE List B Disease
   II.   *Agent: Bacillus anthracis* (Fig. 8.2). Anthrax forms a protective spore under adverse environmental conditions or when exposed to air. Once the conditions improve for the bacteria, the spores germinate to produce the vegetative form. These spores are exceedingly hardy and survive extremes in temperature, dryness, and moisture making eradication nearly impossible. Domestic and wild ruminants are the most frequent source of anthrax. It is the first known bacteria to cause disease in animals and humans. Anthrax is a possible weapon of bioterrorism.
   III.   Affected veterinary species (Table 8.1)
   IV.   *Incubation period:* The incubation period is typically 3–7 days, but it may vary from 1 to 20 days. Human incubation period for ingestion is 1–7 days. For the cutaneous form it is almost immediate of up to a day, but may be as long as 12 days. The inhalation form is usually less than 7 days, but may take as long as 2 months.

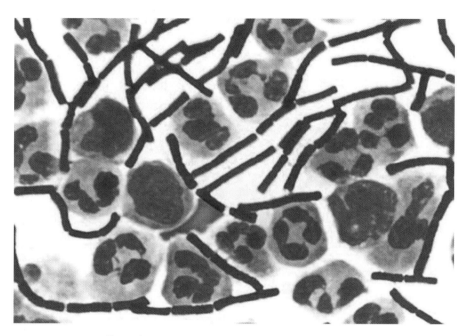

Figure 8.2. *Bacillus anthracis* organisms. (Reprinted with permission from http://commons.wikimedia.org/wiki/Image:Gram_Stain_Anthrax.jpg.)

Table 8.1. Anthrax.

Disease Severity in Potentially Affected Species								
S = Severe D = Moderate M = Mild								
Dogs	**Horses**	**Cattle**	**Sheep**	**Goats**	**Pigs**	**Cats**	**Birds**	**Other Animals**
D	S	S	S	S	D	D	S (raptors)	S Wild herbivores and carnivores; goats, camels, antelope, guinea pigs

V. *Transmission:* Ingestion, cutaneous, or inhalation of anthrax may all be zoonotic.

VI. *Route of transmission:* Spores in contaminated soil are the most frequent source of anthrax in animals. Humans may ingest anthrax through dairy products from infected animals or improperly cooked meat. Humans are primarily exposed through contaminated animal products (wool, meat, hides, furs, bone meal) or open wounds. Biting flies may be another source of anthrax in some areas. Inhalation of spores can also serve as a source of infection in humans (was used to scare the public in the U.S. in 2001).

VII. *Prominent clinical signs:*
A. **Horses:** Illness may be acute with fever and/or chills, colic, septicemia, anorexia, depression, bloody diarrhea, and swelling around the neck, shoulders, and thorax. Death occurs typically in 1–3 days, but some horses will linger for up to 7 days.
B. **Dogs:** Signs include depression, fever, weakness, anorexia, and occasionally death.
C. **Humans:** Symptoms of ingestion of anthrax may include vomiting, nausea, fever, and anorexia. As the disease progresses, there is diarrhea that is usually bloody, extreme abdominal pain, and hematemesis. The inhalation route may have symptoms of a nonproductive cough, low-grade fever, fatigue, myalgia, malaise, sweating, and chest pain without respiratory symptoms. Most humans are exposed by the cutaneous route. There is direct contact with the bacilli or the spores. Initially there is localized itching and a pimple developing into a dry, ulcerated black scab in 48–72 hours. Edema and vesicles appear near the lesion. After about 10 days, the lesion will start to heal and will take 2–6 weeks to completely heal. Although not typical, cutaneous lesions can lead to more severe disease and death if not treated. Severe symptoms of anthrax include prostration, fever, chills, shock, collapse, and death.
D. *Other species:*
Ruminants: Sudden death (peracute) is from septicemia. Trembling and convulsions may be observed prior to death. No signs may be seen except death. Of importance is the lack of rigor mortis and failure of the blood to clot. In acute cases of anthrax, there is rapid onset of fever (107°F) with excitement followed by depression, dyspnea, stupor, convulsions, and death. Blood may be seen emerging from the mouth, nose, and anus. There is edema, especially around the neck, shoulders, and throat. Some of these ruminants may only be found dead or have signs for 2 days before death occurs.

VIII. *Treatment:* Treatment is with antibiotics followed with vaccination 7–10 days afterward.
A. *Penicillin:*
Dogs: Penicillin G potassium: 20,000 units/kg IV, IM, SQ q4h.
Horses: Initially, 22,000 U/kg of aqueous penicillin G (sodium/potassium) IV q6h.
B. *Doxycycline:*
Dogs: 5 mg/kg BID IV or PO.
Horses: NOT recommended for this species.
C. *Ciprofloxacin:*
Dogs: 5–15 mg/kg PO BID.

IX. *Prevention:* Anthrax vaccine (live) is available. To prevent further spread of disease, the recommendations are 1) removal of animals from contaminated areas, 2) quarantine of suspect animals, 3) disposal of dead animals by burning or deep burial, 4) incineration of bedding, manure, or other contaminated materials, 5) disinfection of equipment, instruments, stalls, pens, and barns, 6) reduction of scavengers, 7) maintenance of sanitization of dead animals to decrease exposure to humans, and 8) the use of insecticides.

X. *Decontamination:* Standard decontamination with soap and water should be done. Deep burial or burning of infected carcasses to eliminate the spores. Disposal of bedding, manure, and other contaminated fomites should be done. Formaldehyde 5%–10% is useful in controlling anthrax in the soil. Strong chlorine solutions may be used to destroy the spore.

8.1.2. Brucellosis (contagious abortion, undulant fever, Bang's disease, enzootic abortion, Malta fever, Mediterranean fever)
  I.   CDC category B; OIE List B Disease
  II. *Agents: Brucella abortus, B. ovis, B. suis,* and *B. canis.* These bacteria are responsible for causing serious illness in humans (undulant fever). They can be acquired through drinking raw milk and dairy products. In ruminants, *Brucella* causes abortion and serious economic losses due to treatment not being allowed or practical. Aerosolization of these bacteria may be used as a weapon of bioterrorism.
     A. *Brucella melitensis.* Disease is similar to other *Brucella* species.
  III. Affected veterinary species (Table 8.2)

Table 8.2. Brucellosis.

Disease Severity in Potentially Affected Species
S = Severe   D = Moderate   M = Mild

Brucella abortus, B. ovis, B. suis, B. canis.

Dogs	Horses	Cattle	Sheep	Goats	Pigs	Cats	Birds	Other Animals
D	M	S	S	S	S			S Wild ruminants, buffalo, bison, elk

Brucella melitensis

Dogs	Horses	Cattle	Sheep	Goats	Pigs	Cats	Birds	Other Animals
		M	S	S				Wild ruminants

  IV. *Incubation period:* The incubation period is variable from 5 days to 8 weeks, typically 2 weeks to 5 months in cattle. A variable incubation period of less than 7 days up to several months is seen in humans, but typically it is 2–4 weeks.
  V.   *Transmission:* Direct contact, ingestion, indirect contact, and person-to-person. All routes are zoonotic.
  VI. *Route of transmission:* Animals are exposed through contact with infected animal tissues such as vaginal secretions, placenta, fetal fluids, fetuses, milk, and semen. Fomites that are in high humid environments, no sunlight, or low temperatures are ideal for maintaining *Brucella* for months. This includes contact with feces, equipment, water, clothing, aborted fetuses, feed, and wool. In humans, the usual route is through lesions on the skin and having direct contact with infected animals. Ingestion of unpasteurized milk or dairy products can also occur. Inhalation in the laboratory through aerosolization of *Brucella* has also occurred.

Person-to-person transmission is rare and often associated with importation of contaminated dairy products.

VII. *Prominent clinical signs:*

   A. Horses: There is a suppurative bursitis, also known as poll evil or fistulous withers. This is seen as a thick, straw-colored exudate. The bursa becomes swollen and may burst, leading to inflammation. Abortion is rare in mares.

   B. Dogs: *B. canis* causes infertility, abortion, and stillbirths. Abortion occurs in the last trimester of pregnancy. A vaginal discharge may be prominent for some time after aborting. Male dogs have decreased fertility.

   C. Pigs: Abortion occurs anytime throughout pregnancy. Stillborn or weak new-borns may be seen. Boars will have decreased fertility. Lameness and joint swelling may also occur.

   D. Humans: May display a wide range of symptoms, especially among laboratory workers. Symptoms may include flu-like illness, extended fever, anorexia, malaise, headache, back pain, and sweating (night). More serious or long-lasting symptoms include undulant fever, genitourinary, neurological, chronic fatigue syndrome, arthritis, and depression.

   E. *Other species:*

      1. Cattle: The most frequent signs seen are abortion, stillborn or weak newborns, placentitis, retained placenta, inflammation of the genitals in male animals, arthritis, and lameness. Abortion is most frequent in the second half of pregnancy.

      2. Sheep and Goats: Signs are similar to cattle. Goats may also have mastitis and lameness. Sheep generally do not have arthritis. Abortion occurs late in pregnancy in sheep and during the fourth month of pregnancy in goats. *B. ovis* causes infertility in rams as a result of orchitis and epididymitis.

VIII. *Treatment:* Ruminants should not be treated.

   A. *Doxycycline:*
   Dogs: 5 mg/kg BID IV or PO.
   Horses: NOT recommended for this species.

   B. *Enrofloxacin:*
   Dogs: 5–20 mg/kg PO or IM given BID.
   Horses: 5 mg/kg IV daily.

IX. *Prevention: B. abortus.* A live attenuated vaccine (RB-51) is available for cattle and may have possible use in other ruminants. Identification, quarantine, and slaughter of infected animals are practiced to eradicate the disease. Disinfect areas where infected animals have been. Dogs should not be used for breeding and should be neutered.

X. *Decontamination:* Standard decontamination with soap water. *Brucella* is deactivated by sunlight (requires a few hours) and heat.

8.1.3. Glanders (Farcy, Malleus, Droes)

I. CDC category B; OIE List B Disease

II. *Agent: Burkholderia mallei.* Glanders is a very contagious and often fatal disease in the horse. It is a zoonotic, and it causes painful nodules in humans and can be fatal. Glanders has the potential to be used as a weapon for bioterrorism.

III. Affected veterinary species (Table 8.3)

IV. *Incubation period:* The incubation period is typically 2 weeks, but it may be as long as several months. The incubation period in humans is 1–14 days.

Table 8.3. Glanders.

| Disease Severity in Potentially Affected Species
S = Severe   D = Moderate   M = Mild | | | | | | | | |
Dogs	Horses	Cattle	Sheep	Goats	Pigs	Cats	Birds	Other Animals
M	S			M		D		S Donkeys, mules, camels

V. *Transmission:* Direct contact (zoonotic), indirect contact, or person-to-person.

VI. *Route of transmission:* Direct contact with nasal secretions (ingestion) or the sores (ulcers) on the skin of infected animals. Indirect contact with contaminated water and food (from nasal secretions) is seen. Inhalation of the bacteria is seldom a form of transmission in animals. Carnivorous animals are infected by ingesting infected meat. Humans are infected through contact via the mucous membranes or direct contact with infected animals. Inhalation of infectious aerosols has occurred in laboratory workers. Person-to-person transmission is rare and is thought to occur through family members caring for a patient or via sexual transmission.

VII. *Prominent clinical signs:*

A. **Horses:** Glanders may be either acute (mules and donkeys) or chronic (nasal, pulmonary, and cutaneous forms). Several forms of the disease may be present in an animal at the same time. In the acute form, a high fever (up to 106°F) and septicemia are initially noted. Then, a viscous, mucopurulent discharge from the nose develops and respiratory signs are evident. The nasal form involves the nasal mucosa with the development of nodules that form into deep ulcers. These ulcers leave distinctive star-shaped scars. Nasal secretions are yellowish-green and the submaxillary lymph nodes may be inflamed. The pulmonary form varies from asymptomatic to obvious respiratory signs of coughing and dyspnea. Calcified or caseous nodules develop in the lungs. The cutaneous form is known as "Farcy." Yellowish nodules and ulcers form on the skin, which exude tacky, contagious pus. There is cutaneous lymphatic involvement, especially on the extremities. These lymphatics swell and fill with a purulent exudate (known as "Farcy pipes").

B. **Humans:** Symptoms may be varied, depending on the exposure route. Symptoms include headache, fever, muscle stiffness and pain, and chest pain. In addition, diarrhea, light sensitivity, and increased tear production may be noted. Localized infections occur through skin abrasions or lesions in 1–5 days. Nodules and abscesses are similar to animals. There will be swollen lymph nodes as well as respiratory, ocular and nasal involvement with increased mucus production. Inhaled or pulmonary infection includes pulmonary abscess formation, pneumonia, and pleural effusion. Systemic involvement is fatal within 7–10 days. Chronic infections in humans involve numerous abscesses on the face, arms, legs, nasal mucosa, spleen, or liver. Death occurs in the acute form of the disease in 95% of individuals, in about 3 weeks. If antibiotics are used, survival is greatly improved.

VIII. *Treatment:*
  A. *Tetracycline:*
    Dogs: 10–20 mg/kg PO TID.
    Horses: 5–7.5 mg/kg IV q12h.
IX. *Prevention:* No vaccine is available. Animals need to be identified, quarantined, and humanely euthanized.
X. *Decontamination:* Standard decontamination with soap and water. Most common disinfectants will deactivate the bacteria. Desiccation and sunlight also kills the bacteria. *Burkholderia mallei* thrives in warm, moist environments for several months.

8.1.4. Melioidosis (pseudoglanders, Whitmore disease)

I. CDC category B
II. *Agent: Burkholderia pseudomallei* (formerly *Pseudomonas pseudomallei*). Melioidosis causes abscess formation in the lymph nodes and viscera in a number of animals. It has been called the "mimic" disease because signs of disease can vary. Melioidosis could be used as a weapon for bioterrorism.
III. Affected veterinary species (Table 8.4)

Table 8.4. Melioidosis.

| Disease Severity in Potentially Affected Species S = Severe   D = Moderate   M = Mild | | | | | | | | |
Dogs	Horses	Cattle	Sheep	Goats	Pigs	Cats	Birds	Other Animals
D	D	M	S	S	S	M	D	Rodents, rabbits, zoo animals, fish, nonhuman primates

IV. *Incubation period:* The incubation period is variable and may be longer in pigs. The incubation period in humans is 1–21 days, but it may extend to many years.
V. *Transmission:* Direct contact, inhalation, infected body fluids, wound contamination, ingestion, and person-to-person. Melioidosis is zoonotic.
VI. *Route of transmission:* Direct contact with the bacteria in the surroundings (contaminated water, soil, rodents) is the primary route of exposure. Heavy rain, high humidity, flooding, and high temperatures are ideal for infections as a result of contact with soil. Infected body fluids include milk, urine, and nasal discharges. Melioidosis is much less commonly spread person-to-person.
VII. *Prominent clinical signs:* Signs vary widely with the site of the lesion. There may be suppurative or caseous lesions in the lymph nodes, lungs, and viscera. Fever, nasal discharge, inappetence, gastrointestinal involvement, encephalitis, respiratory signs, or lameness may be seen. The prognosis is grave when there is involvement of a crucial organ and abscess formation is widespread.

A. **Horses:** Predominant clinical signs are neurological, colic, diarrhea, and respiratory.

B. **Humans:** Symptoms may be asymptomatic, localized, systemic, pulmonary, or chronic. Nodules often develop at an exposed skin lesion, and there may be fever, muscle pain, chest pain, cough, pneumonia, septic shock, severe headache, shortness of breath, anorexia, diarrhea, disorientation, numerous abscesses, and skin lesions filled with pus. Chronically, there is skin, lymph node, joint, bone, lung, liver, spleen, brain, or visceral involvement. Compromised individuals are more likely to have systemic infections.

C. *Other species:*

   1. **Cattle:** If signs are seen, there will be pneumonia-like signs or neurological.

   2. **Sheep and Goats:** Pneumonia-like signs, abscess formation in the lungs, nasal discharge, arthritis, encephalitis. Mastitis occurs in goats.

   3. **Pigs:** May have no symptoms or be chronic. They may display inappetence, fever, swollen submandibular lymph nodes, ocular-nasal discharges, and coughing. Reproductive signs of stillbirths, abortion, and orchitis are occasionally seen.

VIII. *Treatment:*

A. *Tetracycline:*

  Dogs: 10–20 mg/kg PO TID.

  Horses: 5–7.5 mg/kg IV q12h.

  Ruminants: Antibiotics have been used, but relapses usually take place when treatment is ended.

IX. *Prevention:* Vaccines are available but not always effective.

X. *Decontamination:* Standard decontamination with soap and water. *B. pseudomallei* is deactivated by heat (moist 250°F at 15 minutes, dry heat 320°–338°F for at least 1 hour). In addition, 70% ethanol, 1% sodium hypochlorite, formaldehyde, and gluataraldehyde may be used to deactivate this organism. *B. pseudomallei* survives in water and soil for months.

8.1.5. Plague (bubonic plague, Black Death, pneumonic plague, pestis minor, septicemic plague, peste, pestis)

I. CDC category A; OIE List B Disease

II. *Agent: Yersinia pestis.* Plague is spread primarily through infected fleas, infected animals, and by aerosol. Plague can be fatal if not recognized early in the course of disease. It has potential as a weapon for bioterrorism.

III. Affected veterinary species (Table 8.5)

Table 8.5. Plague.

Disease Severity in Potentially Affected Species S = Severe D = Moderate M = Mild								
Dogs	Horses	Cattle	Sheep	Goats	Pigs	Cats	Birds	Other Animals
M				M		S Bobcats, mountain lions		S Rodents, rock and ground squirrels, prairie dogs, voles, rabbits

IV. *Incubation period:* The incubation period is variable, typically 1–4 days. Experimentally in cats, 1–2 days. In humans, the incubation is 1–8 days.

V. *Transmission:* Vector, direct contact, aerosol, and person-to-person. Plague is zoonotic (Fig. 8.3).

VI. *Route of transmission:* Fleas feeding on diseased animals are the primary source of infection for animals and humans. Other forms of transmission include contact with tissues from diseased animals, inhalation of infectious aerosols from

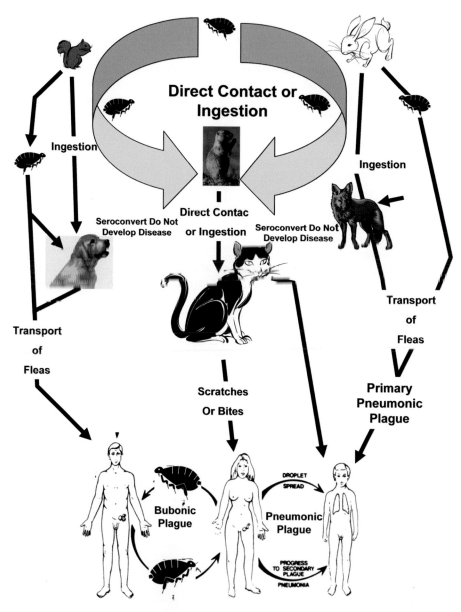

Figure 8.3. Transmission of plague to animals and humans.

either animals or humans, bites from diseased animals, or consumption of diseased rodents (usually animals).

VII.   *Prominent clinical signs:*

 A.   **Dogs:** Generally do not have clinical signs of plague. When they do, lymphadenopathy, depression, coughing, and high fever may be seen.

 B.   **Horses:** Few to no clinical signs.

 C.   **Humans:** Three forms are recognized: bubonic, pneumonic, and septicemic plague.

  1.   *Bubonic:* There is regional lymphadenopathy (bubos), and this form usually involves 80–90% of reported cases. Cervical, axillary, and inguinal lymph nodes are usually involved. There may be draining at the initial site of the infection. Mortality rates may reach 50%–60% in untreated individuals.

  2.   *Pneumonic:* Is the most serious and fatal form of plague; it is not routinely seen. Symptoms include an elevated fever, severe pneumonia, dyspnea, and possibly expectoration of blood. If not treated within 18 hours of respiratory symptoms, fatality is almost certain.

  3.   *Septicemic:* May be seen with the bubonic form or without any lymphadenopathy. In the United States, 50% of individuals with this form died. Only 10% of individuals exposed to plague will present with this form. Death occurs as a result of complications associated with meningitis, consumptive coagulopathy, septic shock, and coma.

 D.   *Other* species:

  1.   **Cats:** The bubonic form is most often seen. Cats will present with a high fever (up to 106°F), extremely swollen lymph nodes ("bubos"), lethargy, dehydration, and anorexia. The lymph nodes may abscess and drain. Other signs include pneumonia, ataxia, sneezing, and hemoptysis. The pneumonic form usually presents as a severe pneumonia with coughing and is associated with the septicemic form in cats. The septicemic form includes fever, lack of appetite, depression, and sepsis (diarrhea, disseminated intravascular coagulopathy, vomiting, and a weak pulse).

  2.   **Cattle and sheep:** Few to no clinical signs.

  3.   **Pigs:** Few to no clinical signs.

VIII.   *Treatment:*

 A.   *Doxycycline:*

  Dogs: 5 mg/kg BID IV or PO.

  Horses: NOT recommended for this species.

 B.   *Enrofloxacin:*

  Dogs: 5–20 mg/kg PO or IM given BID.

  Horses: 5 mg/kg IV daily.

 C.   Cats in general should not be treated because of the high zoonotic risk; also, 50% do not survive infection. If cats are to be treated, use of parenteral antibiotics and strict isolation must be available.

IX.   *Prevention:* There is a vaccine available for at-risk people. Preventative measures should include the use of insecticides on pets, around the house, the premises, and areas known to be infected with plague. Pets should be prevented from roaming and rodent control practiced. Avoid all sick or dead animals, especially in endemic areas. The use of personal protection should be worn when around suspect animals—protective clothing, gloves, mask, and goggles. Deter rodent populations by removing sources of food and water. If an individual is suspected of being exposed to plague, the prophylactic use of antibiotics is recommended.

X. *Decontamination:* Standard decontamination with soap and water. Routine sanitation of equipment, surfaces, and instruments should deactivate these bacteria.

8.1.6. Psittacosis (parrot fever, avian chlamydiosis, ornithosis)

I. CDC category B

II. *Agent: Chlamydophilia psittaci* (formerly *Chlamydia psittaci*). Psittacosis is a contagious disease in birds that ranges from inapparent infection to serious respiratory, septicemic, and gastrointestinal signs. It is zoonotic and can be fatal to humans.

III. Affected veterinary species (Table 8.6)

Table 8.6. Psittacosis.

| Disease Severity in Potentially Affected Species S = Severe   D = Moderate   M = Mild | | | | | | | | |
Dogs	Horses	Cattle	Sheep	Goats	Pigs	Cats	Birds	Other Animals
							M	Parakeets, parrots, love birds, doves, mynah birds, pigeons

IV. *Incubation period:* The incubation period is 3–10 days, up to several weeks. In humans, the incubation period ranges from 4 to 15 days, but it is typically 10 days.

V. *Transmission:* Inhalation, indirect contact, ingestion, and person-to-person (rare). Psittacosis is zoonotic.

VI. *Route of transmission:* Inhalation of dust from infected bird dander, droppings, or secretions is very common. Respiratory secretions and feces contain elementary bodies that remain infective for months and are resistant to desiccation. Mechanical transfer of infection occurs by mites, biting insects, and lice. Ingestion of infected feed is sometimes a source of disease. It is important to note that some birds are asymptomatic carriers. Humans are most often infected by inhalation or contact with infected birds. Person-to-person transmission is thought to be rare, must have an acute infection, and only when forcefully coughing directly into another individual's face.

VII. *Prominent clinical signs:*

  A. Humans: Symptoms may be mild to severe. Humans may display flu-like symptoms which include headache, fever, chills, sore throat, fatigue, nausea, and lack of appetite. Photophobia, sweating, vomiting, diarrhea, and respiratory symptoms (psittacosis) also occur. More severe symptoms of disease are comprised of dyspnea, pneumonia, cough, myocarditis, meningitis, reproductive problems, renal problems, endocarditis, encephalitis, and myelitis. Death may occur if left untreated.

   B.   *Other species:*
       1.   **Birds**: The vulnerability of a bird and potency of the bacterial strain determine the seriousness of the disease. Pigeons, turkeys, and ducks may display sinusitis, conjunctivitis, ocular and nasal secretions, respiratory difficulty, yellow-green or green diarrhea, depression, fever, ruffled feathers, weight loss, and anorexia. There may be a drop in egg production. Pigeons may appear temporarily ataxic, while ducks tend to have an abnormal gait or may shake. Pet birds display similar signs, but there is also sinusitis, yellow diarrhea, and nervous signs. Some birds may be asymptomatic for psittacosis.

VIII.   *Treatment:* Not an important health hazard to the dog or horse.

IX.   *Prevention:* No vaccine available. Quarantine of all infectious birds until treatment is complete. Individuals working with suspect or infected birds should wear protective clothing, gloves, masks, and goggles. Premises should be routinely cleaned and disinfected to minimize feathers and dust. Dead birds should be wetted down with disinfectants or detergents to reduce dust and feather release. Necropsied birds should also be wetted down with detergents or disinfectants.

X.   *Decontamination:* Standard decontamination with soap and water. The use of 1:100 sodium hypochlorite, formaldehyde, 80% isopropyl alcohol, chlorophenols, quaternary ammonium compounds, or iodophore disinfectants is effective for deactivating *C. psittaci.*

8.1.7.   Tuberculosis (TB)

I.   CDC category B; OIE List B Disease

II.   *Agents: Mycobacterium bovis* (cattle), *M. tuberculosis* (human), and *M. avium* (birds). *Mycobacterium* species cause contagious disease in nearly all animals and humans. Most often TB is a debilitating, chronic disease.

III.   *Affected veterinary species:* Primary reservoirs are cattle and humans. Other known reservoirs for TB include bison (and related species), antelope (and related species), red deer, white-tailed deer, mule deer, elk, pigs (and related species), raccoons, ferrets, rats, badgers, opossums, ferrets, Kudu, and llamas (Table 8.7).

Table 8.7.   Tuberculosis.

Disease Severity in Potentially Affected Species S = Severe = Moderate M = Mild								
Mycobacterium tuberculosis								
Dogs	**Horses**	**Cattle**	**Sheep**	**Goats**	**Pigs**	**Cats**	**Birds**	**Other Animals**
D	M				M		M	Non-human primates

Table 8.7. *Continued.*

Mycobacterium bovis

Dogs	Horses	Cattle	Sheep	Goats	Pigs	Cats	Birds	Other Animals
D	M	S	M	M	S	M		Non-human primates, Hoofed animals, deer, elk, elephants, kudu, camels, rhinoceri, oryx, bison

Mycobacterium avium

Dogs	Horses	Cattle	Sheep	Goats	Pigs	Cats	Birds	Other Animals
D	M	S	M		M	M	S	S Non-human primates deer, mink, some cold-blooded animals

IV. *Incubation period:* The incubation period is variable and it may be chronic. In humans, the incubation period is about 15–28 weeks.

V. *Transmission:* Aerosolization, person-to-person, and ingestion. TB is zoonotic.

VI. *Route of transmission:* TB is spread primarily through the respiratory system. Any tissue in the body can be affected, but most often the lungs, lymph nodes, spleen, liver, and intestines are involved. Large numbers of bacteria are released through coughing and picked up by inhalation of the bacteria. Contact with contaminated feed, water, feces, dust, and dried secretions from infected animals can cause disease. Infected milk can also serve as a source of infection.

VII. *Prominent clinical signs:* TB may not be easily identified until it is in the classic advanced case.

   A. **Dogs:** Develop tubercles in the lungs, kidney, peritoneum, liver, and pleura. The nodules are gray, have a necrotic center, and generally are not calcified. A large amount of a straw colored fluid may be found in the thorax.

   B. **Horses:** Generally resistant to TB. When infected, lesions are found in the lungs, liver, mesenteric lymph nodes, and other regions.

   C. **Humans:** TB in humans is seen as pneumonia or lung infection. Immunocompromised individuals are more likely to have more complications of TB. Seldom is there involvement of organs such as the intestines, bones, brain, or kidneys.

D. *Other species:*
1. **Cats:** Consumption of infected milk produced gastrointestinal tract lesions, followed quickly by dissemination to other organs.
2. **Cattle:** Some animals may display only vague to a few signs of disease. Coughing and pneumonia are seen early and as the disease progresses, lymph nodes become swollen (nodular granulomas known as tubercles). Swellings are present on the body, especially around the neck and head. Infrequently, the lymph nodes may break open and drain. Signs of intestinal involvement of TB include diarrhea and constipation, intermittently. In the end stages of disease, dyspnea and weight loss occur. Female genitalia may often be involved, but rarely is the male genitalia involved.
3. **Birds:** Emaciation, lameness, diarrhea, pale skin (face, comb, and wattles), and listlessness are seen in the late stages of the disease. Nodules (yellow to gray) are found along the intestines, spleen, liver, and bone marrow. Multiple organs are involved in advanced illness. In general, the lungs remain unaffected or have limited lesions.
4. **Pigs:** Generally have gastrointestinal tract lymph node involvement.

VIII. *Treatment:*
Dogs and Horses: Treatment not recommended. For the most part, treatment of animals is not recommended because of the potential for drug resistance and human exposure to the disease during the treatment process. Subhuman primates have had some success with medications used in humans.

IX. *Prevention:* Testing and eradication are used to control and eliminate *Mycobacterium* spp. Routine cleaning and disinfection of contaminated premises are recommended. Maintaining good sanitation practices is essential to preventing disease. In addition, routine testing to monitor the status of TB in a herd or flock is advised.

X. *Decontamination:* Thorough, routine cleaning and disinfecting of equipment, troughs, and feeders is recommended. *Mycobacterium* is very resistant to moisture, desiccation, cold, heat, many disinfectants, and changes in pH. It remains stable in soil for months.

8.1.8. Tularemia (rabbit fever, Francis disease, Ohara disease, deer-fly disease)
I. CDC category A; OIE List B Disease
II. *Agent: Franciscella tularensis.* Tularemia is a contagious disease of rabbits and humans. Tularemia could be used as a weapon for bioterrorism (aerosol).
III. Affected veterinary species (Table 8.8)

Table 8.8. Tularemia.

| Disease Severity in Potentially Affected Species S = Severe   D = Moderate   M = Mild | | | | | | | | |
Dogs	Horses	Cattle	Sheep	Goats	Pigs	Cats	Birds	Other Animals
M	D		S		M	S		Rabbits, hares, rodents, aquatic animals, beavers

IV. *Incubation period:* The incubation period is 1–14 days in animals and typically 3–5 days (up to 14 days) in humans.

V. *Transmission:* Arthropod vector, aerosol, ingestion, and direct contact (zoonotic).

VI. *Route of transmission:* Transmission is mainly through arthropods (ticks infective for longer than 2 years, deerflies, other biting flies [flies for 14 days], and mosquitoes). Inhalation of tularemia, eating improperly cooked meat, handling infected animal tissue, or drinking water are other sources for this disease.

VII. *Prominent clinical signs:* Sudden high fever with lethargy, septicemia, stiffness, anorexia, coughing, and diarrhea. Prostration and death occur within hours to days.

  A. **Humans:** Symptoms include sudden fever, chills, muscle pain, headache, dry cough, painful joints, weakness, and diarrhea. Additional symptoms that may be seen include sore throat, mouth ulcers, skin ulcers, painful, enlarged lymph nodes, and painful, swollen eyes.

VIII. Treatment:

  A. *Doxycycline:*

    Dogs: 5 mg/kg BID IV or PO.

    Horses: NOT recommended for this species.

  B. *Enrofloxacin:*

    Dogs: 5–20 mg/kg PO or IM given BID.

    Horses: 5 mg/kg IV daily

IX. *Prevention:* Use of insecticides to decrease exposure to biting insects. Humans should wear a protective clothing, mask, gloves, and goggles when handling potentially infected animals. All foods should be properly cooked to destroy the organism. Drink only from safe sources of water. Frequent hand washing should be done when handling animal carcasses. A live attenuated vaccine is being reviewed by the FDA.

X. *Decontamination:* Standard decontamination with soap and water. Most common disinfectants are effective on tularemia.

8.2. Rickettsiae

The Rickettsiae are intracellular, parasitic microorganisms that are considered intermediate in size between bacteria and viruses. They resemble bacteria in shape and viruses due to their strict growth requirements for living host cells. Most Rickettsiae are parasites of animals and arthropods. They are transmitted to man and other animals by vectors (ticks, fleas, lice, and mites). Rickettsiae are usually easily deactivated by heat, dehydration, or disinfectants.

8.2.1. Query (Q) Fever

I. CDC category B; OIE List B Disease

II. *Agent: Coxiella burnetii.* Q-fever is a highly contagious zoonotic disease that can cause flu-like signs to chronic endocarditis in humans. Q-fever could be used as a weapon for bioterrorism.

III. *Affected veterinary species:* Goats, cattle, and sheep are the main reservoirs for Q-fever (Table 8.9).

IV. *Incubation period:* The incubation period is variable at 1–3 weeks. In humans, the incubation period also varies but is generally 2–3 weeks.

Table 8.9. Query (Q) fever.

Disease Severity in Potentially Affected Species								
S = Severe D = Moderate M = Mild E = Experimental								
Dogs	**Horses**	**Cattle**	**Sheep**	**Goats**	**Pigs**	**Cats**	**Birds**	**Other Animals**
M	M	M	M	M	M	E	M Fowl, geese, pigeons	M Rodents, rabbits, buffalo, camels

V. *Transmission:* Vector, aerosol, ingestion, person-to-person (rare), or direct contact (zoonotic).

VI. *Route of transmission:* Q-fever can be passed on to ruminants by ticks and occasionally to humans. It is highly communicable by aerosol, capable of traveling over a half mile, and is very resilient to the environment. A single viable organism is enough to cause infection in humans. Raw milk from infected animals can cause disease, as well as ingestion of the placenta and reproductive fluids. Q-fever is commonly transmitted in dust from premises contaminated by placental tissues, birth fluids, and excreta of infected animals.

VII. *Prominent clinical signs:* Typically asymptomatic in most animals. Fever and pneumonia may also be present.

  A. **Dogs:** Usually asymptomatic, but may see abortions.

  B. **Humans:** Usually it is sudden onset and includes flu-like symptoms of headache, fever (104°–105°F), chills, sore throat, malaise, nausea, vomiting, diarrhea, and myalgia. Confusion, chest pain, and abdominal pain are also noted. There may be a fever for 7–14 days, loss of weight, pneumonia, and hepatitis. In chronic infections endocarditis occurs. Humans are very susceptible to inhalation of *C. burnetii*. In susceptible individuals, a single inhaled organism is enough to cause disease.

  C. *Other species:*

    1. **Ruminants:** Anorexia, infertility, stillbirths, endometritis, and sporadic late abortion.

    2. **Cats:** Anorexia, transient fever, and listlessness have been seen experimentally.

VIII. *Treatment:*

  A. *Tetracycline:*

   Dogs: 10–20 mg/kg PO TID.

   Horses: 5–7.5 mg/kg IV q12h.

IX. *Prevention:* Heat all foods to destroy the organism. High-temperature pasteurization of milk is necessary before consuming. Protective clothing, mask, gloves, and goggles should be worn by humans handling suspect animals and especially during parturition. Fetal fluids, reproductive discharges, and the placenta have high concentrations of this rickettsia. There is a vaccine for humans, but it is not available in the United States.

X. *Decontamination: C. burnetii* is very resistant to heat, drying, and most common disinfectants. It can be deactivated by 0.05% sodium hypochlorite, 1:100 Lysol solution, or 5% peroxide.

8.2.2. Typhus fever (epidemic typhus, louse-borne typhus)
I.   CDC category: B
II.   *Agent: Rickettsia prowazekii.* Typhus fever is a serious infection in humans and infrequently causes death. Person-to-person contact with body lice has been known to cause large epidemics.
III.   *Affected veterinary species:* Flying squirrels and humans are the only known reservoirs (Table 8.10).

Table 8.10. Typhus fever.

Disease Severity in Potentially Affected Species S = Severe D = Moderate M = Mild								
Dogs	Horses	Cattle	Sheep	Goats	Pigs	Cats	Birds	Other Animals
								M Flying squirrels

IV.   *Incubation period:* The incubation period is 7–15 days in humans.
V.   *Transmission:* Person-to-person, vector (lice, squirrel ticks, and fleas), direct contact, or aerosolization.
VI.   *Route of transmission:* The human body louse, *Pediulus humanus humanus,* is infected by feeding on the blood of a human with an active case of typhus fever. Once the infected louse is transferred to the naïve human, the louse eats and defecates on them. Typhus fever is spread through the infective feces left on the naïve host. Humans become susceptible when feces or crushed lice enter wounds or superficial abrasions, such as scratching. Close person-to-person contact is also a source for typhus fever. Direct contact with flying squirrels or their nests is another source of infection to individuals. Aerosolization of dust or dried feces from either lice or flying squirrels may also serve as a source.
VII.   *Prominent clinical signs:* Domestic animals are asymptomatic.
   A.   **Humans:** Symptoms reported in two individuals were flu-like with fever, chills, headache, vomiting, and joint pain. Hematuria, abdominal pain, confusion, malaise, anorexia, conjunctivitis, ataxia, and myalgia were also seen. Death can occur in some human infections.
VIII.   *Treatment:*
   Dogs and Horses: Not an important health hazard.
IX.   *Prevention:* Use of insecticides and good hygiene. When handling flying squirrels or lice or working in areas where these species may be present, protective clothing, gloves, a mask, and goggles should be worn.
X.   *Decontamination:* Standard decontamination using soap and water.

8.3. Viral Agents

Viruses are all parasites that live in the cells of selected hosts. Once the virus enters a living cell, it is capable of replicating itself by taking over the metabolic processes of the invaded cell. Cells infected with viruses show one of the following responses: 1) degeneration and death or 2) transformation to a nonfunctioning state. In other words, the cell survives without transformation but has the existence of one or more components of the virus. Viruses do not respond to antibiotics.

8.3.1. Viral hemorrhagic fevers (Ebola, Marburg, Lassa, Machupo)

I.   CDC category A

II.   *Agent:* Ebola and Marburg viruses are in the Filoviridae family. Lassa and Machupo (Bolivian hemorrhagic fever) viruses are in the Arenaviridae family. All are RNA viruses that cause hemorrhagic disease and possibly death.

III.   Affected veterinary species (Table 8.11)

Table 8.11. Viral hemorrhagic fevers.

Disease Severity in Potentially Affected Species S = Severe D = Moderate M = Mild								
Dogs	Horses	Cattle	Sheep	Goats	Pigs	Cats	Birds	Other Animals
								S Nonhuman primates, rodents

IV.   *Incubation period:* The incubation period for Ebola is 2–21 days, for Marburg it is 5–10 days, and for Lassa it is 1–3 weeks.

V.   *Transmission:* Person-to-person, zoonotic, and indirect contact (contaminated fomites). Lassa fever and Machupo virus can be spread by infected rodent droppings or urine, inhalation, ingestion of contaminated food, ingestion of the infected rodent, or through abrasions or sores on the skin.

VI.   *Route of transmission:* Body fluids from infected humans are the main source of infection to other humans. It is initially thought that exposure to an infected animal (unknown for Ebola, primates for Marburg, or rodents for Lassa and Machupo) causes disease in humans. Family members, friends, and hospital personnel become infected when caring for the patient. Rodents are responsible for the spread of the Arenavirus (Lassa and Machupo) due to them residing in homes, leaving droppings and urine, or they may be used as a source of food. Contaminated fomites such as needles, syringes, and equipment can also cause disease.

VII.   *Prominent clinical signs:*

A.   **Humans:** Flu-like symptoms are initially seen in humans and may be sudden for Ebola. Vomiting, diarrhea, and stomach discomfort follow. There may be bleeding from the orifices, hiccups, red eyes, and a rash seen in some patients. Marburg is similar to Ebola in that it is sudden and flu-like, initially. After about 5 days of illness, a rash may develop on the trunk of the body. Vomiting, diarrhea, chest and/or abdominal pain, nausea, and a sore throat may be noted. Illness may progress to cause extensive hemorrhaging, organ failure, shock, and weight loss. Signs of Lassa virus include fever, sore throat, vomiting, diarrhea, chest, back, and abdominal pain, coughing, swelling of the face, bleeding mucous membranes, and conjunctivitis. Neurological signs (shuddering, hearing loss) may also occur. Machupo causes mucosal bleeding, fever, epistaxis, tremors, and speech impairment. All of these viral diseases can be fatal.

VIII. *Treatment:*
Dogs and Horses: Not an important health hazard.

IX. *Prevention:* No vaccines are available. Use of protective clothing, mask, gloves, and goggles is required. Sterilization and disinfection of equipment, instruments, and premises where the patient has been is required. Isolation of the infected person and no direct contact with deceased patients is advised.

X. *Decontamination:* Proper sterilization and disinfection should be done to deactivate the viruses.

8.3.2. Viral encephalitis (Venezuelan equine encephalitis [VEE], Eastern equine encephalitis [EEE], and Western equine encephalitis [WEE])

I. CDC category B; OIE List B

II. *Agent:* VEE, EEE, and WEE are all in the Togaviridae family. These viruses are transmitted by mosquitoes and can cause disease in horses, birds, and humans.

III. *Affected veterinary species:* EEE also infects amphibians, bats, and reptiles. VEE can infect marsupials and bats (Table 8.12).

Table 8.12. Viral Encephalitis.

Disease Severity in Potentially Affected Species S = Severe D = Moderate M = Mild								
Dogs	Horses	Cattle	Sheep	Goats	Pigs	Cats	Birds	Other Animals
	S						M	Rodents

IV. *Incubation period:* The incubation period for EEE and WEE is about 5–15 days, while VEE can be as little as 24 hours, but it is usually 2–6 days. In humans, the incubation period for EEE is 4–10 days, WEE is 5–10 days, and VEE is 2–6 days, but can be as little as 24 hours.

V. *Transmission:* Vector (mosquito) and it is zoonotic.

VI. *Route of transmission:* Transmission is through the bite of an infected mosquito. Research and laboratory personnel may be infected through aerosolization of the virus. Human cases typically appear about 2 weeks after horses show signs.

VII. *Prominent clinical signs:*

A. **Horses:** Signs may vary from mild to severe, including death. Signs include neurological dysfunction, depression, fever, altered mentation, impaired vision, head pressing, circling, inability to swallow, ataxia, paralysis, and convulsions. In the late stage of disease, affected horses may have aggressive movement of the head, limbs, eyes, and mouth. Death can occur.

B. **Humans:** Most individuals are asymptomatic. Symptoms may include headache, fever, muscle pain, nausea, anorexia, vomiting, malaise, photophobia, cough, diarrhea, sore throat, neurological involvement (meningitis, altered mental state, disorientation, and encephalitis), convulsions, tremors, and coma. Death can occur occasionally. Permanent neurological deficits have been reported with EEE and WEE. Very young and old individuals have more severe symptoms.

VIII. *Treatment:*

Dogs: Not an important health hazard.

Horses: No specific treatment other than supportive (crystalloid fluids, NSAIDs, and the cautious use of dexamethasone sodium phosphate).

IX. *Prevention:* There is monovalent (EEE), bivalent (EEE and WEE), and trivalent (EEE, WEE, and VEE) vaccine available for horses. Mosquito control should be done to decrease the adult population as well as decrease breeding grounds for the mosquitoes. In addition, horses should be routinely treated with insecticides effective against mosquitoes and housed with screens or fans to deter the insect.

X. *Decontamination:* The viruses can be controlled by heat (80°F) for 30 minutes and the use of standard disinfectants.

8.3.3. Nipah or porcine respiratory and encephalitis syndrome (PRES) (barking pig syndrome [BPS], Hendra-like virus, porcine respiratory and neurologic syndrome)

I. CDC category C

II. *Agent:* Nipah virus is in the Paramyxoviridae family. It is a zoonotic disease that causes sickness and death in both humans and pigs.

III. *Affected veterinary species:* Fruit bats serve as a reservoir (infect pigs or humans) and are usually asymptomatic (Table 8.13).

Table 8.13. Nipah or porcine respiratory and encephalitis syndrome (PRES).

Disease Severity in Potentially Affected Species S = Severe D = Moderate M = Mild								
Dogs	**Horses**	**Cattle**	**Sheep**	**Goats**	**Pigs**	**Cats**	**Birds**	**Other Animals**
D	M		M	D	D	M		M Fruit bats

IV. *Incubation period:* The incubation period is as little as 4 days, but typically is 7–14 days in pigs. In humans, it is 4–18 days.

V. *Transmission:* Direct contact (zoonotic), indirect, ingestion, and possibly person-to-person.

VI. *Route of transmission:* Close direct contact with the secretions (saliva, bronchial, and pharyngeal) or excretions (urine, semen) of infected pigs causes disease in humans and other animals. Aerosolization of respiratory or urinary secretions rarely causes disease. Fomites such as equipment and contaminated needles have been implicated in the spread of Nipah. Humans consuming contaminated fresh date palm sap, which is harvested mid-December through mid-February in Bangladesh, have been infected. Fruit bats are readily found in date palm trees. Possible human-to-human cases have occurred recently in Bangladesh and India.

VII. *Prominent clinical signs:*
   A. Dogs: Have clinical signs comparable to pigs.
   B. Horses: One horse was reported with meningitis.
   C. Humans: Clinical signs include fever, encephalitis, drowsiness, dyspnea, disorientation, severe headaches, myalgia, personality changes, seizures, and death. Severe neurological signs can have death rates that reach 40%–60%.
   D. *Other species:*
   1. **Pigs:** Often have unapparent infections. If clinical signs are present, they include severe respiratory distress, fever, harsh "barking" cough, and open mouth breathing in pigs 1–6 months of age. Possible neurological signs such as twitches, trembling, rear leg weakness, muscle spasms, ataxia when forced to move rapidly, and myoclonus have been seen as well as generalized pain and lameness. Mortality in piglets can be as high as 40%. Neurological disease is more common in older pigs and is seen as head pressing, chomping at the mouth, agitation, seizures, pharyngeal muscle paralysis, and tetanus-like tremors. Older pigs also display fever and respiratory signs as well as a nasal discharge and increased salivation. Abortion has been suspected to occur during the first trimester.
   2. **Goats:** Serious respiratory disease, cough, impaired growth, and death have occurred.

VIII. *Treatment:*
   Dogs and Horses: Supportive care and anti-inflammatory drugs.
IX. *Prevention:* No vaccine is available. Humans should wear protective clothing such as masks, gloves, goggles, and gowns.
X. *Decontamination:* Cleaning and disinfecting with sodium hypochlorite, detergents, Virkon, Lysol, or iodine solutions deactivate this virus.

8.3.4. Hantaviral disease (Hantaan virus, Sin Nombre virus [formerly Muerto Canyon Virus])
   I. CDC category C
   II. *Agent:* Hantavirus is in the RNA virus in the Bunyaviridae family. It is a deadly disease that some rodents can pass to humans. This virus was initially identified in Korea near the Hantan (Hantaan) river during the Korean War.
   III. *Affected veterinary species:* Deer mice and cotton rats are persistently infected and are normally asymptomatic (Table 8.14).

Table 8.14. Hantaviral disease.

				Disease Severity in Potentially Affected Species S = Severe D = Moderate M = Mild				
Dogs	**Horses**	**Cattle**	**Sheep**	**Goats**	**Pigs**	**Cats**	**Birds**	**Other Animals**
								M Rodents

IV. *Incubation period:* Rodents appear to be infected while young and remain carriers throughout life. The incubation period in humans is 7–39 days, with an average of 14–18 days for hantavirus pulmonary syndrome (HPS). The incubation period for hemorrhagic fever with renal syndrome (HFRS) is 2–4 weeks in humans.

V. *Transmission:* Rodent-to-human, indirect contact, ingestion, inhalation, and rarely through rodent bites. It is zoonotic. Person-to-person infection does not occur in the United States.

VI. *Route of transmission:* Contact with infected rodent urine, feces, or saliva. Fomites contaminated with urine, feces, or saliva can be accidentally introduced through the mouth or nose. Food contaminated with urine, feces, or saliva is another source for disease. Aerosolized dried materials such as nests, saliva, droppings, and urine may also cause disease. Although rodent bites rarely occur, hantavirus infection can occur.

VII. *Prominent clinical signs:*

   A. **Humans**: HPS can be fatal in humans if not treated immediately. It is contracted through inhalation of aerosolized rodent urine, feces, and saliva. Nesting material is also a source of infection to humans. HFRS begins with flu-like symptoms that may last for 3–7 days. Renal failure follows, and then recovery.

   B. *Other species:*

      1. **Rodents**: Rodents are asymptomatic carriers.

VIII. *Treatment:*

   Dogs and Horses: Not an important health hazard.

IX. *Prevention:* Rodent control is important. In addition, areas that may attract rodents (food, nesting sites) should be cleaned and kept clean. Humans should wear protective clothing, mask, gloves, and goggles when in areas infested by rodents.

X. *Decontamination:* Standard decontamination with soap and water. Sodium hypochlorite or other disinfectants may also be used deactivate hantavirus. Laundering with detergent is also effective.

8.3.5. West Nile virus (WNV) (West Nile encephalomyelitis, West Nile encephalitis)

   I. CDC category not as yet listed.

   II. *Agent:* West Nile virus is in the Flaviviridae family. It causes illness in horses, birds, humans, and other animals. WNV was introduced into the U.S. in 1999.

   III. *Affected veterinary species:* WNV remains viable primarily through birds and mosquitoes (Table 8.15).

Table 8.15. West Nile virus (WNV).

Disease Severity in Potentially Affected Species S = Severe D = Moderate M = Mild								
Dogs	**Horses**	**Cattle**	**Sheep**	**Goats**	**Pigs**	**Cats**	**Birds**	**Other Animals**
M	S	M	M	M	M	M	S	D Many mammals Some reptiles, and amphibians, bats, rabbits

IV. *Incubation period:* The incubation period is 3–14 days. In humans, the incubation period is 3–15 days.

V. *Transmission:* Vector (zoonotic) and person-to-person.

VI. *Route of transmission:* The WNV vector is primarily the *Culex* species of mosquito, but ticks and other arthropods may cause infection. It is zoonotic in that birds and mosquitoes together serve as a reservoir for WNV (Fig. 8.4). Person-to-person spread is through pregnancy, mother breastfeeding an infant, organ transplants, or blood transfusions.

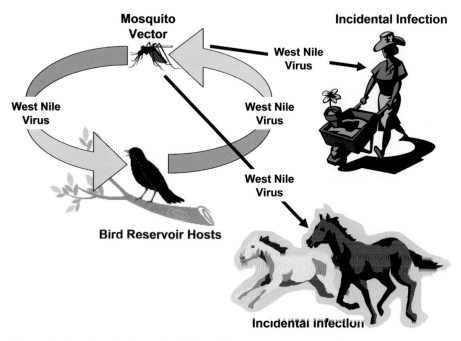

Figure 8.4. Transmission cycle of West Nile virus.

VII. *Prominent clinical signs:* Nearly all animals that are exposed to WNV show no signs or very few signs of illness.

    A. **Horses:** Generally most horses showing illness from WNV will recover. The remaining horses either die from the disease or are euthanized as a result of complications from WNV. Horses with clinical signs tend to have neurological signs. Some signs include ataxia, sleepiness, facial paralysis, listlessness, difficulty eating, muzzle twitching, weakness or paralysis of the hind limbs, head pressing, blindness, encephalitis, circling, muscle tremors, seizures, or coma. Fever is occasionally seen in some horses. Many of these horses display a variety of symptoms, so often the unusual presentation of signs is suggestive of WNV.

    B. **Dogs:** Most often are asymptomatic. Dogs have signs comparable to those of horses, which include depression, fever, weakness, lack of appetite, atypical head posture, tremors, circling, ataxia, flaccid paralysis, inability to stand, hyperesthesia, seizures, diminished or no patellar reflexes, and convulsions.

C. **Humans**: Illness can be asymptomatic to severe. Most humans (80%) will have no symptoms of disease. Less than 20% of exposed humans will have mild symptoms that that are flu-like and include fever, body aches, headache, vomiting, skin rash, nausea, being very tired, and swollen lymph nodes.

D. *Other species:*

    1. **Birds**: Crows, magpies, blue jays, and geese seem to be particularly sensitive to WNV. Often the only sign seen is a dead bird. These birds may have depression, weight loss, neurological signs, or appear to be less active. WNV in chickens and turkeys is unapparent.

    2. **Cats**: Most often are asymptomatic. A few cats have shown mild, nonspecific illness through the first 7 days of disease. Signs included some lethargy, a mild fever, nystagmus, ataxia, hyperesthesia, and seizures.

VIII. *Treatment:*

Dogs: Supportive treatment (crystalloid fluids, NSAIDs, cautious use of dexamethasone SP).

Horses: Supportive treatment (crystalloid fluids, NSAIDs, cautious use of dexamethasone SP).

IX. *Prevention:* Vaccine is available for horses only. Mosquito control is important. Avoid times of the day (at dawn and dusk) when mosquitoes are out. Birds should be removed if living or nesting near animals such as horses. Dead birds should be disposed of properly as dogs and cats are exposed to WNV by consuming the infected birds. Treat or eliminate standing water to decrease mosquitoes. Animals should have mosquito repellants applied to them regularly. Use of fans in barns will help to keep mosquitoes away.

X. *Decontamination:* Standard decontamination with soap and water.

8.3.6. Rift Valley fever (RVF) (infectious enzootic hepatitis of sheep and cattle)

I. CDC category not as yet listed. OIE List A Disease

II. *Agent:* Rift Valley fever virus is an RNA virus in the Bunyaviridae family. It is an arthropod-borne disease of sheep, cattle, and goats that is very contagious to humans. RVF could be used as a weapon for bioterrorism (aerosol).

III. *Affected veterinary species:* Neonates have ≈100% mortality (Table 8.16).

Table 8.16. Rift Valley fever (RVF).

| Disease Severity in Potentially Affected Species S = Severe   D = Moderate   M = Mild | | | | | | | | |
Dogs	Horses	Cattle	Sheep	Goats	Pigs	Cats	Birds	Other Animals
S Puppies		S	S	S		S Kittens		S Water buffalo, camels, monkeys, grey squirrels, rats, mice, voles

IV. *Incubation period:* The incubation period is as little as 12 hours in newborns and up to 3 days in adult sheep, goats, cattle, and dogs. The incubation period in humans is 4–6 days.

V. *Transmission:* Vector or aerosol (zoonotic).

VI. *Route of transmission:* The *Aedes* mosquito is the reservoir for RVF. The *Aedes lineatopinnis* can remain dormant for 5–15 years until heavy rains allow the eggs to hatch. Ruminants serve as the amplifying host; thus, other species of mosquitoes become infected and bite naïve animals. Humans become infected by aerosolization of infected tissue during handling (necropsies or slaughtering animals without a mask). RVF in aerosols may be viable for longer than 1 hour when conditions are optimal. Such conditions include temperatures of 77°F. In addition, at neutral alkaline pH and combined with protein or serum, RVF survives at 39°F for 4 months and below 32°F for 8 years. RVF is suitable for weaponization. An "animal abortion storm" would be the indication of disease.

VII. *Prominent clinical signs:*
  A. **Horses:** Appear to be viremic only.
  B. **Dogs:** Newborn puppies have high death rates due to acute disease. Older dogs are generally viremic without severe disease.
  C. **Humans:** Signs range from none to flu-like to more serious. Headache, fever (100°–104°F), nausea, dizziness, photophobia, weakness, muscle pain, back pain, and severe weight loss. Humans may also display vomiting, photophobia, and a stiff neck. Serious signs of illness (usually less than 1%) with RVF include hemorrhagic fever, ocular disease, hematemesis, encephalitis, melena, and jaundice.
  D. *Other species:*
    1. **Sheep:** Lambs less than 1 week old have fever (104°–107°F), weakness, and loss of appetite. Death occurs roughly 36 hours after initial exposure. Adult animals have a fever (104°–106°F) as well as thick nasal secretions. Vomiting and death may be noted in them. Abortion is frequently the only indication of disease. Cattle: Calves and adults have a fever (104°–106°F). Death rates may be high in calves. Adults may have weakness, foul-smelling diarrhea, anorexia, increased salivation, icterus, and regurgitate. Abortion is frequent in pregnant cows.
    2. **Cats:** Newborn kittens have high death rates due to acute disease. Older cats are generally viremic without severe disease.

VIII. *Treatment:*
  Dogs: Supportive care.
  Horses: Not an important health hazard.

IX. *Prevention:* A vaccine is available for both animals and humans. Mosquito control is helpful but is not as efficient as vaccination. Carcasses of diseased animals should be burned or buried. No RVF-infected animal should be slaughtered due to potential exposure to humans. Protective clothing, gloves, mask, and goggles should be worn.

X. *Decontamination:* Chloroform, ether, and sodium or calcium hypochlorite (chlorine content greater than 5000 ppm) can be used to deactivate this virus. Most detergents, lipid solvents, and solutions with pH < 6.8 will also deactivate RVF.

8.3.7. Hendra (equine morbillivirus pneumonia, Hendra virus disease, acute equine respiratory syndrome)
  I. CDC category not as yet listed.

II. *Agent:* Hendra virus is in the Paramyxoviridae family. Initially found in Hendra, Australia, where both horses and humans had shown respiratory and neurological signs. Hendra is not very contagious.

III. *Affected veterinary species:* Fruit bats (flying foxes) serve as the natural reservoir for Hendra (Table 8.17).

Table 8.17. Hendra.

Disease Severity in Potentially Affected Species S = Severe D = Moderate M = Mild E = Experimental								
Dogs	Horses	Cattle	Sheep	Goats	Pigs	Cats	Birds	Other Animals
	S					E		M Guinea pigs

IV. *Incubation period:* The incubation period in horses is 6–18 days. Experimentally it can be 5–10 days. In humans, the incubation period is 4–18 days and up to 3 months.

V. *Transmission:* Direct contact (zoonosis) and ingestion of contaminated feed.

VI. *Route of transmission:* Direct contact. It is suspected that fruit bats infected horses through either the aborted fetuses or urine of the fruit bat. The fruit bat is asymptomatic for Hendra. Horses have become ill after eating feed contaminated by infected fruit bats. The virus has been found in the urine and the oral cavity of horses and in experimentally infected cats. In fruit bats, the virus has been found in urine, blood, and fetal tissue. Humans became ill when exposed to excretions and body fluids from infected horses. Handling of infected tissues may also be a source of disease.

VII. *Prominent clinical signs:*

A. **Horses:** Hendra in horses usually causes a fever (up to 106°F), acute respiratory distress, anorexia, depression, nasal discharge (blood tinged or frothy), pneumonia, ataxia, and sweating. Additional signs that may be noted include dependent edema, neurological signs (head pressing, muscle fasiculations), and jaundiced or cyanotic mucous membranes. Disease is acute in horses and death occurs 1–3 days after initial signs are seen.

B. **Humans:** Appear to have a severe form of the flu that includes a fever, respiratory illness, and myalgia. Renal failure and pneumonia killed a horse trainer while another individual came down with meningitis and died as a result of complications from progressive encephalitis. Hendra killed two of three individuals known to be exposed to this virus.

C. *Other species:*

1. **Cats:** Death usually occurs within a day after signs of elevated respiration, fever, and serious illness are noted.

VIII. *Treatment:*

Dogs: Not an important health hazard.

Horse: Symptomatic treatment.

IX. *Prevention:* No vaccine is available. Protective clothing, gloves, mask, and goggles should be worn. Identification of infected animals, quarantine, and humane euthanasia were done in Australia to control this disease.

X. *Decontamination:* Hendra is an enveloped virus that is readily deactivated by formaldehyde, heat, lipid solvents, oxidizing agents, and nonionic detergents.

8.3.8. Monkeypox

I. CDC category not as yet listed.

II. *Agent:* Monkeypox virus belongs to the genus Orthopoxvirus. This genus also includes the smallpox virus (variola), the virus used in the manufacture of smallpox vaccine (vaccinia), and the cowpox virus. Monkeypox is contagious and looks very similar to smallpox in humans.

III. *Affected veterinary species:* Rodents are probably the reservoir for monkeypox. It is likely that other animals may be susceptible to monkeypox, but they are unknown at this time (Table 8.18).

Table 8.18. Monkeypox.

Disease Severity in Potentially Affected Species S = Severe D = Moderate M = Mild									
Dogs	**Horses**	**Cattle**	**Sheep**	**Goats**	**Pigs**	**Cats**	**Birds**	**Other Animals**
								Rodents, prairie dogs, Gambian giant rats, rabbits, squirrels, nonhuman primates

IV. *Incubation period:* The incubation period is 6–7 days in cynomolgus monkeys that were experimentally infected with a fatal aerosol dose of monkeypox. Current recommendations by the CDC are that any animal exposed to monkeypox be quarantined for 6 weeks. The incubation period is approximately 12 days for humans.

V. *Transmission:* Uncertain in animals. Direct contact, aerosol, or cutaneous routes (zoonotic) can infect humans. Less often, monkeypox is spread person-to-person.

VI. *Route of transmission:* It is suspected that animals become infected through the oropharynx, nasopharynx, eating infected tissue, or through wounds. Humans are infected through direct contact with body fluids, respiratory droplets (aerosols), wounds, blood, fomites, handling, bites, and handling bedding or cages of infected animals. The monkeypox outbreak in the United States in 2003 was mostly the result of cutaneous exposure to the virus. The spread of monkeypox person-to-person is unusual, but does occasionally occur. The virus is spread through contaminated fomites, aerosolization, or body fluids of infected individuals.

VII. *Prominent clinical signs:*

    A. **Humans:** It is usually a milder disease than smallpox. Initially fever, swollen lymph nodes, chills, malaise, headache, sore throat, weariness, cough, and myalgia are noted. A rash with papules is seen 1–3 days or more after fever develops. The papules turn to pustules, crust, and fall off. More serious signs of monkeypox include respiratory signs and death.

B. *Other species:*

    1. Rodents and Rabbits: Clinical signs of disease include fever, cough, nasal secretions, inappetent, conjunctivitis, depression, and lymphadenopathy. In addition, there is a nodular rash that develops into pustules ("pocks"), patches of hair loss, and pneumonia may be seen. Monkeypox can be fatal in some animals. Gambian rats showed only mild clinical signs when infected.

    2. Nonhuman Primates: Typically a self-limiting rash is reported in these animals. Fever and papules are seen first. The papules become pustules that crust (pocks). The pocks generally cover the extremities, but may also be found on the rest of the animal. Once the crusts fall off, scars remain. More serious signs of disease include anorexia, dyspnea, coughing, facial edema, nasal secretions, lymphadenopathy, and oral ulcers. Experimental aerosol exposure of monkeypox has been shown to cause pneumonia. Death can occur and is usually more common in infant monkeys.

VIII. *Treatment:*

Dogs and Horses: Not an important health hazard. Supportive treatment is suggested for other animals, although there is no safe treatment for animals without exposing humans.

IX. *Prevention:*

Humans: Vaccination with smallpox in humans may reduce disease incidence in humans. Protective clothing using a mask, goggles, gloves, and disposable gown is recommended.

X. *Decontamination:* Recommendations by the CDC are to use an EPA-approved detergent or disinfectant or sodium hypochlorite solution. Laundering should be done with sodium hypochlorite, if possible. Autoclaving or incineration may be used to deactivate monkeypox. Contaminated objects (clothing, bedding, towels, toys, water and food bowls, etc.) should not be thrown away, disposed of in a landfill, or buried until proper disinfection has been done on them.

8.4. Toxins

Toxins are poisonous byproducts of living organisms. They essentially interfere with the host's cells by inhibiting protein synthesis, damaging cell membranes, activating immune responses, activating second messenger pathways, or are proteases. They are very stable in the environment. Some toxins are susceptible to heat and light, while others are heat stable. Toxins are able to produce mild to severe illness when ingested, inhaled, or injected into the body. They also have the potential to cause death.

8.4.1. Botulinum toxins (botulism, limberneck, shaker foal syndrome, Western duck sickness, toxicoinfectious botulism, bulbar paralysis, loin disease, Lamziekte)

  I.   CDC category A

  II. *Agent: Clostridium botulinum.* Botulinum toxins are comprised of seven types of toxins. The spores of this bacterium are everywhere and they develop into vegetative bacteria that create toxins under anaerobic conditions. There are three naturally occurring forms of botulism: a) food borne, b) infantile, and c) wound. Botulinum toxin is the most potent neurotoxin known. It is 15,000 times more toxic than VX (the most toxic of the nerve agents) and 100,000 times more toxic than sarin. It is considered a weapon of bioterrorism.

III.   Affected veterinary species (Table 8.19)

Table 8.19.   *Botulinum toxins.*

Disease Severity in Potentially Affected Species S = Severe D = Moderate M = Mild								
Dogs	**Horses**	**Cattle**	**Sheep**	**Goats**	**Pigs**	**Cats**	**Birds**	**Other Animals**
D	S	S	S	S	D	M	S	Foxes, mink, fish

A.   *Toxins:* There are seven types (A through G) of botulinum toxins. In humans, types A, B, E, and F (rarely) may bring about disease. In animals, type C is the most frequent source of botulism. Horses may be affected by type B. Cattle and dogs will occasionally be affected by type D. Birds and mink may be affected by types A and E. Type G toxin has occasionally been noted in animals and humans, but apparently does not cause disease. Botulinum toxins all cause the same disease. Effective treatment will depend on the use of antiserum for the specific type of toxin.

IV.   *Incubation period:* The incubation period ranges from 2 hours to 14 days. Most often illness is seen within 12–72 hours. In humans, the incubation period is usually 12–36 hours after consuming the toxin, but can range from 6 hours to 10 days.

V.   *Transmission:* Wounds, food borne, and intestinal (all are zoonotic). There is also the adult colonization form in humans.

VI.   *Route of transmission:* The botulinum toxin is not contagious. Wound contamination (the toxicoinfectious form) with botulinum toxins results when a wound is anaerobic. Such infections are usually associated with the intestinal tract, deep muscle or skin wounds, navel infections, and lung or liver abscesses. The "shaker foal syndrome" is thought to result from this type of an infection. Chickens also exhibit this form of botulisum. Transmission is also from consuming contaminated food (raw meat, garbage, flesh, ensilage), decaying vegetation, or infected carcasses. (Herbivores may ingest feed contaminated by carcasses.)

A.   **Humans:** Botulinum toxins can enter through wounds that are not properly cleaned or are contaminated with soil. (Spores are routinely present in soil.) Ingestion of the toxins is typically the result of improper handling of food or not heating food thoroughly. Children under 1 year of age are most susceptible to the intestinal form of botulinum. Honey and other foods that may contain spores from soil are a source of infection. The adult colonization form is common in individuals with a history of intestinal illness (inflammatory bowel disease) or recent gastrointestinal surgery. This form of botulinum is extremely rare. Aerosolization of the toxin may be used for weaponization.

VII.   *Predominant clinical signs:*

A.   **Horses:** Signs may include incoordination, drooling, paralysis of the tongue, restlessness, and knuckling. Muscle paralysis is common (and seen in most

RORO

species of animals). The paralysis is progressive and ascending. These animals lose the ability to swallow or chew and death results from respiratory or cardiac paralysis. "Shaker foal syndrome" is seen in very young foals (less than 4 weeks). They are unable to stand for more than a few minutes, muscle tremors are present, and they appear stiff when moving. Often times these foals show no signs before death. Other signs that may be noted include constipation, repeated urination, dysphagia, and dilation of the pupils. Respiratory paralysis is most often the cause of death in these foals in 1–3 days.

B. **Dogs:** Signs may include incoordination, drooling, paralysis of the tongue, restlessness, and knuckling. Muscle paralysis is common. The paralysis is progressive and ascending. These animals lose the ability to swallow or chew and death results from respiratory or cardiac paralysis. Other signs that may be noted include constipation, repeated urination, dysphagia, and dilation of the pupils. Respiratory paralysis is most often the cause of death.

C. **Humans:** Display drooping eyelids, altered voice, double vision or blurred vision, difficulty in speaking or swallowing, and dry mouth. Infected individuals may have a descending, symmetrical flaccid paralysis. Other symptoms that may be seen include vomiting, diarrhea, nausea, and abdominal pain. Impaired respiratory function due to the toxin may cause paralysis of the respiratory muscles. Infants will display lack of appetite, constipation, decreased crying and sucking, weakness in the neck and periphery (known as "floppy baby"), and have respiratory failure.

D. *Other species:*
   1. **Ruminants:** Signs seen in cattle are incoordination, dysphagia, drooling, inability to urinate, restlessness, and sternal recumbency. Sheep display a nasal discharge (serous), incoordination, drooling, and stiffness. The disease can be progressive in ruminants, causing paralysis and death.
   2. **Birds:** Usually a flaccid paralysis is seen that involves the neck, legs, eyelids, and wings. Occasionally diarrhea may be noted with the toxic infectious form.
   3. **Mink and Foxes:** Often the only sign seen is dead animals. One may also see dyspnea and various stages of paralysis.
   4. **Pigs:** Signs include vomiting, muscle paralysis, anorexia, not wanting to drink, and dilation of the pupils. Pigs are generally resistant to botulism.

VIII. *Treatment:* Cl. botulinum C + D antitoxin may be used to decrease or stop the signs of disease. Supportive care with respiratory support provides the best means of treatment. If botulinum antitoxin can be administered early, it may slow the progression of disease and diminish the symptoms. In cases of food-borne illness, the levels of toxin in the intestinal tract may be decreased with the use of stomach lavage and enemas. Infected wounds are best treated through debridement and the use of antibiotics. The use of antibiotics in food-borne illness has been done intermittently and is usually not advised. Antitoxins are used only in the treatment of botulinum toxin and not the prevention of it.

IX. *Prevention:*
   Dogs and Horses: Supportive care. Vaccination with C and D toxoid has proved useful in cattle, sheep, goats, pheasants, and mink.

X. *Decontamination:* Botulinum toxins are proteins that are easily denatured. Toxins that are exposed to sunlight are inactivated within 1–3 hours. It can also be deactivated by 0.1% sodium hypochlorite, heating to 176°F for 30

minutes or 212°F for 10 minutes, and 0.1N sodium hydroxide. Water can be
treated with chlorine or other disinfectants to deactivate the toxin. The vegetative
form of *Cl. botulinum* is deactivated by 1% sodium hypochlorite, 70% ethanol,
and other disinfectants. The spores are deactivated by moist heat at 248°F for a
minimum of 15 minutes.

8.4.2. *Clostridium perfringens* toxins

I.   CDC category B
II. *Agent: Clostridium perfringens.* It is a common anaerobic bacillus that
produces at least 12 exotoxins. In animals, *Cl. perfringens* is a normal inhabitant
of the intestinal microflora and also found in the soil. Some of the exotoxins
produce enterotoxemias (A, B, C, and D) which can cause necrosis and death of
the host. It is uncertain if type E plays a role in disease.
III. Affected veterinary species (Table 8.20)

Table 8.20. *Clostridium perfringens* toxins.

| Disease Severity in Potentially Affected Species S = Severe   D = Moderate   M = Mild | | | | | | | | |
Dogs	Horses	Cattle	Sheep	Goats	Pigs	Cats	Birds	Other Animals
S	S	S	S	S	S	S	S	Nonhuman primates

IV. *Incubation period:* The incubation period is 1–6 hours, but one may only find
dead animals. In humans, the incubation is usually 10–12 hours but ranges from 6
to 24 hours.
V.   *Transmission:* The consumption of contaminated food, contact with sewage, or
an altered intestinal tract.
VI. *Route of transmission: Cl. perfringens* is in the soil and the intestinal tract of
normal healthy animals and people. Most cases of enterotoxemia in animals are the
result of food contaminated with these bacteria or spores. The bacteria can also
proliferate suddenly in the altered intestinal tract, which allows for production of
toxin. In humans, the route of transmission is through improperly cooked food or
food that is not adequately stored or kept at proper temperature.
VII. *Prominent clinical signs:*
   A. Animals: The young appear more severely affected and often it is the
   animal on full feed. In lambs, calves, and pigs the clinical sign is of a healthy
   animal that died suddenly and for no apparent reason. There is often
   abdominal pain, depression, not eating, bloody diarrhea or diarrhea with no
   blood, recumbency, convulsions, and opisthotonus. There is septicemia prior to
   an acute death. A necrotic enteritis, excitement, and incoordination may also
   be noted.
   B. Humans: *Cl. perfringens* is also called the "food-service germ." It results
   from raw food that is not properly cooked, not heated and maintained at proper
   temperature, or food that is not properly cooled. Most often food poisoning is
   the result of food served in large quantities and left out either at room

temperature or on steam tables for several hours. The typical history is a large quantity of individuals displaying the same symptoms after eating a particular food. Clinical signs are most often sudden and include cramping, abdominal pain and gas, as well as watery diarrhea. Fever, dehydration, and vomiting may occur in a few cases. The duration of illness is usually less than a day and is not serious in most healthy individuals.

VIII. *Treatment:*

Dogs and Horses: In animals with severe clinical signs, it may be too late to treat. Supportive care should be provided along with *Cl. perfringens* antitoxin and large doses of penicillin.

IX. *Prevention: Cl. perfringens* antitoxin in very young animals (if mothers are unprotected) for immediate protection, followed with the toxoid product when older. Reduce the amount of concentrate and increase the roughage provided to animals in feedlot situations.

X. *Decontamination:* Decontaminate with soap and water.

8.4.3. Ricin

I. CDC category B

II. *Agent:* Ricin. It is a potent cytotoxin derived from the beans of the castor plant (*Ricinus communis*) (Fig. 8.5). The ricin toxins are potent inhibitors of DNA replication and protein synthesis. Ricin may be used as a weapon of bioterrorism.

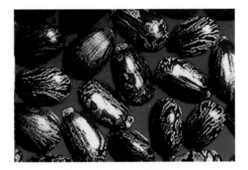

Figure 8.5. Castor beans are the source of ricin. (Source: Public domain. http://www.ars. usda.gov/is/AR/archive/jan01/plant0101.htm.)

III. Affected veterinary species (Table 8.21)

IV. *Incubation period:* The incubation period in animals is a few hours up to 48 hours. In humans, the incubation period is less than 6 hours if ingested and 8 hours if inhaled.

Table 8.21. Ricin.

| Disease Severity in Potentially Affected Species S = Severe   D = Moderate   M = Mild | | | | | | | | |
Dogs	Horses	Cattle	Sheep	Goats	Pigs	Cats	Birds	Other Animals
S	S	S	S	S	S	S	S	S Nonhuman primates, most if not all species of animals

V.   *Transmission:* Ingestion, inhaled, or by injection.

VI.   *Route of transmission:* Ricin is found in the castor bean plant and the seeds contain the highest concentration of this toxin. Large quantities of the plant or bean must be consumed to cause illness. It is not very palatable, so animals will eat it if hungry, fed as castor bean meal, or if it has been accidentally introduced into feed. Transmission by inhalation of toxin occurs during industrial operations (extraction of oils from the plant). Ricin has been used as a terrorist weapon in humans when the product was injected via a modified umbrella into an individual in Great Britain.

VII.   *Predominant clinical signs:*

A.   **Animals:** May have a fever, abdominal pain, muscular twitching, vomiting, diarrhea, convulsions, coma, and death. Shock and anaphylaxis (allergic reaction) may occur due to ricin being a cytotoxin. Horses may die within 24–36 hours after ingestion of ricin.

B.   **Humans:** Accidental exposure may happen through the consumption of castor beans. Ricin exposure is usually the deliberate use as a poison. Violent vomiting and diarrhea is initially seen and may contain blood in it. Dehydration, flu-like symptoms, hypovolemic shock, weakness, seizures, hallucinations, and multiple organ system failure occur. Inhaled exposure of ricin is not well documented. A few symptoms that may be seen, or all, may include flu-like symptoms, respiratory distress, cough, bronchoconstriction, pulmonary edema, nausea, weakness, multiple organ failure, cyanosis, respiratory failure, and death. Individuals exposed to dust from the castor bean may have an allergic reaction, hives, tightness in the chest, watery itchy eyes, or wheezing. Information on exposure to ricin by injection is limited. Symptoms varied some, but included flu-like signs, dizziness, nausea, weakness, vomiting, anorexia, pain at the injection site, mylagia, shock, and death. If the individual survives 3–5 days, they generally recover. There are only four reported cases to date; two of the individuals died.

VIII.   *Treatment:*

Dogs and Horses: Supportive care, laxatives, antihistamines, and gastrointestinal protectants (fats or oils are best). Sedatives may be used to control signs.

IX.   *Prevention:* There is currently no vaccine or prophylactic antitoxin available at this time.

X. *Decontamination:* Use of copious amounts of soap and water to rinse ricin off of skin. All clothing and personal belongings are removed, double bagged, and sealed for proper disposal. Environmental decontamination is done with soap and water and deactivated with 0.1% hypochlorite solutions or EPA-registered disinfectants.

8.4.4. Staphylococcal enterotoxin B (SEB) (Staph enterotoxicosis)

I. CDC category B

II. *Agent: Staphylococcus aureus.* It can produce seven types of toxin that exert their effects on the intestinal tract and is most often the source of food poisoning. It may be a possible weapon of bioterrorism (aerosol).

III. Affected veterinary species (Table 8.22).

Table 8.22. Staphylococcal enterotoxin B (SEB).

Disease Severity in Potentially Affected Species S = Severe D = Moderate M = Mild								
Dogs	Horses	Cattle	Sheep	Goats	Pigs	Cats	Birds	Other Animals
S	S	S	S	S	S	S	S	S Nonhuman primates

IV. *Incubation period:* The incubation period if ingested is typically 2–4 hours but may range from ½ hour to 12 hours. The incubation period for inhalation is 3–4 hours; 8–20 hours in nonhuman primates. Humans may experience symptoms ½ hour to 6 hours after consuming contaminated food. When SEB is inhaled by humans, the incubation is 3–12 hours.

V. *Transmission:* Ingestion, direct contact, or aerosolization.

VI. *Route of transmission:* The usual route is through food that is not properly handled. Direct contact with infected animals (mastitis in cattle and sheep; rodents may be a reservoir). Humans do not transmit the disease to other humans. Aerosolization of SEB (use as a weapon) was done by the United States in the 1960s.

VII. *Predominant clinical signs:* When contaminated food is ingested, signs include vomiting, abdominal pain, nausea, weakness, hypotension, drop in body temperature, and diarrhea.

    A. **Humans:** Clinical signs of SEB food poisoning include vomiting, abdominal pain, diarrhea, and nausea. Symptoms usually last 1–3 days and are generally mild in humans. Symptoms of inhalation exposure to SEB include dyspnea, fever, nonproductive cough, acute respiratory difficulty, myalgia, vomiting, diarrhea, nausea, headache, anorexia, hypotension, and pulmonary edema. Illness may last up to 14 days in humans.

    B. *Other species:*

        1. **Nonhuman Primates:** Inhalation exposure of nonlethal SEB caused abdominal pain less than 24 hours, with signs beginning in about 8–20 hours. Fever is seen only with inhalation of SEB. In addition, sudden hypotension, nonproductive cough (for up to 4 weeks), and myalgia were noted. The primates were ill for 3–4 days. If SEB was inhaled at a lethal dose, signs were noted within 2 days. Signs of pulmonary edema, dyspnea, and gastrointestinal were noted. Death within 3–4 days resulted from multiple organ failure.

VIII.   *Treatment:*

  Dogs and Horses: Supportive care for ingestion of SEB includes fluids, electrolytes, and medications to ease abdominal discomfort. Inhalation SEB exposure may require oxygen, mechanical ventilation, atropine, antihistamines, and cough suppressants.

IX.   *Prevention:* Keep foods at proper temperature and use good hygiene will help prevent food poisoning. No vaccine is currently available. A toxoid vaccine and a vaccine with toxins have or are being developed, respectively.

X.   *Decontamination:* Decontaminate with soap and water. Five percent sodium hypochlorite can be used to deactivate SEB on surfaces. When handling dead carcasses, use protective clothing, mask, gloves, and goggles. Dispose of carcasses by incineration or deep burial.

8.4.5.   T-2 Mycotoxins

I.   CDC category not as yet listed.

II.   *Agent: Fusarium* spp. It is a fungus that produces the trichothecene (T-2) mycotoxins, and they are often found on grain products. These mycotoxins are unique in that they are dermally active. T-2 mycotoxins must be suspected when any aerosol occurs in the form of "yellow rain." The yellow rain will contain droplets of pigmented oily fluids that contaminate hair coats of animals and the surrounding environment. Mycotoxin T-2 has been used as a weapon of bioterrorism.

III.   Affected veterinary species (Table 8.23)

Table 8.23.   T-2 Mycotoxins.

| Disease Severity in Potentially Affected Species S = Severe   D = Moderate   M = Mild | | | | | | | | |
Dogs	Horses	Cattle	Sheep	Goats	Pigs	Cats	Birds	Other Animals
?	S	S	?	?	S	?	S	S Poultry, invertebrates

IV.   *Incubation period:* The oral incubation period is 3–12 hours, respiratory route is less than 1 hour, dermally it is 6–12 hours, and ocular exposure is less than 5 minutes.

V.   *Transmission:* Ingestion, aerosol, dermal, or injection.

VI.   *Route of transmission:* In domestic animals, ingestion is most often through moldy food such as corn, corn silage, wheat, legumes, sorghum grain, barley, pelleted feed, rice meal, groundnuts, cottonseed meal, tall fescue grass, standing corn, and maize. Humans may be infected by consuming contaminated cereals and grains. A terrorist event would result in the spraying of the oily agent, which would affect the hair coat and skin.

VII. *Predominant clinical signs:*

A. **Animals:** Signs of ingestion of T-2 mycotoxins include inappetence, decreased milk and egg production, hypotension, staggering, diarrhea, shock, vomiting, lesions in the mouth and upper GI tract. There may be death of some animals. Dermal exposure causes inflammation and cutaneous necrosis, while eye exposure may result in damage to the cornea.

B. **Humans:** Ingestion results in vomiting and diarrhea relatively quickly. Skin exposure results in redness, pain, pruritus, necrosis, blisters, and sloughing. Blurred vision is often the result of ocular exposure. Inhalation causes nasal secretions, itching, irritation in the nose and throat, blindness, coughing, bleeding, sneezing, chest pain, and seizures. High levels of T-2 mycotoxins cause ataxia, weakness, shock, prostration, and death.

VIII. *Treatment:*

Dogs and Horses: Supportive care. Bathe the dermally exposed animal with soap and water. Activated charcoal given within an hour of ingestion may help. Animals being fed contaminated feed or grazed on affected pastures should be immediately removed from the source. Flush eyes with copious amounts of water following ocular exposure.

IX. *Prevention:* Prevent mold contamination of feed. No vaccine is available.

X. *Decontamination:* Decontaminate with soap and water. Individuals should wear protective clothing, gloves, mask, and goggles when handling animals with dermal exposure to these mycotoxins. Environmental decontamination can be done with 5% sodium hypochlorite to deactivate contaminated equipment. T-2 mycotoxins are deactivated by heating at 900° for 10 minutes or 500° for 30 minutes. Dermal lesions can result if contaminated clothing is touched.

8.5. Prions

Prions or transmissible spongiform encephalopathies (TSEs) are infectious pieces of protein and are smaller than any known virus. They are capable of causing neurodegenerative disease in both animals and humans. They are unique in that they have long incubation periods of months to years before clinical signs are seen. They are almost always fatal, extremely hardy, and often difficult to transmit. At one time, it was believed that the TSEs were unique to each species. Apparently, some of these TSEs are capable of infecting other species. Normal cell protein is transformed by the abnormal prion protein, causing disease in the brain. When these abnormal proteins insert themselves into brain cells, they are capable of altering the normal proteins in the cell into prions. The altered brain cell dies and releases the prions to infect other brain cells.

Prions or TSEs became of interest to the public when the mad cow epidemic (or BSE) affected Great Britain in 1996. To date, there is no known treatment for prion diseases. There are multiple TSEs which affect different species of animals including kuru in humans, scrapie in sheep, transmissible mink encephalopathy (TME, mink scrapie), feline spongiform encephalopathy (FSE), chronic wasting disease (CWD) in deer and elk, and a spongiform encephalopathy of exotic ruminants (Fig. 8.6).

8.5.1. Bovine spongiform encephalopathy (BSE) (mad cow disease)

I. CDC category not as yet listed: OIE List B Disease

II. *Agent:* BSE. It is a fatal, nonfebrile, progressive disease of cattle. The BSE outbreak is responsible for FSE in cats and spongiform encephalopathy in exotic

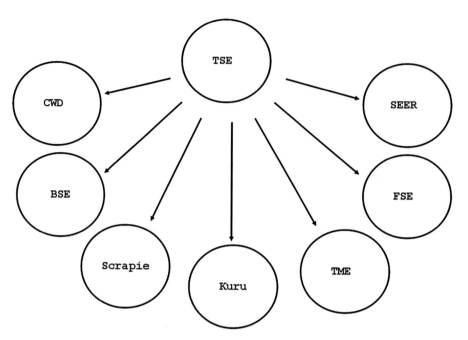

Figure 8.6. Transmissible spongiform encephalopathies (TSEs) affect cattle (bovine spongiform encephalopathy, BSE, mad-cow disease); sheep, goats, Moufflon, rodents, monkeys (scrapie); white-tailed deer, black-tailed deer, mule deer, elk, moose (chronic wasting disease [CWD]); mink (transmissible mink encephalopathy [TME]); cats (feline spongiform encephalopathy [FSE]); humans (Kuru); and exotic ruminants (spongiform encephalopathy of exotic ruminants [SEER]).

ruminants. A variant of Creutzfeldt-Jakob disease (CJD) that occurs in humans is apparently related to BSE.

III.   Affected veterinary species (Table 8.24)

Table 8.24. Bovine spongiform encephalopathy (BSE).

| | | | Disease Severity in Potentially Affected Species | | | | | |
| | | | S = Severe   D = Moderate   M = Mild   E = Experimental | | | | | |
Dogs	Horses	Cattle	Sheep	Goats	Pigs	Cats	Birds	Other Animals
?		S	E	E	E	E		E Mink, Cynomologus monkeys, mice, marmosets

IV.   Incubation period: The incubation period of BSE is greater than a year (usually 2 years) to a number of years. Typically, cattle are affected at 4–5 years of age. The incubation period is unknown in humans (years to decades?).

V.   *Transmission:* Ingested (zoonotic).

VI.   *Route of transmission:* BSE is transmitted through the ingestion of
nervous tissue or bone meal from infected animals. There are several theories as to
how BSE was introduced into cattle. It may be a genetic mutation that occurred as
early as the 1970s, it may be a mutation of scrapie in sheep (cattle were fed
infected sheep tissue), or a human TSE mutation. BSE was noted in Great Britain
during the 1980s. In November 1986, scientists became aware of the problem in
cattle. At this time period, cattle were being fed meat-and-bone meal (MBM) that
had been added to their rations. The MBM came from animal carcasses that were
in all probability infected with the BSE agent. Cattle that acquire BSE through
natural means have this agent in the spinal cord, brain, and retina. Experimentally,
it can also be found in the distal ileum of infected calves. Cows infected with BSE
are more likely to produce calves that are at increased risk of having BSE. At
present, the mode of transmission of the agent to these higher risk calves is
unknown.

VII.   *Predominant clinical signs:*

   A.   **Humans:** Symptoms are only seen in some individuals, and it appears to be
a variant of Creutzfeldt-Jakob disease (vCJD). It is more common in young
individuals (death occurs at about 28–29 years), symptoms persist for about 14
months, and it is probably linked to food contaminated with the BSE agent. CJD
is more common in 65-year-olds and illness lasts about $4\frac{1}{2}$ years. Initial clinical
presentation of vCJD involves sensory or behavioral changes. Neurological
symptoms occur weeks to months later. Symptoms are ataxia, dementia, and
myoclonus. The final, fatal progression of vCJD causes inability to speak or
move followed by death.

   B.   **Cattle:** BSE is progressive and insidious. Once clinical signs become evident,
the disease progresses fairly rapidly. Death is usually 3 months after signs are
initially noted. Neurological signs predominate this disease. At the outset, these
animals demonstrate sneezing, rubbing and tossing of the head, decreased
rumination, increased licking of the nose or crinkling it, and bruxism. As the
disease progresses, they may have hyperesthesia, head shyness, kicking, be easily
startled, ataxia of the hind limbs, tremors, fall down, and appear nervous.
Animals with advanced disease tend to have a fixed facial appearance, stand with
a lowered head for extended periods of time, lose weight, have reduced milk
production, become recumbent, lose consciousness, and then die. Unlike scrapie,
there is no pruritus in BSE-infected cattle.

VIII.   *Treatment:*

   Dogs and Horses: Not an important health hazard.

   Cattle: No treatment other than supportive. Humane euthanasia recommended
      when illness incapacitates the animal.

IX.   *Prevention:* No vaccine is available. Humane euthanasia of any adult bovine
demonstrating neurological signs and "downer" cows should be done. Animals that
die on the owner's premises or are negative for rabies also should not enter the
food chain. A ban of all ruminant animals and their products from countries
known to have BSE has been used to control the disease. In addition, the "animal
feed rule" was implemented, which forbids feeding animal proteins or animal
protein products, especially spinal cord, brain, and eyes to domestic ruminants.
Once BSE has been identified in an animal, the herd is quarantined, and trace
backs are performed to identify all animals that are related or had contact with the
positive animal.

X. *Decontamination:* BSE appears to be resistant to heating at normal cooking temperatures, pasteurization, freezing, sterilization, and drying. Scrapie, which is a similar disease, is very resistant to heat, ionizing radiation, disinfectants, formalin, and ultraviolet radiation. Scrapie is very resistant to destruction if it is in desiccated organic material or tissue. Autoclaving for a minimum of 273°–280°F for 18 minutes may deactivate this protein. Incineration or autoclaving contaminated tissue is recommended. Disinfectants that may be used to deactivate BSE include sodium hydroxide, sodium hypochlorite, and sodium hypochlorite with 2N sodium hydroxide or 2% available chlorine for at least 1 hour at 68°F (overnight for equipment) is recommended. It is unclear if these procedures will completely deactivate this prion, but they may reduce the titer of this agent. Great Britain disposes of contaminated carcasses by heating to 271°F at 3 millibar pressure for at least 20 minutes. The prevailing thought in the medical field of neurosurgery is to use disposable instruments if CJD is highly suspected in a patient. In Great Britain, equipment that is used in brain biopsies is quarantined until a final diagnosis has been made. This is due to the high risk for CJD in the country.

8.5.2. Chronic wasting disease (CWD)

I. CDC category not as yet listed: OIE List B Disease
II. *Agent:* CWD is a contagious, fatal disease of deer, moose, and elk. Deer, moose, and elk are the only known animals to serve as a natural host for this disease. In 1967, it was identified as a "wasting" syndrome in mule deer at a wildlife research facility in northern Colorado. It was subsequently recognized as a transmissible spongiform encephalopathy (TSE) in 1978. CWD is most likely caused by a prion.
III. *Affected veterinary species:* Experimentally mice, squirrel monkeys, mink, domestic ferrets, and hamsters (Table 8.25).

Table 8.25. Chronic wasting disease (CWD).

Disease Severity in Potentially Affected Species S = Severe D = Moderate M = Mild E = Experimental								
Dogs	**Horses**	**Cattle**	**Sheep**	**Goats**	**Pigs**	**Cats**	**Birds**	**Other Animals**
		E	E	E				**S** Mule deer, white-tailed deer, elk

IV. *Incubation period:* The incubation period ranges from 1½ to 3 years. Most animals with CWD are older than 16 months, and it has been found in animals greater than 15 years.
V. *Transmission:* Direct contact (animal-to-animal) or indirectly through contaminated water and food (zoonotic?).
VI. *Route of transmission:* Lateral transmission (animal-to-animal) appears to be the main source of CWD infection. Maternal transmission may also happen, but is not significant. It is suspected that the naïve animal may ingest the protein through contaminated food and water. To date, it has not been proven there is a

risk in humans and it would be considered low if there is one. A few cases possibly suggest eating venison in endemic areas may increase the risk of CJD.

VII.   *Predominant clinical signs:*

A.   Humans: Information is limited and has not been confirmed that CWD can cause disease in humans. There have been just a few cases to date that suggest CJD or a prion disease in humans who had no family history of CJD and had consumed venison. Symptoms seen in these humans may include seizures, depression, fatigue, memory loss, speech abnormalities, headaches, social withdrawal, combative behavior, anger outbursts, vision problems, photophobia, confusion, ataxia, incontinence, and coma. Documented illness lasted from 5–6 months up to 22 months prior to death. Death was due to a degenerative neurological disorder or a prion disease.

B.   *Other species:*

1.   **Cervids:** CWD is progressive and fatal in adult animals. Initially there may be subtle loss of weight and changes in behavior. As the disease becomes more obvious, there may be persistent walking, change in interactions with other animals (and caregivers), less wary, head tremors, polydipsia, polyuria, difficulty swallowing, ataxia, and drowsiness. In the final stages of disease, there may be excess salivation, bruxism, fixed gaze, droopy ears, and lowered head. Aspiration pneumonitis should always raise the suspicion of CWD in adult cervids. The most prevalent and consistent sign of CWD is weight loss. Elk may also display hyperexcitability and nervousness. Some affected animals may not show any weight loss. Death usually results from stress or cold weather.

VIII.   *Treatment:*

Dogs and Horses: Not an important health hazard.

Cervids: No treatment other than supportive. Humane euthanasia recommended when illness incapacitates the animal.

IX.   *Prevention:* No vaccine is available. Humans should avoid tissues that are known to contain CWD (brain, spinal cord, eyes, tonsils, lymph nodes, spleen) from deer or elk in areas endemic with the disease. Any animal that is suspected of the CWD disease or is abnormal should be avoided for consumption by animals and humans. All utensils (knives, tables, saws) used to cut up a cervid carcass should be disinfected with 50% sodium hypochlorite. The animal should then be tested for CWD prior to consuming the meat. Humans should wear protective clothing, mask, gloves, and goggles when any cervid is being harvested for the meat.

X.   *Decontamination:* There are limited methods for deactivating prion proteins. The use of 50% sodium hypochlorite for at least 30–60 minutes is beneficial in deactivating CWD. There may be other disinfectants that may prove useful for deactivating CWD, but they are not known at this time. Alkaline digestion and incineration may be done to dispose of carcasses and infected tissue. It has been suggested to dispose of these remains in landfills, but this may not be practical as scavenger animals will seek these tissues out.

Suggested Reading/Websites

All about hantaviruses, Special Pathogens Branch, 2004. www.cdc.gov/ncidod/ diseases/hanta/hps/noframes/transmit.htm.

American Association of Avian Pathologists. *Avian Disease Manual*, ed 2.

Arenavirus fact sheet, 2005. www.cdc.gov/ncidod/dvrd/mnpages/dispages/arena.htm.

Basic information about monkeypox, 2003. www.cdc.gov/ncidod/monkeypox/factsheet.htm.

Belay ED, Maddox RA, Williams ES, Miller MW, Gambetti P, Schonberger LB. Emerg Infect Dis 2004;10:977–983.

Bioterrorism agents: Implications for animals. www.mda.state.md.us/pdf/animlimp.pdf.

Botulism: Background Information for Clinicians, 2006. http://emergency.cdc.gov/agent/Botulism/clinicians/Background.asp.

Bovine spongiform encephalopathy, 2002. www.who.int/mediacentre/factsheets/fs113/en/print.html.

Brucellosis (*Brucella melitensis, abortus, suis,* and *canis*), Division of Bacterial and Mycotic Diseases, 2005. www.cdc.gov/ndidod/dbm/diseaseinfo/brucellosis_t.htm.

Brucellosis outbreak at a pork processing plant—North Carolina, 1992. Morbid Mort Wkly Rep MMWR 1994;43(07):113–116. www.cdc.gov/mmwr/preview/mmwrhtml/00024911.htm.

Canadian Centre for Occupational Health and Safety. Psittacosis, 1998. www.ccohs.ca/oshanswers/diseases/psittacosis.html.

Case Definition: Trichothecene Mycotoxin, Emergency Preparedness and Response, 2006. http://emergency.cdc.gov/agent/trichothecene/casedef.asp.

CDC Health Advisory, Emergency Preparedness and Response, 2008. http://emergency.cdc.gov/agent/ricin/han_022008.asp.

CDC Information on arboviral encephalitides, 2005. www.cdc.gov/ndidod/dvbid/arbor/arbdet.htm.

Center for Emerging Issues, Emerging disease notice update Nipah virus, Malaysia, 1999. www.aphis.usda.gov/vs/ceah/cei/taf/emergingdiseasenotice_hles/nipahupd.htm.

Center for Emerging Issues, Nipah Virus, Malaysia, May 1999, emerging disease notice, 1999. www.aphis.usda.gov/vs/ceah/cei/taf/emergingdiseasenotice_files/nipah.htm.

Clostridium perfringens: Not the 24 Hour Flu, 1998. http://ohioline.osu.edu/hyg-fact/5000/5568.html.

Compendium of measures to prevent disease associated with animals in public settings, 2007. MMWR Recommend Rep 2007;56(RR-5):5. www.cdc.gov/mmwr/PDF/rr/rr5606.pdf.

Dvorak GD, Spickler AR. Glanders. JAVMA 2008;233:570–577.

Ebola hemorrhagic fever information packet, 2002. www.cdc.gov/ncidod/dvrd/spb/mnpages/dispages/fact_sheets/ebola_fact_booklet.pdf.

Fact sheet *Clostridium perfringens* food poisoning, 1998. www.johnson-county.com.

Fact sheet: Anthrax information for health care providers, March 8, 2002. www.emergency.cdc.gov/agent/anthrax/anthrax-hcp-factsheet.asp.

Facts About Ricin, 2008. http://emergency.cdc.gov/agent/ricin/facts.asp.

Foreign Animal Diseases, The Gray Book. 1998. Committee on Foreign Animal Diseases of the United States Animal Health Association. Suite 114, 1610 Forest Avenue, P.O. Box K227, Richmond, Virginia 23288.

Glanders (*Burkholderia mallei*), 2008. www.cdc.gov.nczved/dfbmd/disease-listing/glanders_gi.html.

Glaser A. West Nile encephalitis: A new differential for neurological illness in dogs and cats. DVM Newsmagazine 2003;June:16–19.

Glynn MK, Lynn TV. Brucellosis. JAVMA 2008;233:900–908.

Guidelines for conducting surveillance for hantavirus in rodents in California, 2004. www.dhs.ca.gov.

Hanta virus, 2000. www.hantaviru.net.

Hantavirus. http://en.wikipedia.org/wiki/Hantavirus.

Hantavirus pulmonary syndrome (HPS): What you need to know, 2006. www.cdc. gov/ncidod/diseases/hanta/hps/noframes/FAQ.htm.

Hendra and Nipah viruses. www.health.vic.gov.au/ideas/bluebook/hendra.

Hendra virus disease and Nipah virus encephalitis, 2007. www.cdc.gov/ncidod/dvrd/ spb/mnpages/dispages/nipah.htm.

Henipavirus. http://en.wikipedia.org/wiki/Henipavirus.

Howard JL, editor: Current Veterinary Therapy, 2: Food Animal Practice. Philadelphia, WB Saunders.

Hulbert LC, Oehme FW. Plants Poisonous to Livestock, ed 3. Manhattan, KS, Kansas State University Printing Service, 1981.

International Notes: Bolivian hemorrhagic fever—El Beni Department, Bolivia. Morbid Mort Wkly Rep MMWR 1994;43:943–946.

Key facts about tularemia, 2003. www.emergency.cdc.gov/agent/tularemia/facts.asp.

Krishanan S, Biswas K. Nipah outbreak in India and Bangladesh. Commun Dis Dept Newslett 2007;4(2):June. www.searo.who.int/en/Section10/Section372_13452.htm.

Laboratory-acquired human Glanders—Maryland, May 2000. Morbid Mort Wkly Rep MMWR 2000;49(24):532–535. www.cdc.gov/mmwr/preview/mmwrhtml/ mm4924a3.htm.

Lassa fever fact sheet, 2004. www.cdc.gov/ncidod/dvrd/spb/mnpages/dispages/lassaf. htm.

Luby SP, Rahman M, Hossain MJ, Blum LS, Husain MM, Gurley E, Khan R, Ahmed B, Rahman S, Nahar N, Kenah E, Comer JA, Ksiazek TG. Foodborne transmission of Nipah virus, Bangladesh. Emerg Infect Dis 2006;12(12). www.cdc.gov/ncidod/ eid/vol12no12/pdfs/06–0732.pdf.

Marburg hemorrhagic fever fact sheet, 2007. www.cdc.gov/ncidod/dvrd/spb/mnpages/ dispages/marburg.qa.htm.

Melioidosis, Division of Foodborne, Bacterial and Mycotic Diseases (DFBMD). 2008. www.cdc.gov/nczved/dfbmd/disease_listing/melioidosis_gi.html.

Monkeypox infections in animals: Updated interim guidance for veterinarians, 2003. www.cdc.gov/ncidod/monkeypox/animalhandlers.htm. Nipah, 2004. www.cfsph. iastate.edu/Factsheets/pdfs/nipah.pdf.

Orriss GD. Animal diseases of public health importance. Emerg Infect Dis 1997;3(4).

Prevention of plague: Recommendations of the Advisory Committee on Immunization Practices (ACIP). MMWR Recommend Rep 1996;45(RR-14):1–15. www.cdc.gov/ mmwr/preview/mmwrhtml/00044836.htm.

Psittacosis (ornithosis, parrot fever, chlamydiosis), 2006. www.health.state.ny.us/ disesases/communicable/.

Q-fever, viral and rickettsial zoonoses branch, 2003. www.cdc.gov/ndidod/ddvrd/ qfever/.

Reynolds MG, Krebs JW, Comer JA, Sumner JW, Rushton TC, Lopez CE, Nicholson WL, Rooney JA, Lance-Parker SE, McQuiston JH, Paddock CD, Childs JE. Flying squirrel-associated typhus. Emerg Infect Dis 2003;9(10).

Ricin: Clinical Description, Emergency Preparedness and Response, 2008. http:// emergency.cdc.gov/agent/ricin/clinicians/clindesc.asp.

Ricin: Control Measures Overview for Clinicians, Emergency Preparedness and Response, 2006. http://emergency.cdc.gov/agent/ricin/clinicians/control.asp.

Ricin: Treatment Overview for Clinicians, Emergency Preparedness and Response, 2006. http://emergency.cdc.gov/agent/ricin/clinicians/treatment.asp.

Rift Valley Fever Fact Sheet. www.cdc.gov.

Rift Valley Fever, National Agricultural Biosecurity Center. http://nabc.ksu.edu.

Schmitt CK, Meysick KC, O'Brien AD. Bacterial toxins: Friends or foes? Emerg Infect Dis 1999;5(2). www.cdc.gov/ncidod/eid/vol5no2/schmitt.htm.

Shadomy SV, Smith TL. Anthrax. JAVMA 2008;233:63–72.

Spicler AR, Roth JA. *Emerging and Exotic Diseases of Animals*, ed 3. 2006.

Staphylococcal food poisoning, 2006. www.cdc.gov/ncidod/dbmd/diseaseinfo/staphlococcus_food_g.htm.

Su HP, Chou CY, Tzeng SC, Feng T, Chen YL, Chen YS, Chung TC. Possible typhoon-related melioidosis epidemic, Taiwan 2005. Emerg Infect Dis 2006;12(11). www.cdc.gov/eid,

T-2 mycotoxin. http://en/wikipedia.org/wiki/T-2_mycotoxin.

Ten Asbroek AH, Borgdorff MW, Nagelkerke NJ, Sebek MM, Deville W, van Embden JD, van Soolingen D. Estimation of serial interval and incubation period of tuberculosis using DNA fingerprinting. Int J Tuberc Lung Dis 1999;3:414–420.

The Merck Veterinary Manual, ed 6. Rahway, NJ, Merck and Company.

The Merck Veterinary Manual, ed 8. Rahway, NJ, Merck and Company.

Tuberculosis: What you need to know, 1997. www.fsis.usda.gov/OPHS/tbbroch.htm.

Typhus Fever—Frequently Asked Questions, Bureau of Emergency Preparedness and Response Home Page. 2005. www.azdhs.gov.

Venezuelan Equine Encephalitis (Profile for Healthcare Workers), 2005. www.azdhs.gov.

Vial PA, Valdivieso F, Mertz G, Castillo C, Belmar E, Delgado I, Tapia M, Ferres M. Incubation period of hantavirus cardiopulmonary syndrome. Emerg Infect Dis 2006;12:1271–1273.

West Nile virus. www.healthpet.com.

West Nile virus. www.nsc.org/resources/Factsheets/environment/west_nile_ virus.aspx.

West Nile virus and dogs and cats, 2003. www.cdc.gov/ncidod/dvbid/westnile/qa/wnv_dogs_cats.htm.

West Nile virus fact sheet, 2005. www.cdc.gov/ncidod/dvbid/westnile/wnv_factsheet.htm.

West Nile virus in horses: Diagnosis and prevention tips.www.michigan.gov/documents/MDA_WNVHorses_8938_7.pdf.

Western Equine Encephalitis (Profile for Healthcare Workers), 2005. www.azdhs.gov.

What horse owners should know about West Nile virus, 2006. www.ohioline.osu.edu/wnv-fact/1007.html.

Yagupsky P, Baron EJ. Laboratory exposures to Brucellae and implications for bioterrorism. Emerg Infect Dis 2005;11(8). www.cdc.gov/eid.

Young JC, Hansen GR, Graves TK, Deasy MP, Humphreys JG, Fritz CL, Gorham KL, Kan AS, Ksiazek TG, Metzger KB, Peters CJ. The incubation period of hantavirus pulmonary syndrome. Am J Trop Med Hygiene 2000;62:714–717.

CHAPTER 9
SELECTED ANIMAL PATHOGENS

Sherrie L. Nash, MS, DVM

The following animal pathogens have been selected because of the importance of the role they play in causing disease in various animals. Many of the pathogens listed in this chapter are foreign animal diseases (FADs). These diseases become important because they can either be introduced accidentally or intentionally into the United States. Animal agriculture would be quickly impacted by any FAD and the consequences are not only economic but also psychological. Millions to billions of dollars would be needed to eradicate the disease or to immunize the affected animals. Thousands to millions of animals would have to be destroyed or would be lost due to disease. In addition, livelihoods of livestock owners would be severely impacted or destroyed, as well as the trust lost by the public in animal agriculture. As veterinarians and animal responders, it is important to promptly recognize an unusual disease presentation or FAD. In addition, methods of controlling and preventing the spread of disease should be readily available. Some of the diseases listed here are also capable of causing serious illness in working dogs and horses as well as humans. It is imperative to know when extra precautions should be put in place when dealing with a suspicious pathogen.

The Office International des Epizooties (OIE) was established in 1924. In 2003, the OIE became the World Organization for Animal Health, but it is still recognized as the OIE. Many diseases in this chapter are listed according to how they should be reported. An OIE List A Disease requires immediate reporting to state and federal authorities. An OIE List B Disease requires reporting to state and federal authorities. Other diseases that are listed as reportable in the United States may vary by state, but they should always be reported to state and federal authorities.

9. Selected Animal Pathogens

9.1. African Horse Sickness (AHS) (La Peste Equina, Pestis Equorum, Peste Equina Africana, Perdesiekte)

9.1.1. *Agent:* AHS is a highly fatal arthropod-borne virus of Equidae. It is an orbivirus (double-stranded RNA) with nine serotypes. Four forms of the disease are present: Peracute (pulmonary), acute (mixed—both pulmonary

193

and cardiac), subacute (cardiac), and mild (fever). Horses and mules are considered indicator hosts for AHS.

9.1.2. *Affected species:* Horses (death rates of 70%–95%) and mules (death rates of 50%) are very susceptible to AHS. Donkeys (0% for African, 5%–10% for European and Asian), zebras (0% and permanent carrier), camels, and elephants appear resistant to the disease. Dogs get the disease by eating infected raw meat. Dogs appear to be a dead-end host for the disease. Cattle and sheep are resistant to AHS (Table 9.1).

Table 9.1. African Horse Sickness.

Disease Severity in Potentially Affected Species S = Severe D = Moderate M = Mild								
Dogs	**Horses**	**Cattle**	**Sheep**	**Goats**	**Pigs**	**Cats**	**Birds**	**Other Animals**
S	S Mules							M Donkeys, zebras, camels, elephants

9.1.3. *Incubation period.* The incubation period is 3–5 days for the pulmonary form, 1–2 weeks for the cardiac form, and 4–14 days for the fever form of the disease.

9.1.4. *Transmission:* AHS is spread primarily by gnats and midges. Biting flies and mosquitoes may also play a role in the spread of the disease. Transmission is seasonal, so the disease only occurs when the weather is warm and moist. It is not spread by direct contact.

9.1.5. *Occurrence:* AHS is endemic in Africa and is also present in Spain, most of the Middle East, Pakistan, and India.

9.1.6. *Predominant clinical signs:* The peracute or pulmonary form has a mortality rate in horses approaching 95%. A high fever (104°–106°F) is present for 1–2 days. Increased respiration with severe dyspnea occurs. Horses will stand with their necks extended, nostrils dilated, front legs apart, have uncontrolled coughing, and copious sweating. These horses die from severe hypoxia within hours of being dyspneic. Prior to death or at death, there is a copious amount of frothy discharge from the nose. The subacute edematous or cardiac form has a mortality rate of 50%–70%. A fever (103°–106°F) is present for 3–6 days. There is swelling of the supraorbital fossa (pathognomonic), head, neck, chest, and shoulders. Some horses may develop colic before death. Death occurs as a result of cardiac failure 4–8 days after the fever. The acute or mixed form is usually diagnosed after death, on necropsy. Respiratory signs are typically mild and swelling of the head, neck, and chest occurs. Death is a result of cardiac failure. Many of these horses will clinically show signs of the cardiac form of the disease before the respiratory form. The mild or fever form (horsesickness fever) of AHS will have a fever (up to 104°F) that may last 3–8 days. Fever may be the only sign seen and is usually higher in the afternoon versus earlier in the day. Other signs that may be seen with the fever form of the disease include depression, anorexia, and congested mucous membranes. This form of AHS is seen in zebras, donkeys, and horses that have had immunity to a different serotype of AHS. Nearly all of these horses survive. **Dogs** infected with AHS have the pulmonary form of the disease.

9.1.7. *Treatment:* There is no treatment available. There are vaccines for all of the nine serotypes. Mouse-brain attenuated vaccine provides longer lasting immunity, but occasionally causes encephalitis in horses and mules. An inactivated vaccine requiring two doses (3 weeks apart) is available, but protection is short lived.

9.1.8. *Prevention:* The most important means of preventing disease in countries without AHS is strict quarantine and testing of all equine species. The United States has mandatory 60-day quarantine in an insect-proof facility of all equidae from Africa, the Mediterranean, and Asia. In countries where the disease occurs or areas known to have had the disease should be identified and movement of equide should be stopped. All equidae should be monitored for signs of disease. Equidae should be housed from dusk to dawn to limit exposure to arthropods. In addition, animals should be sprayed with an insecticide. Rectal temperatures should be taken twice daily and any animals with a fever should be isolated and placed in an insect-proof facility until AHS can be ruled out. Vaccination with the appropriate serotype should be performed on all susceptible equine. AHS is a reportable disease in the United States and an OIE List A Disease.

9.1.9. *Control:* Control of arthropod populations will decrease the risk of disease. Planes flying from endemic regions to AHS-free countries should be sprayed with insecticide.

9.1.10. *Zoonotic potential:* Humans are not susceptible to AHS other than exposure to the neurotropic forms of vaccine via intranasal route, which may cause encephalitis and retinitis.

9.2. African Swine Fever (ASF) (Pesti Porcine Africaine, Maladie de Montgomery, Fiebre Porcina Afticana)

9.2.1. *Agent:* ASF is a tick-borne, highly contagious, and usually fatal disease of swine only caused by Asfarviridae family. It is the only DNA virus transmitted by arthropods and is probably a tick virus with pigs as the accidental host. Three different strains are present: highly virulent (causes peracute and acute disease), moderately virulent (subacute disease), and low virulent (chronic disease).

9.2.2. *Affected species:* Domestic swine, European wild boar, and African wild swine (Wart hog, Giant forest hog, and Bush pig). All ages of pigs are susceptible to the disease (Table 9.2).

Table 9.2. African Swine Fever.

Disease Severity in Potentially Affected Species **S = Severe D = Moderate M = Mild**								
Dogs	**Horses**	**Cattle**	**Sheep**	**Goats**	**Pigs**	**Cats**	**Birds**	**Other Animals**
					S European boar			M Wart hog, bush pig

9.2.3. *Incubation period:* The incubation period is 5–15 days by contact and less than 5 days by tick bite. The acute form has an incubation of 5–7 days.

9.2.4. *Transmission:* Mode of transmission is primarily by direct contact (between sick and healthy animals). Direct contact is most likely through the oral-nasal route. All tissues and body secretions are infectious, especially blood. Indirect contact occurs through Ornithodorus soft ticks, vehicles, equipment, boots, clothes, and feeding unprocessed or uncooked garbage with infected meat. Another potential source of ASF is sausage that is often smuggled into the United States.

9.2.5. *Occurrence:* It occurs in sub-Saharan Africa and on the island of Sardinia, Italy. It has occurred in Europe (Spain, Portugal, Belgium, the Netherlands), the Caribbean (Cuba, Dominican Republic), and Brazil.

9.2.6. *Predominant clinical signs:* There are four basic forms of the disease: peracute, acute, subacute, and chronic. Mortality rates may reach 10% in the peracute and acute forms (highly virulent strain). Survivors of the peracute and acute forms are carriers for life. The peracute form causes sudden death. The acute form is characterized by high fever (105–108°F), depression, red to purplish skin discoloration, diarrhea, and vomiting. There may be loss of appetite, huddling, as well as coughing and dyspnea. Abortion can occur at any stage of pregnancy, with these animals dying a few days after aborting. Death usually occurs within 4–10 days. In the subacute form of the disease (moderately virulent strain), death occurs in 30%–70% of the affected pigs. The chronic form of ASF (low virulent strain) is characterized by skin ulcers, transient fever (may be recurrent), and joint lesions. Pneumonia, lack of growth and emaciation are common. There is low mortality and these pigs can transmit the virus for 1 month or longer. Pigs that survive from the less virulent strains of ASF are apparently persistently infected for life, although they do not appear to transmit the virus to their offspring or other pigs.

9.2.7. *Treatment:* There is no treatment available. Attempts at developing a vaccine have not been successful due to the inability to neutralize the vaccine with antibodies.

9.2.8. *Control:* Slaughter and disposal of all acutely infected pigs, along with widespread testing and elimination of all seropositive animals is recommended. Good herd isolation and sanitary practices can accomplish control and eradication of ASF in developed countries. It is suggested that control of rodent populations may help. ASF is a reportable disease in the United States and is an OIE List A Disease.

9.2.9. *Decontamination:* ASF is very stable in the environment. It is stable at a pH of 4–13. It can survive in pork products for 6 months, 15 weeks in chilled meat, and up to 15 years in frozen carcasses. Parma Hams are commonly smuggled into the United States and ASF lasts up to 300 days in this product. Pig pens that are contaminated with ASF remain so for up to 1 month. ASF is present in purified blood for 15 weeks. Disinfectants that can be used include bleach (5.25% chlorine): 0.1%–3% chlorine, Betadine, 1% Virkon S, and 1% One Stroke Environ.

9.2.10. *Zoonotic potential:* Humans are not susceptible to ASF.

9.3. Aujeszky's Disease (AJD) (Pseudorabies, Mad Itch, Infectious Bulbar Paralysis)

9.3.1. *Agent:* AJD is caused by a porcine DNA alphaherpesvirus in the family Herpesviridae. It causes an acute respiratory infection in older pigs and it may be fatal in young pigs.

9.3.2. *Affected species:* Pigs are the main host, but sporadic cases have occurred in cattle, sheep, goats, horses, dogs, cats, and rodents. Almost all mammals, except for humans and tailless apes, can naturally be infected by AJD (Table 9.3).

Table 9.3. Aujeszky's Disease.

Disease Severity in Potentially Affected Species S = Severe D = Moderate M = Mild								
Dogs	**Horses**	**Cattle**	**Sheep**	**Goats**	**Pigs**	**Cats**	**Birds**	**Other Animals**
S	M	S	S	S	S	S	M?	S Rodents, skunks, raccoons, foxes, opossums

9.3.3. *Incubation period:* Death in newborn pigs can occur as early as 1 day of age. The incubation period is thought to be about 48 hours in older pigs.

9.3.4. *Transmission:* AJD is highly contagious and is principally spread via the respiratory route from infected pigs. Pigs transmit the disease via oral-nasal secretions, fecal-oral contact, inhalation, milk, breeding boars, and the placenta. AJD diseased tissue of pigs used for food is another source of infection. Other mammals (dogs, cats, rodents) may also spread the disease.

9.3.5. *Occurrence:* This disease is endemic in the swine of many countries including Mexico, Cuba, Venezuela, Brazil, Europe, Asia, Samoa, and New Zealand. The United States has been free of the disease since May 2005.

9.3.6. *Predominant clinical signs:* The death rate is very high among younger pigs (can be up to 100%) versus older pigs (40%–60% in 3- to 4-week-old pigs) who may have mild to no signs present. Rapid onset of signs is seen in young pigs where neurological signs are more prominent. Signs include depression, fever, vomiting, paddling, tremors, ataxia, convulsions, and death. The most prominent signs seen in weaned pigs are sneezing and dyspnea. Intense itching may be observed. Abortion occurs in the sow. The most distinctive sign seen in cattle, sheep, and goats is severe biting, rubbing, and licking. The illness is usually short in duration (1–2 days). Along with the itching, there is fever, vocalization, stomping, paralysis of hind limbs, staggering, and aggression. For the most part, AJD is fatal in ruminants. Dogs and cats are most susceptible to AJD through the oral route. They will suddenly become ill and die before any swine on the farm are showing signs of illness.

9.3.7. *Treatment:* No treatment is available.

9.3.8. *Prevention:* Vaccination with a modified live virus (MLV) may be useful in reducing signs seen in some age groups of pigs. It may help losses in herds in which the disease is a continuing problem. The vaccine does not necessarily prevent infection or shedding of the virus. AJD is a reportable disease in the United States and is an OIE List B Disease.

9.3.9. *Decontamination:* AJD is a fairly stable virus in the environment. Disinfection can be done with bleach, 1%–2% sodium hydroxide, 5% phenol, ether, chloroform, and quaternary ammonia. It is easily inactivated by sunlight, high temperature, and drying.

9.3.10. *Zoonotic potential:* Humans are not susceptible to Aujeszky's disease.

9.4. Avian Influenza (AI) (Fowl Plague, H5N1)

9.4.1. *Agent:* AI is a virus in the Orthomyxoviridae family with type A influenza being significant. The virus ranges from a mild or even asymptomatic infection to an acute, fatal disease of chickens, turkeys, ducks, guinea fowls, and other avian species. Migratory waterfowl are also affected. The virus is found in the intestinal tract of wild birds.

9.4.2. *Affected species:* Most avian species appear to be affected by AI, including imported pet birds, birds at live markets, ratites, and apparently normal sea birds. Ducks appear to have a less virulent form of the disease. Type A influenza viruses will usually have specificity for a particular species. (Bird virus will infect the same type of birds; human virus infects other humans.) Pigs located near turkeys appear to be a reservoir for swine influenza in the turkeys. Humans have also been infected by AI. Recent strains of AI (2003–2004) in Asia have been found in dogs, cats, and other mammals (Fig. 9.1).

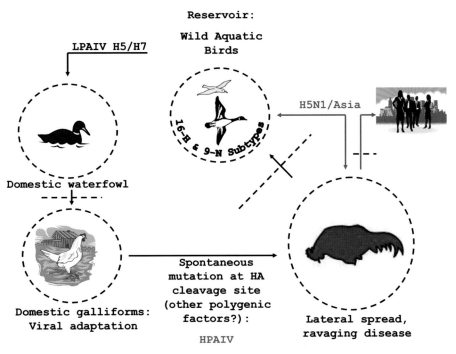

Figure 9.1. Avian influenza pathogenesis and epidemiology. LPAIV, low pathogenic avian influenza virus; HPAIV, highly pathogenic avian influenza virus; HA, hemagglutinin protein; dotted lines with arrows represent species barriers.

Domestic and large cats, as well as dogs, have been infected with high pathogenic AI by consuming raw meat or carcasses. Both cats and dogs have died as a result of eating the infected meat. Transmission in cats appears to occur from domestic cat-to-cat. There is no evidence at present that these infected cats or dogs are contagious to humans, but precautions should be taken because the possibility exists (Table 9.4).

9.4.3. *Incubation period:* A variable incubation period of 1–7 days.

Table 9.4. Avian Influenza.

Disease Severity in Potentially Affected Species S = Severe D = Moderate M = Mild								
Dogs	Horses	Cattle	Sheep	Goats	Pigs	Cats	Birds	Other Animals
S					S	S Big cats	S Turkeys, chickens, quail, pheasants	M Possible?

9.4.4. *Transmission:* Current thought is that waterfowl, sea birds, and shore birds are responsible for introducing the virus into poultry. Most common methods of transmission are aerosol and fecal-oral in birds. Once AI has been introduced to a flock, the virus is easily spread by infected birds, equipment, personnel, feed trucks, flies, and other fomites. Transmission is usually bird-to-bird, human-to-human, or pig-to-pig, although interspecies transmission is possible. Low pathogenic AI does have the ability to mutate to the high pathogenic form.

9.4.5. *Occurrence:* Highly pathogenic AI viruses (H5 and H7 subtypes) have been found worldwide—in recent years, in Australia, Cambodia, China, Korea, Indonesia, Thailand, Vietnam, Malaysia, Mongolia, the Netherlands, England, Ireland, Scotland, Italy, South Africa, Pakistan, Romania, Turkey, Croatia, Russia, Ukraine, Chile, Mexico, and the United States.

9.4.6. *Predominant clinical signs:* Signs can be variable with AI—low (LP) to high pathogenicity (HP). HP AI is sudden onset and quickly spreads throughout the flock. Mortality is high with the HP form of AI (H5 and H7 subtypes). Depression, inappetence, and respiratory signs are commonly seen. There is often cyanosis and edema of the head, comb, and waddle. Blood-tinged nasal and oral discharges, greenish-to-white diarrhea, discolored shanks and feet may also be noted. Egg production decreases and eggs may be laid without shells as the disease progresses. Turkeys, ducks, and quail may have a sinusitis. Death can occur within 24 hours of the first signs seen, although usually within 48 hours. Some birds may survive up to 1 week before dying. A few birds may even survive the disease.

9.4.7. *Treatment:* A vaccine is available but it must be the same strain present in the flock to be effective. The control of secondary bacteria with broad-spectrum antibiotics and raising the temperature of the house may help to reduce losses.

9.4.8. *Control:* The practice of strict sanitation and biosecurity procedures in the raising of poultry is of the utmost importance. Restricting access to the houses is another way to decrease the possibility of introducing disease. The all-in, all-out management of birds is recommended. Areas where waterfowl, shore birds, or sea birds are prevalent should be avoided if possible, since these birds can serve as a source of infection. Cleaning and disinfection procedures are critical. In the face of an outbreak, the best measure may be to test and euthanize birds on all affected premises. AI is reportable in the United States and high pathogenic avian influenza is an OIE List A Disease.

9.4.9. *Decontamination:* Strict sanitation and restricting access to poultry houses will help in preventing the spread of disease.

9.4.10. *Zoonotic potential:* Humans are susceptible to AI. Avian influenza is a type A influenza virus, which can potentially mutate and become infective to other mammals, including humans. The infection and the subsequent deaths of 6 of 18 humans infected with an AI virus in Hong Kong in 1997 has raised the question of the role the avian species plays in influenza in humans. Humans in direct contact with infected birds or contaminated fomites are at risk. Handling of infected meat, such as in cooking, may be another source of infection. Signs in humans include flu-like symptoms, respiratory disease, pneumonia, ophthalmia (eye infections), and serious complications, including death. At present, AI is rarely spread from person to person, but because influenza is a highly mutative virus, the potential is there for it to become more virulent.

9.5. Babesiosis (Piroplasmosis, Texas Cattle Fever, Redwater Disease, Tick Fever, Texas Fever)

9.5.1. *Agent:* Babesiosis is an infectious, intraerythrocytic protozoan in the *Babesia* genus. It is of primary economic importance in the cattle industry, although other animals as well as humans can be infected with it. There are about six strains of *Babesia* that cause disease in cattle. Only two of these strains are of importance in the United States—*B. bovis* and *B. bigemina*. Ticks are the main source of infection.

9.5.2. *Affected species:* In addition to infecting cattle, Babesiosis infects sheep, horses, pigs, goats, and dogs. Humans may also be infected (Table 9.5).

Table 9.5. Babesiosis.

Disease Severity in Potentially Affected Species S = Severe D = Moderate M = Mild								
Dogs	Horses	Cattle	Sheep	Goats	Pigs	Cats	Birds	Other Animals
S	S	S	M	M	S			S Water buffalo, African buffalo

9.5.3. *Incubation period:* The incubation period is typically 2–3 weeks from the initial tick contact. Once *Babesia* spp. has been introduced into the blood, the incubation period is probably no longer than 4–5 days with *B. bigemina* and 10–14 days with *B. bovis* in cattle.

9.5.4. *Transmission:* The *Boophilus* spp. tick (one host) is the primary tick in cattle. Transovarial transmission (from the ovary to the eggs in ticks) occurs. Other species of ticks are also capable of causing the disease in cattle and other animals. These ticks include *Rhipicephalus, Ixodes, Haemaphysalis, Hyalomma,* and *Dermacentor.* Mechanical transfer of infected blood can occur through fomites and biting flies. Rarely does intrauterine infection cause disease. Babesiosis is spread when ticks feed on infected animals. The now *Babesia*-infected tick transmits the disease to the developing larvae of the tick. The larvae become infected nymphs and adults that then feed on naïve animals. Thus, the transfer of *Babesia* occurs.

9.5.5. *Occurrence:* Babesiosis is found worldwide and is mostly a disease of the subtropics and lowland tropics. In North and South America, it predominantly affects cattle. It was first described in the United States in 1814. The first serious outbreak did not occur until 1868, when 15,000 cattle died. It has since been eradicated in the United States, where it was endemic in the southern regions. Babesiosis occasionally occurs along the United States and Mexican borders. It may still be found from Mexico to Argentina.

9.5.6. *Predominant clinical signs:* Fever (105.8°–106.7°F) is the initial sign seen and remains throughout the course of the disease. Loss of appetite followed by rumen stasis is noted. The affected animal will seek shade, isolate itself, and appear uncomfortable. The *Babesia* organism infects and damages the erythrocytes, causing them to rupture, which leads to anemia (Fig. 9.2).

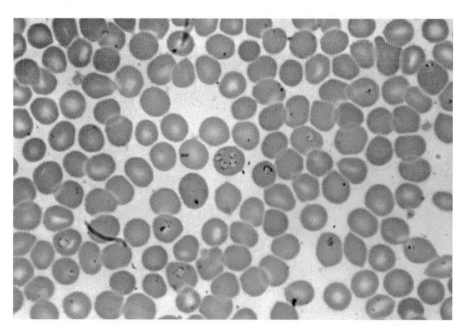

Figure 9.2. The *Babesia* organism parasitizes red cells as shown in this blood film. (Source: Public Domain, Image ID# 5943; http://phil.cdc.gov/phil/details.asp.)

In the later stages of disease, hemoglobinemia and hemoglobinuria will occur once lysis of 75% or more of the red blood cells occurs. Other initial signs of disease include a poor hair coat, lack of an appetite, depression, icterus, increased respiratory and heart rate, weight loss, muscle tremors, dehydration, diarrhea or constipation, and abortion (late term). CNS signs consist of convulsions, arched back, and coma, all of which are more common with *B. bovis* than *B. bigemina*. The CNS signs are a result of destruction of the red blood cells and/or blockage of the brain capillaries by the infected red blood cells. Death usually results from severe anemia, the discharge of vasoactive substances, and the buildup of toxins. Mortality may be as high as 50%, especially if the animal is stressed.

9.5.7. *Predominant clinical signs:* Clinical disease in endemic areas is dependent on calves having immunity owing to colostrum that protects them for about 6 months. Their resistance decreases with age. Commonly, cattle in endemic regions rarely show signs of disease. They become infected as calves and become carriers of Babesiosis. Generally, *B. bigemina* is not as pathogenic as *B. bovis*, but strains of the protozoa vary in virulence. *B. bigemina* in Africa is a serious pathogen versus *B. bigeminia* in Australia, which seldom causes clinical signs.

9.5.8. *Treatment:* Supportive care includes fluids, blood transfusions, corticosteroids, anti-inflammatories, antioxidants, or no treatment if easily agitated. These animals may become anoxic, so care should be performed when handling them. The medications Diminazene aceturate and imidocarb dipropionate are most often used. Their use may be restricted in some countries or availability may be limited. The use of long-acting tetracyclines shortly after infection or prior to infection may decrease the severity of the disease.

9.5.9. *Prevention:* Live, attenuated vaccines are available and very effective. The vaccine has the potential to cause disease in cattle, so vaccination is only recommended in endemic areas. Some animals may need to be treated after vaccination to help control the disease since it is a modified-live vaccine. Control of ticks should be done, but is not always very effective. If the ticks are eradicated or substantially decreased, such as *Boophilis* spp. in the United States, cattle and other animals become susceptible. Tick numbers need to be maintained in endemic areas to cause a low infection rate for immunization of animals to occur. This is a blood-borne disease so disinfection is only effective when equipment, instruments, or needles contaminated with blood are cleaned. Sanitizing or disinfecting does little to control Babesioses. Babesiosis is reportable in the United States.

9.5.10. *Zoonotic potential:* Humans are susceptible to babesiosis. Individuals who are immunocompromised or who have had splenectomies may have fatal infections. Infections in humans are the result of either infected ticks biting them or receiving infected blood from a transfusion.

9.6. Bluetongue (BT) (Sore Muzzle, Muzzle Disease, Pseudo Foot-and-Mouth Disease)

9.6.1. *Agent:* Bluetongue is an acute, noncontagious, arthropod-borne disease of sheep, goats, cattle, wild ruminants, and carnivores caused by an Orbivirus in the Reoviridae family. There are 24 serotypes of BT. Sheep are most affected with lesions being on the mucous membranes and swelling of the coronary band.

9.6.2. *Affected species:* Sheep and wild ruminants are most susceptible to BT. Cattle and goats with unapparent infections are important reservoirs of the virus (Table 9.6).

Table 9.6. Bluetongue.

Disease Severity in Potentially Affected Species S = Severe D = Moderate M = Mild								
Dogs	**Horses**	**Cattle**	**Sheep**	**Goats**	**Pigs**	**Cats**	**Birds**	**Other Animals**
M		M	S	M				S Wild ruminants (big horn sheep, pronghorn antelope, white-tailed deer)

9.6.3. *Incubation period:* The incubation period is about 5–10 days in sheep. Cattle usually have no signs but may have viremia 4 days after being exposed. The incubation period in deer is 7–12 days.

9.6.4. *Transmission:* BT is a seasonal disease, being present only during the warmer months. It may be present year-round in warmer climates. Gnats (*Culicoides*) are the major biological vector in the United States for transmitting the disease. Sheep keds and ticks may occasionally serve as mechanical vectors for the disease. Needles and surgical equipment may also serve as mechanical vectors.

9.6.5. *Occurrence:* Occurrence is worldwide.

9.6.6. *Predominant clinical signs:* Signs of BT in cattle are subclinical. If it is seen, it may affect only up to 30% of cattle. Signs of disease may include oral vesicles and ulcers, nasal exudate and erosions, salivation, fever, lacrimation, hyperesthesia, and dermatitis with vesicles and ulcers. The skin may have crusty, dry exudates, and it becomes thickened, especially in the cervical area. There may be decreased fertility in cows. Some bulls may have transitory infertility when acutely infected with BT. Infection during fetal development (between 60 and 140 days) may cause cerebral cysts and hydranencephaly. In sheep, signs may be subclinical, mild, or severe depending on the strain of BT. Mortality rates may reach 30%–50%. Signs include dyspnea, fever (up to 107.5°F), depression, weight loss, hyperemia and edema of the lips, muzzle, and ears. Nasal discharge often causes crustiness of the muzzle. The tongue may be swollen and cyanotic ("blue tongue"). Erosions and ulcers can be seen on the oral mucosa and dental pad. Lameness is due to coronitis of the hooves. Abortion and congenital defects occur in susceptible pregnant sheep. Goats are similar to cattle, they typically are asymptomatic. Pregnant dogs will abort their pups or have stillborn pups and then die 3–7 days later. White-tailed deer and pronghorn antelope can suddenly die from the severe hemorrhagic form of the disease.

9.6.7. *Treatment:* Treatment is supportive. Minimize animal stress and administer broad-spectrum antibiotics to reduce secondary infections.

9.6.8. *Prevention:* A modified-live attenuated (MLV) vaccine is available for use in sheep in the United States. Due to multiple serotypes of BT, the vaccine is effective only when the serotype is the same as that causing disease. The MLV vaccine is not recommended for use during the vector season as there is debate as to whether the vaccine can reassort to infect other animals with the vaccine strain. BT is reportable in many states in the United States.

9.6.9. *Control:* Use of insecticides (sprays, fly tags, back rubbers), housing animals indoors from dusk to dawn, and water management all decrease exposure to the arthropod. Vector control will help decrease incidence of the disease. Common disinfectants are only useful when cleaning instruments and equipment. They are ineffective in controlling virus spread between animals.

9.6.10. *Zoonotic potential:* Humans are not typically susceptible to BT. However, caution should be used as there is one documented human infection (a laboratory worker).

9.7. Canine Influenza (CI)

9.7.1. *Agent:* CI is an emerging disease of dogs caused by a type A Orthomyxovirus. This disease appears to have resulted from the horse influenza virus mutating and becoming a virus that is specific to infecting dogs. The importance of this disease is that it is very similar to kennel cough. Because CI is a relatively newly identified disease, nearly all dogs are vulnerable.

9.7.2. *Affected species:* Virtually 100% of dogs exposed to CI will become infected with CI and 80% of dogs will show mild signs of disease. Dogs that have been exposed to CI but do not show signs of disease can shed the virus and spread the disease. Fatality rate is less than 8% (Table 9.7).

Table 9.7. Canine Influenza.

Disease Severity in Potentially Affected Species S = Severe D = Moderate M = Mild								
Dogs	**Horses**	**Cattle**	**Sheep**	**Goats**	**Pigs**	**Cats**	**Birds**	**Other Animals**
S								

9.7.3. *Incubation period:* The incubation period appears to be about 2–5 days (experimentally as little as 1–2 days). CI infected dogs may be contagious for 7–10 days after signs are first seen.

9.7.4. *Transmission:* CI is spread primarily by aerosolization and direct contact with secretions of infected dogs (discharges from the nose, eyes, and coughing). Any fomite (bowls, cages, leashes, and bedding) that an infected dog has been in contact with or humans who have been in contact with infected dogs, also serves as a source of infection. No humans have become ill when exposed to CI, but precautions to limit exposure should be practiced.

9.7.5. *Occurrence:* CI was first recognized in Florida in 2004 in racing greyhounds. Since that time, CI has been reported in other states where racing greyhounds reside and in other breeds of dogs. All exposed dogs were located in animal shelters, boarding facilities, humane societies, pet stores, rescue groups, and veterinary clinics. Therefore, animals that are in close proximity to other dogs (boarding facilities, animal shelters, sports, shows, etc.) are at an increased risk of exposure to CI.

9.7.6. *Predominant clinical signs:* Two forms of CI exist—the mild form and the severe form. The mild form of CI resembles kennel cough and may be mistaken for it. There can be a soft, moist cough for 10–30 days. In addition, a thick discharge from the nose may be present, usually resulting from secondary bacterial infections (*Pasteurella multocida, Mycoplasma*). A low grade fever might also be noted. The severe form of CI presents as a fever (104°–106°F). Breathing will be difficult due to pneumonia. Dogs with kennel cough generally have a dry, harsh cough that lessens after 5 days. Coughing may last up to 10–20 days with CI. Dogs with kennel cough will gag, retch, and lose their appetite. Dogs with CI have worsening of signs (fever) and a discharge from the nose. Respiration increases and requires more effort to breathe. Death is due to hemorrhaging and high fever.

9.7.7. *Treatment:* Treatment for CI is supportive. Supportive care usually consists of antibiotics and good nutrition. Because CI is a virus, there are no effective antiviral medications available or a vaccine. The severe form of CI possibly will require hospitalization and intravenous fluids.

9.7.8. *Control:* No vaccine is currently available. Strict sanitation and biosecurity procedures should be performed to decrease the spread of disease.

9.7.9. *Decontamination:* Most disinfectants will clean equipment and surfaces. People handling animals should wash with soap and water or use personal sanitizers between animals to decrease the spread of infection. Laundry detergent will clean clothing and any infected bedding. Disposable gloves and gowns should be worn if handling numerous animals.

9.7.10. *Zoonotic potential:* At present, CI does not appear to be infectious to humans. People handling infected dogs should limit their exposure and practice biosecurity measures.

9.8. Caprine Arthritis and Encephalitis (CAE)

9.8.1. *Agent:* CAE is an enveloped single-stranded RNA lentivirus in the Retroviridae family. Most infections with CAE are not recognized (subclinical). It causes a polyarthritis in adult goats and occasionally a progressive paresis in kid goats. Many dairy goats in North America carry the disease and therefore cannot be exported.

9.8.2. *Affected species:* Dairy goats are susceptible to CAE while meat and wool-producing goats are not as susceptible. Lambs that suckle from infected goats become persistently infected with CAE (Table 9.8).

Table 9.8. Caprine Arthritis and Encephalitis.

Disease Severity in Potentially Affected Species S = Severe D = Moderate M = Mild								
Dogs	Horses	Cattle	Sheep	Goats	Pigs	Cats	Birds	Other Animals
			M Lambs	M				

9.8.3. *Incubation period:* Infection occurs while the goats are young. Clinical signs take months to years to be seen.

9.8.4. *Transmission:* CAE is spread through infected milk or colostrum. A common dairy goat practice is to pool the colostrum or milk and feed it to the kids. Therefore, one or several infected does can infect a large number of kids. Direct contact with infected animals, equipment, instruments, feeding utensils, and waterers is also a source of infection.

9.8.5. *Occurrence:* CAE is more common in countries such as the United States, Canada, France, Norway, and Switzerland. Greater than 65% of goats in these countries have been exposed to CAE. Developing countries with their own goat breeds do not have the problem unless imported goats have come into contact with the native breeds.

9.8.6. *Predominant clinical signs:* Arthritis is the main clinical sign seen in adult goats. Onset of arthritis may be progressive or abrupt. The carpal joints are most often affected and the disease becomes progressively worse. Swelling and lameness become more pronounced. These goats over time will lose weight and have poor quality hair coats. Chronic interstitial pneumonia may be seen in some adults as well as "hard udder" syndrome. Encephalitis is more common in kids 2–4 months of age but can occur in older kids and goats. Neurological signs include ascending paralysis, difficulty moving or standing, lameness, and paralysis. Additional neurological signs may include opisthotonos, circling, depression, head tilt, paddling, and torticollis.

9.8.7. *Treatment:* None other than supportive care.

9.8.8. *Control:* Four recommendations should be followed to decrease/eliminate CAE in a herd. a) Remove the kids at birth from their mothers, especially if the doe is seropositive for CAE. b) Colostrum should be heat-treated (60 minutes at 132.8°F) and milk should be pasteurized. c) Twice yearly testing of the herd, separating the seronegative animals from the seropositive. d) Culling of all the seropositive goats.

9.8.9. Disinfection: Phenolic or quaternary ammonium products may be used to disinfect equipment, instruments, feeders, etc.

9.8.10. *Zoonotic potential:* Humans are not susceptible to CAE.

9.9. Contagious Bovine Pleuropneumonia (CBPP)

9.9.1. *Agent:* CBPP is caused by *Mycoplasma mycoides mycoides* small colony type bacteria and affects primarily cattle. It is considered to be highly contagious and more common when cattle are closely confined. It can cause acute, subacute or chronic disease and principally affects the lungs and occasionally the joints. *M. mycoides mycoides* large-colony type does not cause disease in cattle, but affects both sheep and goats. Mortality ranges from 10%–70% in cattle.

9.9.2. *Affected species:* Bos cattle such as the European breeds (*Bos taurus*) and zebu (*Bos indicus*) are more susceptible than African cattle and zebra. Younger cattle, less than 3 years old, appear to be more susceptible than older cattle. Yak and bison in zoos and water buffalo have also been infected with CBPP. Camels and wild bovine appear not to be susceptible (Table 9.9).

9.9.3. *Incubation period:* Incubation is variable, 3 weeks to 4 months (most occurring in 3–8 weeks) after exposure.

9.9.4. *Transmission:* The principal mode of infection is by inhalation from coughing CBPP infected cattle. Saliva, fetal tissues, uterine secretions, and

Table 9.9. Contagious Bovine Pleuropneumonia.

	**Disease Severity in Potentially Affected Species** **S = Severe D = Moderate M = Mild**
Dogs	**Horses**	**Cattle**	**Sheep**	**Goats**	**Pigs**	**Cats**	**Birds**	**Other Animals**
		S	D	D				S Antelope, bison, reindeer, water buffalo, Yak

urine may also contain the bacteria. It is thought that cattle that survive the disease can become active carriers.

9.9.5. *Occurrence:* The disease occurs in Africa and some regions of Asia (especially India and China) and the Middle East, and occasionally there have been several outbreaks in Europe. CBPP was introduced in New York in 1843. It was the first disease to have an eradication program in the United States. The United States was declared CBPP free in 1893, and the Western Hemisphere is currently CBPP free.

9.9.6. *Predominant clinical signs:* There are three forms of CBPP: acute, subacute, and chronic. Acute and subacute forms of disease include anorexia, fever (up to 107°F), depression, dyspnea and painful breathing (may be open mouthed), and coughing. Animals stand with their elbows out to relieve the thoracic pain. Calves may have pneumonia as well as a polyarthritis, which causes swollen, painful joints. They become unwilling to move and may stand with an arched back. The chronic form of the disease may last 3–4 weeks. It can manifest itself as a low-grade fever, weight loss, lack of thriftiness, and coughing when forced to exercise. There can be asymptomatic carriers.

9.9.7. *Treatment:* Treatment is generally ineffective for this pathogen. Oxytetracycline, Tylosin, chloramphenicol, and streptomycin have been used, but these antimicrobials may slow the progression of the disease and cause sequestra (dead bone).

9.9.8. *Prevention:* Eradication of CBPP is done through quarantine, testing, and slaughter. A live attenuated vaccine is used in areas where eradication is not feasible. CBPP is a reportable disease in the United States and is an OIE List A Disease.

9.9.9. *Decontamination:* CBPP survives in the environment for only a few days. CBPP survives freezing, but it does not thrive in meat or meat products. Most disinfectants are effective against it.

9.9.10. *Zoonotic potential:* Humans are not susceptible to CBPP.

9.10. Contagious Equine Metritis (CEM) (Contagious Equine Metritis Organism)

9.10.1. *Agent:* CEM is a highly contagious gram-negative coccobacillus, *Taylorella equigenitalis*, that causes venereal disease in horses. There are differences in strains of the coccobacillus. The most prominent sign of disease is a mucopurulent vaginal discharge and decreased fertility in mares with initial exposure.

9.10.2. *Affected species:* Horses appear to be the only species susceptible to the disease. Thoroughbreds seem to be at higher risk for CEM. Donkeys have been experimentally infected with CEM (Table 9.10).

Table 9.10. Contagious Equine Metritis.

| Disease Severity in Potentially Affected Species S = Severe D = Moderate M = Mild | | | | | | | | |
Dogs	Horses	Cattle	Sheep	Goats	Pigs	Cats	Birds	Other Animals
	S							

9.10.3. *Incubation period:* Inflammation from CEM occurs as early as 24 hours postbreeding. Clinically, the first signs of the disease are seen 10–14 days postbreeding when the mare shows signs of being in estrus.

9.10.4. *Transmission:* Primary transmission is through breeding. Fomites (equipment) can also serve as a source of infection. Stallions infected with CEM are asymptomatic with the organism found on the external genitalia. Stallions and asymptomatic carrier mares can transmit the disease.

9.10.5. *Occurrence:* It has been reported mostly in Great Britain and parts of Europe including Italy, France, Ireland, Germany, Belgium, Denmark, Czechoslovakia, the Netherlands, Norway, Sweden, Luxembourg, and Switzerland. It has also been found in Australia and Japan. CEM has been eradicated from the United States.

9.10.6. *Predominant clinical signs:* Oftentimes the only sign of CEM in mares is an abbreviated estrus cycle or return to estrus. Mares with clinical signs will have a profuse vaginal discharge or evidence of a vaginal discharge approximately 10–14 days postbreeding. The discharge is present for only a few days, but the mare will remain chronically infectious for several months. These mares do not show any sign of the disease. Mares typically do not breed while infected with CEM. If the mare does get bred, the fetus is often aborted, infected in utero, or infected shortly after birth. These foals may become carriers. Morbidity is high as virtually every mare bred by an infected stallion will get CEM. Stallions are asymptomatic.

9.10.7. *Treatment:* Treatment of mares with antimicrobial drugs is not always effective, even though the disease-causing organism is generally susceptible to most antibiotics. The external genitalia of both the mare and stallion can be cleaned with soap and water, followed with chlorhexidine surgical scrub, and rinsed with water once daily for 5 days. Nitrofurazone ointment is then applied to the genitalia. The stallion should be retested 10 days after treatment. Mares usually clear up several weeks after the infection. Clitoral sinuses and fossa (depressed area) can remain a source of infection and are difficult to treat and clean. The clitoral sinuses can be surgically excised to help clear up the infection in mares.

9.10.8. *Prevention:* Some natural immunity is conferred and vaccination is not recommended because of the possibility of carriers.

9.10.9. *Control:* Detection, treatment, and quarantine of infected animals should be performed. Attempts should be made to eliminate actively infected animals and identify positive carriers. Most common disinfectants will deactivate *T. equigenitalis*. CEM is reportable in the United States and is an OIE List B Disease.

9.10.10. *Zoonotic potential:* Humans are not susceptible to CEM.

9.11. Dourine (el Dourin, Covering Disease, Mal de Coit, Slapsiekte, Beschalseuche, Morbo Coitale Maligno, Sluchnaya Bolyezn)

9.11.1. *Agent:* Dourine is one of the oldest diseases recognized in horses. It is a chronic, contagious venereal disease in horses caused by the protozoa *Trypanosoma equiperdum*.

9.11.2. *Affected species:* Horses, mules, and donkeys may be affected. Thoroughbred horses and other improved breeds seem to be more vulnerable than native donkeys, ponies, and mules. Donkeys are asymptomatic or latent carriers of Dourine. Zebras that have shown exposure to Dourine (via testing) do not appear infected or able to transmit the disease (Table 9.11).

Table 9.11. Dourine.

Disease Severity in Potentially Affected Species S = Severe D = Moderate M = Mild								
Dogs	Horses	Cattle	Sheep	Goats	Pigs	Cats	Birds	Other Animals
	S							M Donkeys, native ponies, mules

9.11.3. *Incubation period:* Dourine is a venereal disease that typically takes a few weeks to several months after initial exposure for clinical signs to occur. It can take up to several years before the disease becomes evident.

9.11.4. *Transmission:* Dourine is strictly a venereal disease that is found in the vaginal discharge of the mare or the urethra, sheath, penile exudates, and seminal fluid of the stallion. Dourine also causes disease by passing through intact mucous membranes. Although an animal may be infected with the protozoa, it may not always be present in the vagina or the urethra. There may be periods of weeks to months where the animal is not considered infectious. The noninfectious intervals happen more commonly in the later stages of disease. Foals may be infected through the mare either at birth or through consumption of the infected milk. These infected foals will transmit the disease as adults. Passive immunity passed in the colostrum may protect some foals until they are 4–7 months old.

9.11.5. *Occurrence:* Dourine was eradicated in the United States in 1949. It is still present in South America, the Middle East, southeastern Europe, northern and southern Africa, and most of Asia.

9.11.6. *Predominant clinical signs:* Signs of disease differ depending on the virulence of strain of the infectious protozoa. In addition, the level of stress and nutritional plane of the animal are important as to the severity of the disease. The strain of Dourine that was present in the United States and the Americas along with southern Africa appears to be more chronic and less virulent than that found in Europe, northern Africa, or Asia. Early in the disease, mares will have a mucopurulent discharge from the vagina and the discharge may be observed on the tail and hind legs. In stallions, the initial sign is edema of the prepuce, penis, and perineum. Swelling may then spread to the scrotum, ventral abdomen and the thorax. Distension and edema of the vulva in mares occurs with progression of the disease. The perineum, mammary gland, and ventral abdomen may also become distended and edematous. Vaginitis and vulvitis may be observed along with polyuria. Often, the mare will raise her tail due to discomfort. Only mares with the more virulent strains of Dourine will abort. Stallions can have paraphimosis with distention that is sporadically present. Leukodermic patches (permanent white scars) are the result of ulcers and vesicles on the genitals that have healed. Pathognomic transient plaques or "silver dollar plaques" (2–10 cm in diameter) may form on the skin, but not in all cases. Keratitis and conjunctivitis may also occur. There will be loss of weight as the disease progresses despite little to no change in the appetite. Lameness and weakness of the hind legs may also be noted. With time, the weakness progresses, incoordination occurs, and recumbency results from paralysis. Anemia may also occur. If left untreated, mortality rates reach nearly 50%–100% in Dourine-infected horses.

9.11.7. *Treatment:* Treatment with trypanocidal medications has been done, but is not recommended in endemic areas. The treated animals may still be asymptomatic carriers of the disease. The more virulent strains of Dourine may benefit from treatment. Vaccination for Dourine is not currently available because of sporadic changes in the surface antigens of the protozoa.

9.11.8. *Prevention:* Prevention is done by bleeding, testing, and quarantine of animals. Infected animals should be humanely destroyed or neutered. Some gelded stallions may still attempt to breed, so they need to be isolated from other animals.

9.11.9. *Control:* Dourine is strictly a venereal disease, so cleanup and disinfection of the premises does little to affect this disease. Dourine is reportable in the United States.

9.11.10. *Zoonotic potential:* Humans are not susceptible to dourine.

9.12. Equine Infectious Anemia (EIA) (Coggins Disease, Swamp Fever, Mountain Fever, Slow Fever, Equine Malarial Fever)

9.12.1. *Agent:* EIA is an equine lentivirus in the Retroviridae family. It causes infection in horses, donkeys, and mules. The virus is related to the viruses that cause leukemia in cats, cattle, and mice. EIA is only transferred to other equidae. Several forms of the disease exist including acute, chronic, and inapparent infection. Horses infected with the EIA virus carry it for life and are a source of infection to other equine.

9.12.2. *Affected species:* Horses, donkeys, and mules and other Equidae (Table 9.12).

Table 9.12. Equine Infectious Anemia.

			Disease Severity in Potentially Affected Species S = Severe D = Moderate M = Mild						
Dogs	Horses	Cattle	Sheep	Goats	Pigs	Cats	Birds	Other Animals
	D							D

9.12.3. *Incubation period:* The incubation period for EIA is as little as 7 days to greater than 45 days.

9.12.4. *Transmission:* Transmission is primarily from the bites of horse flies, deer flies (*Stomoxys* spp.), and tabanids that feed on blood and then transfer the infection from one horse to another. It is thought that the painful bite of many of these insects causes them to be shaken off quickly by the host horse. The insect will immediately seek another horse to bite, thus passing the virus on. The EIA virus is carried in the insect mouth for 30 minutes and up to 4 hours after a blood meal. Transmission of the virus also occurs by infected needles, equipment, or instruments that have not been properly disinfected. The virus is found in semen and can cross the placental barrier in chronically infected mares.

9.12.5.   *Occurrence:* Worldwide and in the United States.

9.12.6.   *Predominant clinical signs:* Signs of EIA usually occur 1 to 4 weeks after exposure to the disease. The acute form of EIA may have a fever that comes and goes, along with loss of appetite. More often, if the horse is in a pasture, the owner may never see any signs of illness. Horses that survive the acute form of the disease generally become chronic. Infrequently, horses may die from the acute form of EIA. Often the first indication of an EIA infection is when these horses are tested for EIA. The chronic or classic form is the most common form of the disease. Chronic signs include intermittent signs of illness. Episodes of fever, depression, weight loss, anemia, small hemorrhages, listlessness, and edema of the lower parts of the body, and weakness may be seen. Death can also occur. Other signs that may be noticed include abortion, diarrhea, urinating frequently, paralysis of the hindquarters, and/or rapid breathing. The unapparent form is one where the owner is not aware that the animal has the disease. These animals are carriers for EIA and, thus, are a source of infection to the rest of the herd. Depending on the strain of virus and the immune status of the animal, EIA can cause an inapparent infection, clinical disease, or even death. Times of stress—extremes in weather, workload, pregnancy, and certain medications can cause the animal to display signs of illness. Pregnant mares with the acute form of EIA may abort the fetus or give birth to EIA-positive foals. These foals often become carriers of EIA.

9.12.7.   *Treatment:* There is no specific treatment for horses showing signs of EIA. If these horses are kept, they should be treated symptomatically. EIA infected horses need to be isolated/quarantined at least a minimum of 200 meters from other equidae to prevent the spread of the disease.

9.12.8.   *Prevention:* At present, there is no vaccine available.

9.12.9.   *Control:* Testing horses (Coggins test) is used to control the spread of disease. Any horse that tests positive for EIA must be quarantined from other horses (especially during the fly season) if the horse is not to be euthanized. EIA-positive horses should be lip tattooed, marked with a brand, or freeze-branded to indicate that they are a reactor. These horses cannot cross state lines unless they go to slaughter, their home place, or to a research facility. Control of arthropod populations will decrease the risk of disease, so a good insect control program should be in place. It is important to keep instruments, equipment, and needles disinfected to prevent disease spread. Most disinfectants that have a detergent in them will inactivate the virus. It is recommended that after cleaning equipment, instruments, etc. that they be soaked for 10 minutes in the disinfectant. Instruments should be cleaned and sterilized for a minimum of 15 minutes in boiling water before reusing. Minimize use of equipment to only one horse (bridle, brushes, saddle, etc.) to prevent the spread of disease. Whenever there is an addition of a new horse to a farm, the new horse should always be quarantined for at least 30 days and tested for EIA. EIA is a reportable disease in the United States and an OIE List B Disease.

9.12.10. *Zoonotic potential*: Humans are not susceptible to EIA.

9.13. Equine Viral Arteritis (EVA) (Equine Typhoid, Epizootic Cellulitis-Pinkeye, Rotlaufseuche, Epizootic Lymphangitis Pinkeye)

9.13.1. *Agent*: EVA is a contagious equine RNA enveloped virus in the Arteriviridae family. Although a single serotype has been identified, there are differences in the strains of virus causing disease. Illness ranges from fever, conjunctivitis, dependent edema to abortion and death in young foals.

9.13.2. *Affected species*: EVA is strictly a virus of Equidae. Standardbreds and warmbloods appear to be more affected than other breeds of horses. Wild equine display little evidence of infection (Table 9.13).

Table 9.13. Equine Viral Arteritis.

Disease Severity in Potentially Affected Species S = Severe D = Moderate M = Mild								
Dogs	Horses	Cattle	Sheep	Goats	Pigs	Cats	Birds	Other Animals
	M							

9.13.3. *Incubation period*: The incubation period for EVA is typically 1 week, but it can range from 3–14 days.

9.13.4. *Transmission*: Transmission is venereal, respiratory, indirect by fomites (such as tack, equipment, instruments, handling an infected animal and not changing clothes or washing between animals), or congenital. Aerosol is the primary mode of infection in acute cases. It is most common in places where horses congregate (sales, racetracks, shows, breeding farms, etc.). Mares that are acutely infected or chronically infected (carrier) stallions can cause disease during breeding. EVA is shed continuously in the semen and has the capability to infect greater than 85% of unexposed mares to the virus. Collected semen for artificial insemination purposes also serves as a source of EVA. Carrier or persistently infected stallions may harbor EVA for years without showing decreased fertility or clinical signs. Some carrier stallions have been known to recover from EVA.

9.13.5. *Occurrence*: The primary countries affected include the United States, Canada, Great Britain, Switzerland, Poland and Austria. Japan and Iceland are EVA free.

9.13.6. *Predominant clinical signs:* Horses with EVA may show clinical signs or none. Any animal that is compromised such as the ill, the young, or the old tend to have more clinical signs than healthy animals. The virus strain, the amount of virus exposed to, and environmental factors all play a role in the severity of EVA. Signs of EVA may include depression, fever lasting for 2–9 days, edema of the limbs (predominant in the hind limbs), edema of the scrotum and prepuce, and anorexia. Other signs that may be seen include nasal discharge, rhinitis, conjunctivitis, photophobia, lacrimation, supraorbital or periorbital swelling, ventral edema, urticaria, dyspnea, stiffness, ataxia, and diarrhea. Abortion may occur from 3–10 months of gestation and be as high as 50% in a group of animals. Abortion is typically the result of a pregnant mare that has been exposed to an acutely infected animal. Mares can breed and become pregnant despite the semen being infected with EVA. If a mare is exposed to EVA in late pregnancy, the foal is usually congenitally infected with EVA. Stallions that are acutely infected with EVA have decreased fertility due to fever and swelling of the scrotum.

9.13.7. *Treatment:* Nothing specific other than supportive treatment in the more acutely affected animals. There is no treatment to eradicate the carrier state. A modified-live vaccine is available. The vaccine should not be used in pregnant mares, particularly after 10 months of gestation and should not be used in foals under 6 weeks of age.

9.13.8. *Prevention:* Good breeding practices such as testing for EVA, vaccinating, and identifying stallions that are carriers. If carrier stallions are to be used, they should be kept separate from the rest of the animals and bred only to mares that have also been exposed to EVA or have good immunization to the virus.

9.13.9. *Control:* EVA is destroyed by most common disinfectants as it is an enveloped virus. EVA is reportable in the United States.

9.13.10. *Zoonotic potential:* Humans are not susceptible to EVA.

9.14. Enterovirus Encephalomyelitis (PEV) (Teschen Disease, Talfan Disease, Porcine Polioencephalomyelitis, Benign Enzootic Paresis, Poliomyelitis Suum, Benign Enzootic Paresis)

9.14.1. *Agent:* This neurological disease of pigs is caused by several closely related enteroviruses in the Picornaviridae family. There are at least nine serotypes present. Usually mild disease is found in young pigs. Teschen disease is caused by porcine enterovirus serotype 1 (PEV-1), it affects all ages of pigs and is the most severe form.

9.14.2. *Affected species:* PEV occurs only in pigs and affects all ages (Table 9.14).

Table 9.14. Enterovirus Encephalomyelitis.

				Disease Severity in Potentially Affected Species S = Severe D = Moderate M = Mild				
Dogs	Horses	Cattle	Sheep	Goats	Pigs	Cats	Birds	Other Animals

9.14.3. *Incubation period:* Incubation period of PEV is about 14 days. Teschen disease in piglets may manifest neurological signs 5–7 days after the virulent "Zabreh" strain is inoculated experimentally.

9.14.4. *Transmission:* Transmission is by the oral-fecal route, direct contact, indirect contact (fomites), or feeding uncooked infected pork products. Virus can be shed for up to 7 weeks in recovering pigs.

9.14.5. *Occurrence:* PEV-1 is found in central and eastern Europe, Madagascar, and Uganda. In the past, PEV had been found worldwide. Recently, mild disease has been reported and only intermittently in most countries. In the United States, disease is seen only intermittently.

9.14.6. *Predominant clinical signs:* Pigs with Teschen disease (PEV-1) typically have ataxia followed by fever, anorexia, and depression. Convulsions, opisthotonos, nystagmus, stiffness, muscle spasms or tremors, loss of voice or change in quality, and coma may also be seen. Pigs may be painful and hypersensitive, and ascending paralysis occurs as the disease progresses. Paralysis of the respiratory muscles frequently causes death. Death occurs by day 3–4 and typically within 2 weeks. Teschen disease has a mortality rate of 70%–90%, affecting pigs less than 90 days more severely. Pigs that survive usually recover in 3–4 weeks. Older pigs may not fully recover from paralysis. Other strains of PEV cause a milder form of disease comprised of ataxia and paresis. Paralysis may be seen infrequently.

9.14.7. *Treatment:* No treatment is available for this pathogen. Supportive care may help prevent secondary infections.

9.14.8. *Prevention:* Live attenuated vaccine and inactivated vaccines are effective in controlling the disease in endemic areas. Quarantine and hygienic measures should be applied. PEV/Teschen disease is a reportable disease in the United States.

9.14.9. *Decontamination:* Enteroviruses (nonenveloped) are resistant to most chemicals. Sodium hypochlorite and 70% alcohol appear to be effective against the enteroviruses. PEV is heat resistant and not affected by lipid solvents. These viruses can survive for months in the environment. Virus-laden manure should be removed and rendered inactive (anaerobic digestion, aeration, or ionizing radiation).

9.14.10. *Zoonotic potential:* Humans are not susceptible to PEV.

9.15. Exotic Newcastle Disease (END) (Newcastle Disease, Velogenic Newcastle Disease, Asiatic Newcastle Disease, Avian Pneumoencephalitis)

9.15.1. *Agent:* END is a highly contagious RNA virus of poultry and birds in the Paramyxoviridae family. It is likely the most critical disease of poultry throughout the world. END can cause mild to severe disease, especially in chickens.

9.15.2. *Affected species:* Most poultry, caged birds, waterfowl, and wild birds are affected. All age of birds are susceptible. Chickens appear to more vulnerable to END than turkeys. Ducks and geese are least vulnerable (Table 9.15).

Table 9.15.   Exotic Newcastle Disease.

Disease Severity in Potentially Affected Species S = Severe D = Moderate M = Mild								
Dogs	**Horses**	**Cattle**	**Sheep**	**Goats**	**Pigs**	**Cats**	**Birds**	**Other Animals**
							S	

9.15.3. *Incubation period:* The incubation period is ranges from 2 to 15 days. Chickens with the velogenic form of END have an incubation period of 2–6 days.

9.15.4. *Transmission:* Transmission is by aerosolization (respiratory discharges, coughing), direct contact with feces, indirect contact with fomites (water, food, equipment, clothing, tools, racks, manure, etc.), flies, and mice. All parts of the bird carry virus when acutely infected, including carcasses present in garbage that may be used as feed for birds. Psittacine and some other birds may be asymptomatic or be carriers of END.

9.15.5. *Occurrence:* Worldwide. END is frequently brought into the United States, usually illegally, through imported birds and fighting cocks. The last outbreaks of END in the United States were in 2002 (California) and 2003 (Arizona, Texas, Nevada, and New Mexico).

9.15.6. *Predominant clinical signs:* There are several clinical forms of END that are recognized: velogenic (virulent), mesogenic (intermediate), lentogenic or respiratory (mild), and asymptomatic enteric (subclinical). The velogenic form has two subcategories: neurotropic form (respiratory and neurological components) and viscerotropic form (hemorrhagic lesions of the intestinal tract, hemorrhages on the head, edema). There can be mixed infections of both the neurotropic and viscerotropic forms. The velogenic form is indicated by a drop in egg production, followed with morbidity rates near 100% and mortality rates as high as 90% in susceptible chickens.

Death may be the first sign seen with no evidence of prior illness. Dyspnea may be obvious, conjunctivitis, severe diarrhea (viscerotropic form), paralysis, and death can all occur within 1–3 days. Swelling and hemorrhaging of the eyes may be noted as well as a discharge from the eyes and nose. Birds that survive the velogenic form of END (12–14 days) may have permanent neurological signs (circling, tremors, head and neck twisting, paresis, and paralysis) and lowered egg production. The mesogenic form of disease is common among young chickens. Respiratory signs with or without neurological involvement and a high mortality rate is seen. Laying hens may only show a abrupt drop in egg production, few signs, and very low mortality. The lentogenic form may have few to no signs of disease and low to no mortality. END possibly serves as an unknown source for infection. The asymptomatic enteric form is usually subclinical. Pigeon and psittacines tend to have neurological signs with the viscerotropic form of END.

9.15.7. *Treatment:* There is no treatment for END.

9.15.8. *Prevention:* The establishment of a strict quarantine and destruction of all infected and exposed birds must be performed to eradicate END where not endemic. Thorough cleaning and disinfection of the building with no poultry present for a minimum of 30 days is also necessary to eradicate the virus. Control of mice and insects should be done prior to depopulating a flock. Live and killed vaccines are available. END is a reportable disease in the United States and is an OIE List A Disease.

9.15.9. *Control:* After all organic material has been removed, a high pressure spray system and use of a disinfectant such as phenolics or cresylics should be employed. END has been recovered from effluent water for as long as 21 days and from carcasses for 7 days when the daytime temperatures were over 90°F.

9.15.10. *Zoonotic potential:* Humans have become infected with END, which is usually limited to conjunctivitis. Conjunctivitis is usually temporary and virus cannot be isolated in eye fluids after 4–7 days. Infections are commonly seen with first time exposure to the virus (laboratory workers, vaccinating crews, and poultry handlers). Humans do not contract the disease from handling or the consumption of poultry products. Individuals with conjunctivitis from END virus should be quarantined from poultry buildings and birds.

9.16. Foot-and-Mouth Disease (FMD) (Fiebre Aftosa) (Hoof and Mouth Disease)

9.16.1. *Agent:* FMD is a highly contagious viral disease of the Picornadviridae family of cloven-hoofed animals. Seven serotypes exist and immunity to one serotype does not grant immunity to another serotype. The morbidity is essentially 100 percent, with a mortality of less than 1%.

Worldwide, FMD is the most important livestock disease. Great economic loss results from the effects of this disease which also causes lameness, low milk production, weight loss, mastitis, debilitation, and abortion.

9.16.2. *Affected species:* Domesticated and wild cloven-hoofed animals are susceptible. Armadillos, buffalo, elephants, grizzly bears, hedgehogs, mice, and rats are also susceptible. Cats, dogs, chickens, chinchillas, guinea pigs, and rabbits have been experimentally infected (Table 9.16).

Table 9.16.   Foot-and-Mouth Disease.

Disease Severity in Potentially Affected Species S = Severe D = Moderate M = Mild								
Dogs	**Horses**	**Cattle**	**Sheep**	**Goats**	**Pigs**	**Cats**	**Birds**	**Other Animals**
M		S	D	D	S	M	M Chickens	S Buffalo, deer, camels, armadillos, mice, rats, hedgehogs, grizzly bears, elephants

9.16.3. *Incubation period:* Incubation can be very short—as little as 12 hours and up to 14 days depending on the strain of virus and nativity of the host animal. Typically, signs are seen 2–6 days after exposure. Recovery takes 8–15 days.

9.16.4. *Transmission:* Transmission is by direct or indirect contact, aerosolization, feeding infected garbage (meat, milk, milk products, blood, bone, and glands), fomites, vehicles, artificial insemination, and biologicals contaminated with FMD. All secretions, tissues, and excretions are contagious. Carrier state lasts 3.5 years in cattle, 9 months in sheep, 4 months in goats, and 3–4 weeks in pigs.

9.16.5. *Occurrence:* FMD is endemic in Africa, the Middle East, and parts of South America. Europe has had sporadic outbreaks (United Kingdom in 2001). FMD is endemic in Asia except for Indonesia, Japan, and Korea. Australia, New Zealand, and North and Central America are FMD free. The United States had the last outbreak of FMD in 1929.

9.16.6. *Predominant clinical signs:* Initial signs of FMD in cattle include fever (103°–107°F), anorexia, depression, drooling, and movement of the feet. Vesicles form on the nose, muzzle, tongue, dental pad, lips, feet, utter, and on the teats. Animals become very painful at the area of the vesicles, which eventually rupture.

 Weight loss and unthriftiness (decreased milk production and growth rate) are seen in animals that survive FMD. Many animals never fully recover. Pregnant cattle may abort and calves may die before any signs of disease are seen. Sheep and goats have fewer signs than cattle or pigs. Lameness is the predominant sign. Vesicles are usually smaller than in cattle. Pregnant sheep and goats can also abort. The very young may die before any signs are seen. Pigs may have vesicles on the mouth, nose, tongue, and feet. Fever (104°–105°F) may be present as well as anorexia, vocalization when moved, and lameness. Sows may abort and the very young may die before any signs are seen.

9.16.7. *Treatment:* Treatment is supportive and antibiotics are used to decrease secondary bacterial infection.

9.16.8. *Prevention:* A number of inactivated vaccines, including those prepared in cell cultures containing the appropriate types or subtypes are used in countries where the disease is endemic. The duration of immunity may be as short as 6 months.

9.16.9. *Control:* In FMD-free countries, a policy of rapid identification, quarantine, and slaughter is usually practiced with the goal of complete eradication. Regulation of garbage feeders is also important. Vaccine is available, but it protects for only about 6 months. It does not cross protect against the other serotypes. Vaccinated animals are permanently identified from nonvaccinates. Most FMD-free countries do not vaccinate. FMD is a reportable disease in the United States and an OIE List A Disease.

9.16.10. *Zoonotic potential:* Humans may be susceptible to FMD. In a review of the zoonotic aspects of FMD in 1997, it was reported that since 1921, the FMD virus has been isolated and typed from slightly over 40 human cases. The cases occurred on three continents: Europe, Africa, and South America. Although humans are seldom infected with FMD, precautions should be taken to decrease exposure to the virus. Currently, FMD is not a public health concern.

9.17. Heartwater (Cowdriosis, Blacklung, Daji Enguruti, Kabowa, Khadar, Magak, Pericardite Exsudative Infectieuse, Idropericardite Dei Ruminanti, Malkopsiekte, Hidrocarditis Infecciosa)

9.17.1. *Agent:* Heartwater is a noncontagious, infectious disease of ruminants caused by the rickettsia *Ehrlichia ruminantium* (formerly *Cowdria ruminantium*) that is transmitted by ticks in the *Amblyomma* genus. The name heartwater comes from hydropericardium, which is often found with this disease. There are four forms of heartwater: peracute, acute, subacute, and mild. In Africa, heartwater is a significant disease in livestock.

9.17.2. *Affected species:* Cattle, sheep, goats and antelope are susceptible to infection. African cattle appear to be more resistant than other breeds of cattle. Some species of African antelope have an inapparent infection. A few animals with subclinical infection may serve as a source of infection. The blesbok and wildebeest are known sources of infection. Other known sources of infection include the leopard tortoises, scrub hare, and guinea fowl. The white-tailed deer in the United States is experimentally susceptible to heartwater (Table 9.17).

Table 9.17. Heartwater.

Disease Severity in Potentially Affected Species **S = Severe D = Moderate M = Mild**								
Dogs	**Horses**	**Cattle**	**Sheep**	**Goats**	**Pigs**	**Cats**	**Birds**	**Other Animals**
		S Water buffalo	S	S				M African sheep and goats, blesbok, black wildebeest, eland, springbok. white-tailed deer, mice, ferret

9.17.3. *Incubation period:* The incubation period in cattle is 10–16 days and is usually shorter for sheep and goats. If inoculated intravenously, cattle show signs in 7–10 days and sheep and goats show signs after 10–16 days. It can take up to 28 days in some animals.

9.17.4. *Transmission:* Only *Amblyomma* ticks (12 species) transmit heartwater (Fig. 9.3). These ticks may take from 5 months to 4 years to

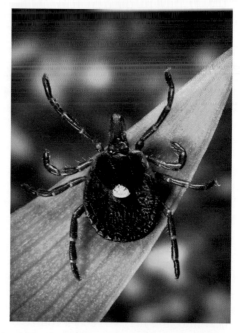

Figure 9.3. Female adult of *Amblyomma americanum* (Lone Star) tick. (Source: Public Domain; Image # 8683 http://phil.cdc.gov/phil/details.asp; Photograph by: James Gathany, Center for Disease Control and Prevention.)

complete their life cycle. They are three-host ticks. The major tick in Africa is the tropical bont tick (*A. variegatum*).

9.17.5.   *Occurrence:* It occurs in Africa, Madagascar, Mauritius, Reunion, Zanzibar, Antigua, Guadeloupe, Marie Galante, and other islands of the Caribbean.

9.17.6.   *Predominant clinical signs:* The peracute form of heartwater is not generally seen. Clinical signs may be present for about 36 hours prior to sudden death. Fever is present followed by dyspnea, lacrimation, hyperesthesia, prostration, convulsions, collapse, and death. Pregnant cows are more prone to this form of heartwater. The peracute form is more common in nonnative ruminants (cattle, sheep, and goats) brought to an endemic area of Africa. The acute form is usually seen in all ruminants. Fevers (up to 107°F) can occur within 12 hours. Anorexia, depression, and difficulty breathing are observed. Nervous system signs comprise of chewing movements, licking and frothing at the mouth, an extended tongue, excessive eyelid movement, unsteady movement, prostration, convulsions, and death. Diarrhea (more common in cattle than in sheep and goats) and abortion may also occur. Most animals die within 2–6 days of showing signs. If they survive, recovery is slow. The subacute form of heartwater is infrequently seen. Animals show less severe signs for 1–2 weeks. There is an extended fever, coughing, milder nervous system signs, collapse, and death. The mild or subclinical form is also known as "heartwater fever." The only sign seen is a transient fever. Cattle and sheep that have partial immunity, native breeds of cattle and sheep with a naturally high immunity, calves less than 3 weeks old, and antelope have the mild form. These animals are important as they serve as a reservoir of infection for ticks.

9.17.7.   *Treatment:* Treatment is effective if antibiotics are given early in the course of the disease. Tetracycline, oxytetracycline, doxycycline, rifampin, and many sulfonamides are effective. Supportive therapy should be given as needed.

9.17.8.   *Control:* Preventive measures include control of ticks. Because the *Amblyomma* tick is a three-host tick, eradication is difficult and may never be possible. Maintaining a controlled population of ticks seems to be the best way to maintain immunity in the ruminant. Immunity only lasts 6–18 months, so continuous reexposure to heartwater maintains immunity. The "infection and treatment method" is used in older animals. Susceptible animals are injected with infected blood (from sheep), monitored, and treated with antibiotics as needed. Simultaneous infection with infectious blood and treatment with tetracyclines provides protection against some strains. Calves that are less than 4 weeks and goats less than 6 weeks of age have natural protection. Most strains of heartwater cross-protect. Heartwater is a reportable disease in the United States and an OIE List B Disease.

9.17.9.   *Control:* The use of acaricides to control ticks as well as to prevent infected animals from being exposed to ticks should be done. *E. ruminantium* does not survive off the host for more than a few hours. In addition, blood transfer between animals should be prohibited.

9.17.10.   *Zoonotic potential:* Humans are not susceptible to heartwater.

9.18. Hog Cholera (CSF) (Classical Swine Fever, Swine Fever, Peste du Porc, Virusschweinepest, Colera Porcina)

9.18.1. *Agent:* Hog cholera is an extremely contagious disease caused by the enveloped RNA virus Pestivirus in the Flaviviridae family. It is characterized as having a high mortality in fully susceptible pigs, both domestic and wild. There are five forms of CSF: peracute, acute, subacute, chronic, and persistent. It was first noted in the United States during the early 19th century.

9.18.2. *Affected species:* The pig and wild boar are susceptible. The Collard Peccary is somewhat susceptible (Table 9.18).

Table 9.18. Hog Cholera.

								Disease Severity in Potentially Affected Species S = Severe D = Moderate M = Mild
Dogs	**Horses**	**Cattle**	**Sheep**	**Goats**	**Pigs**	**Cats**	**Birds**	**Other Animals**
					S			M Collared Peccary

9.18.3. *Incubation period.* The incubation period is typically 2–6 days, but it can range from 2 to 15 days.

9.18.4. *Transmission:* Pigs are the major source of infection. Direct contact (secretions, excretions, all tissues, blood, semen), uncooked pork products (feeding improperly cooked garbage), and indirect contact (people, equipment, vehicles, insects) are all sources of infection.

9.18.5. *Occurrence:* The disease is endemic in Central and South America, Asia, and in some of the Caribbean Islands. It can also be found in China, India, East and Central Africa, Eastern Europe, and Germany. It has been eradicated in Australia, Canada, New Zealand, the United States, and most of Europe.

9.18.6. *Predominant clinical signs:* Pigs with the peracute form of CSF are either dying or found dead. The acute or classic disease has a mortality of nearly 100%. Initial signs include depression, arched back, drooped heads, and drowsiness. A fever (106°–108°F), conjunctivitis with crusty eyelids (often seen), inappetance, vomiting (yellow fluid), seeking warmth, piling up on each other, and constipation. As the disease progresses, there is diarrhea, emaciation, staggering, purplish discoloration of the skin, convulsions, and death in 10–20 days. The subacute form of CSF is milder than the acute form. The fever is lower (105°–106°F) and may last 2–3 weeks. Death occurs in 30 days. The chronic form of CSF has a low mortality rate and death occurs 1–3 months later. A fever occurs, followed by an improvement in signs, and then a relapse of signs. Depression, fever, anorexia, constipation, diarrhea, and weight loss are seen. Pigs with the chronic form become carriers. These pigs have a large head compared to their body. The chronic form of CSF usually results in death due to other infections and immunosupression by CSF. The persistent or "carrier sow syndrome" occurs in pregnant sows. Very few signs of illness (mild fever) are seen in the sows. Piglets are infected *in utero* and are aborted or die shortly after birth. Congenital defects, mummies, stillborn pigs, and "shaker pigs" occur. Some pigs are persistently infected and shed the virus. These pigs will look healthy for several months before becoming ill with CSF. Death occurs within 6–12 months. CSF is analogous to bovine viral diarrhea (BVD) in cattle in that it suppresses the immune system and can cause diarrhea. Piglets infected *in utero* with BVD can appear to have signs resembling CSF.

9.18.7. *Treatment:* There is no treatment available for CSF.

9.18.8. *Prevention:* A strict regimen of vaccination in endemic areas will reduce the number of outbreaks. Once the incidence of disease has been lowered, vaccination is discontinued and sanitary measures should be implemented to eradicate CSF. CSF is a reportable disease in the United States and an OIE List A Disease.

9.18.9. *Control:* CSF is inactivated by heat, bleach, cresol, 2% sodium hydroxide, and detergents. It can survive in chilled pork for 85 days and for greater than 4 years if frozen. CSF survives for months to greater than 1 year in cured hams. Lack of sanitation allows CSF to survive for months in pens and up to 15 days in liquid manure.

9.18.10. *Zoonotic potential:* Humans are not susceptible to CSF.

9.19. Johne's Disease (Paratuberculosis)

9.19.1. *Agent:* Johne's is caused by *Mycobacterium avium paratuberculosis* (previously known as *M. paratuberculosis, M. johnei*) and it is believed to infect all ruminants. Johne's is a chronic, debilitating disease that causes diarrhea, loss of weight, and death.

9.19.2. *Affected species:* All ruminants appear to be affected including some omnivores and carnivores. Dairy cattle in dairy-producing countries seem to be the largest group of animals affected with 20%–50% of herds being infected. Little is known about the infection rate of *M. avium paratuberculosis* in other animal species. Experimentally, dogs and horses have been infected (Table 9.19).

9.19.3. *Incubation period:* The incubation period is long. Cattle are usually exposed shortly after birth and may not show signs of disease until 2 years of age of older. Adults are less likely to succumb to the disease.

Table 9.19. Johne's Disease.

Disease Severity in Potentially Affected Species S = Severe D = Moderate M = Mild								
Dogs	**Horses**	**Cattle**	**Sheep**	**Goats**	**Pigs**	**Cats**	**Birds**	**Other Animals**
M	M	S	S	S	S			S Llamas, deer, elk, buffalo, alpaca, camels, foxes, moose, reindeer, nonhuman primates, wild rabbits, weasels

9.19.4. *Transmission:* The usual route of transmission is the fecal-oral route. One of the most common routes is when the calves nurse on the contaminated teats of the mother. *M. avium paratuberculosis* is found in contaminated colostrum, milk, feed, water, or consumed during the normal licking and grooming activities of animals.

9.19.5. *Occurrence:* Worldwide. Infected sheep in Australia and goats in Spain are of economic concern. The United States, Australia, Norway, the Netherlands, Iceland, and Japan have national plans in place to manage the disease. Sweden is Johne's free.

9.19.6. *Predominant clinical signs:* Affected animals may not show signs for months to years. Once clinical signs are seen in cattle, quite a bit of weight has been lost and diarrhea is usually continuous. As the disease progresses, weight loss continues and the diarrhea becomes more constant. Dependent edema may be noted due to protein-losing enteropathy and the hair coat may be lighter in color or rougher. Appetite and attitude are usually good, but increased water intake may be noted. There is usually a drop in milk production. Goats and sheep generally do not have diarrhea with Johne's. They will have inferior wool and shed it in the later stages of illness. Other ruminants tend not to have diarrhea and may show a faster course of illness. Ultimately, the animal dies as a result of the infection, dehydration, and poor physical health.

9.19.7. *Treatment:* No treatment other than supportive.

9.19.8. *Prevention:* If a herd is known to have Johne's, routine testing should be done and positive animals sent to slaughter. Testing should be done annually once the herd prevalence of Johne's is manageable. Good management practices should include feed and water that is not easily contaminated by feces. Feces should be kept to a minimum. It may take 5 years to bring the problem under control once it has been introduced into a herd. Most disinfectants are ineffective against *M. avium paratuberculosis*. Thorough cleaning with soap and water, followed with detergents will be helpful.

9.19.9.   *Control:* Strict sanitation and good management practices should be in place. Calves, lambs, and kids should be birthed in areas that are kept clean and that are cleaned between birthings. Manure is the main source of infection to the young, so it should be kept picked up at all times. In dairy herds that have Johne's present, it is recommended that newborns be removed from their mothers and that colostrum be either free of Johne's or is heat treated. The calves should then be raised separate from the herd to avoid exposure. All milk provided to the calves should either be pasteurized or substituted with milk replacer. Johne's is a reportable disease in the United States.

9.19.10.   *Zoonotic potential:* It is uncertain if *M. avium paratuberculosis* causes Crohn's disease in humans. The bacterium has been documented in nonhuman primates. Therefore, humans should be considered at risk, especially if immunocompromised. Crohn's disease causes chronic enteritis in humans.

9.20. Leishmaniasis (Visceral Leishmaniasis, Black fever, Dum-dum Fever, Shahib's Disease, Infantile Splenic Fever, Kala-azar, Sikari Disease, Febrile Tropical Splenomegaly, Burdwan Fever)

9.20.1.   *Agent:* Leishmaniasis is caused by the protozoan species *Leishmania*. *L. chagasi*, *L. braziliensis*, *L. mexicana* are found in Central and South America, while *L. infantum* and *L. donovani* are in the Middle East and the Mediterranean. Leishmaniasis causes a chronic disease with weight loss, skin lesions, lameness, and lymphadenopathy.

9.20.2.   *Affected species:* Leishmaniasis is most often seen in dogs (foxes, jackals). Rodents, sloths, marsupials, anteaters, and hyraxes may also be serious affect. Cats, horses, and other domestic animals usually develop cutaneous ulcers. Humans are susceptible to leishmaniasis (Table 9.20).

Table 9.20.   Leishmaniasis.

Disease Severity in Potentially Affected Species S = Severe D = Moderate M = Mild								
Dogs	**Horses**	**Cattle**	**Sheep**	**Goats**	**Pigs**	**Cats**	**Birds**	**Other Animals**
S Foxes, jackels	**M** Equidae					**M**		**M** Rodents, anteaters, sloths, marsupials, hyraxes

9.20.3. *Incubation period:* The incubation period may range from 3 months to several years in dogs. Some incubation periods have been as long as 7 years.

9.20.4. *Transmission:* Leishmaniasis is a seasonal disease. It is transmitted indirectly by the *Phlebotomidae* sandfly. These sandflies generally stay within an area of only a few kilometers to complete their lifecycle. The female sandfly sucks the blood of vertebrates. Their most active feeding times are at dusk and dawn. The female sandfly will ingest the amastigote (an aflagellate) and/or the infected cells from the host. The Leishmania protozoa transforms in the sandfly to the promastigote (flagellated form) of the protozoa. The promastigote, once transferred to the host, is swallowed up by the macrophages. Once inside the macrophage they become the amastigote. The protozoa then spread throughout the body—skin, lymph nodes, kidneys, bone marrow, liver, and spleen. Rarely, horizontal transmission occurs between dogs and is thought to be through biting.

9.20.5. *Occurrence:* North, Central, and South America; Africa; the Middle East; the Mediterranean; and Asia. Greater than 90% of visceral leishmaniasis is found in Nepal, Bangladesh, India, Brazil, and the Sudan. Greater than 90% of cutaneous leishmaniasis is found in Peru, Brazil, and the Middle East. Old World Leishmaniasis refers to the disease in the Eastern Hemisphere while New World Leishmaniasis refers to the disease in the Western Hemisphere. Leishmaniasis in the United States is found in the northeastern part of the country in dogs (especially foxhounds), but not in humans. Other states in the United States have also had leishmaniasis cases reported.

9.20.6. *Predominant clinical signs:* Usually a chronic disease in dogs, but it may be inapparent. Signs of disease are highly inconsistent. Often a history of traveling to an endemic area in the last 6–7 years will help identify this disease. Visceral and cutaneous forms of the disease occur. When a dog displays the cutaneous form of leishmaniasis, it is assumed he also has the visceral form. The visceral form consists of loss of weight, loss of appetite, muscle atrophy, reduced exercise intolerance, and skin lesions. Other signs that may be seen include lymphadenopathy, fever, splenomegaly, and anemia. Less often there may be renal or liver failure, lameness, ocular lesions, epistaxis, diarrhea, vomiting, polyuria-polydipsia, sneezing, chronic colitis, and ascites. The cutaneous form is seen in nearly 90% of dogs with the leishmaniasis. The skin lesions involve alopecia with a very dry, nonpruritic exfoliation or ulceration that typically starts on the head (eyes, ears, and face) and expands to the rest of the body (feet). These dogs may also have long, brittle nails, hyperkeratosis of the nose or digits, ulcers between the digits, and loss of temporal muscle mass. In severe leishmaniasis, scabs, ulcers, and nodules may be pruritic. Leishmaniasis is often asymptomatic in wild animals and rodents. *L. braziliensis* causes systemic signs while *L. mexicana* causes cutaneous signs. Horses and other Equidae will often display cutaneous signs. Cats seldom become infected with leishmaniasis. If they do, signs are usually cutaneous.

9.20.7.   *Treatment:* N-Methylglucamine antimoniate or sodium stibogluconate (must be obtained from the CDC in the United States) along with allopurinol or Amphotericin B in dogs. Unfortunately, despite the treatment method used, relapses are common.

9.20.8.   *Prevention:* No vaccine is available for dogs.

9.20.9.   *Control:* Control of the insect vector and immediate treatment of dogs that have the disease is advised in endemic areas. In addition, the stray and feral dog population should be reduced. In nonendemic areas, treatment may be questionable. Dogs serve as a reservoir for human infection. *Leishmania spp.* can be deactivated with formaldehyde, 1% sodium hydroxide, heat (50–60°C), or 2% glutaraldehyde. Leishmaniasis is reportable in the United States.

9.20.10.   *Zoonotic potential:* Humans are susceptible to leishmaniasis. Visceral or cutaneous forms of the disease occur depending on the species of Leishmania that infects the individual. A mucocutaneous form (a papule that can spread to other mucocutaneous areas on the body) has also been described in people. In humans, the incubation period can be 2–6 months and possibly several years.

9.21. Lumpy Skin Disease (LSD) (Pseudo-urticaria, Exanthema Nodularis Bovis, Neethling Virus Disease, Knopvelsiekte)

9.21.1.   *Agent:* LSD is an acute to chronic virus in the Poxviridae family that causes disease in cattle. There is only one virus type and it can survive in skin nodules for 1–3 months. LSD is closely related to sheep and goat pox.

9.21.2.   *Affected species:* Cattle are susceptible to LSD as well as domestic buffalo. African buffalo are suspected of being carriers. It is not certain whether water buffalo can be infected with LSD. Other animals that can be infected with LSD include zebu, giraffes, impala and the Oryx. Experimentally, sheep and goats can be infected with LSD (Table 9.21).

Table 9.21.   Lumpy Skin Disease.

Disease Severity in Potentially Affected Species S = Severe D = Moderate M = Mild								
Dogs	**Horses**	**Cattle**	**Sheep**	**Goats**	**Pigs**	**Cats**	**Birds**	**Other Animals**
		S Domestic buffalo	M	M				D African buffalo, zebu, giraffe, impala, oryx, water buffalo?

9.21.3. *Incubation period:* The incubation period for LSD is 2–5 weeks.

9.21.4. *Transmission:* The major mode of transmission is through biting insects (flies, mosquitoes). LSD is more common during the warm, wet months of the year. Direct contact plays a lesser role in transmission. Virus may be found in saliva, nasal secretions, skin lesion, milk, lymph nodes, semen, muscles, and the spleen. LSD endures for 35 days in desiccated skin crusts.

9.21.5. *Occurrence:* LSD was first seen in Northern Rhodesia. It has since become endemic throughout most of Africa. Kuwait, Egypt, and Israel have had outbreaks of LSD.

9.21.6. *Predominant clinical signs:* Morbidity ranges from 3% to 85%, with a mortality of up to 10% (especially in calves). Nonclinical to severe disease can be seen, with the younger animals being much more affected. The first clinical sign seen is a fever (104°–107°F) of several days duration up to 4 weeks. Painful nodules of 1–5 cm usually appear on the skin, respiratory tract, GI tract, and genital tracts 1–2 days after the onset of fever. There is enlargement (4–10 times normal) of the superficial lymph nodes, depression, an ocular-nasal discharge, excessive drooling, loss of appetite, dyspnea, decreased milk production, and weight loss that follow. Nodules (1–7 cm) appear on the body, especially the back, legs, eyelids, nose, muzzle, ears, mouth, perineum, udder, scrotum, and tail. Lameness can result from inflammation and edema. Secondary bacterial infections can cause permanent damage to the joints and tendon sheaths. Mastitis, abortion (from prolonged fevers), and delayed breeding can occur. Sterility may be temporary or permanent in bulls. Lesions remain for up to 4–6 weeks and take 2–6 months to heal. Sit fasts are nodules that become hard, raised, and necrotic. The sit-fasts slough, ulcerate, heal, and then scar. Nodules may be present for up to 2 years. Economic loss is in damage to the hide, lameness, infertility, and decreased milk production.

9.21.7. *Treatment:* Treatment is usually supportive and prevention of secondary bacterial infections. Immunity appears to be less than 1 year.

9.21.8. *Prevention:* Vaccination is used to control the disease in endemic areas. Control of insects and movement of infected hides should be performed. If LSD is introduced to an area, quarantine, identification of exposed and infected animals should be made. The animals are slaughtered and the premises and equipment should be cleaned and disinfected. Control of insects does not eliminate the disease, but may still be helpful in controlling LSD. It is a reportable disease in the United States and an OIE List A Disease.

9.21.9. *Control:* It is a very stable virus and is resistant to many chemical and physical agents. It survives a pH 6.6–8.6 and a temperature of 37°C for 5 days.

9.21.10.   *Zoonotic potential:* Humans are not susceptible to lumpy skin disease.

9.22.   Malignant Catarrhal Fever (MCF) (Malignant Head Catarrh, Malignant Catarrh, Catarrhal Fever, Gangrenous Coryza, Snotsiekte)

9.22.1.   *Agent:* MCF is an infectious and often fatal viral gamma herpes viral disease of cattle, buffalo, and exotic ruminants. It has been suggested that up to 70% of MCF is not identified.

9.22.2.   *Affected species:* Cattle, buffalo, bison, antelope, white-tailed deer, red deer, and a few other deer species, water buffalo, wapiti, banteng, gaurs, greater kudus, gnus, and sida deer are susceptible. Wildebeest, hartebeest, and topi are carriers of alcelphine herpesvirus 1 (wildebeest associated). The addax and Oryx may serve as reservoirs. Domestic and wild sheep and goats are reservoirs of ovine herpesvirus 2 (sheep/goat associated) (Table 9.22).

Table 9.22.   Malignant Catarrhal Fever.

Disease Severity in Potentially Affected Species S = Severe D = Moderate M = Mild									
Dogs	Horses	Cattle	Sheep	Goats	Pigs	Cats	Birds		Other Animals
		S	M	M					S Buffalo, bison, deer, antelope, water buffalo, wapiti, banteng, gaur, greater kudu,gnu

9.22.3.   *Incubation period:* The incubation period is unknown with other forms of MCF, but it may be up to 200 days. It is thought that some animals have the infection subclinically and only break with the disease under stressful conditions.

9.22.4.   *Transmission:* Transmission is of the cell-free virus through direct or indirect contact. Direct contact occurs by inhalation, ingestion of contaminated water or feed, secretions (ocular, nasal), and feces. MCF is a problem at calving time because it is readily shed by calves. Indirect contact is by fomites or by insects. Adult cattle rarely infect other adults because the virus is cell associated.

9.22.5.   *Occurrence:* The sheep-associated MCF occurs worldwide, including in the United States and Europe. The wildebeest associated MCF only occurs in Africa.

9.22.6. *Predominant clinical signs:* There are several different forms of MCF. The peracute form is most often seen in deer. There is fever, acute inflammation of the mucosa of the mouth and nose, and hemorrhagic gastroenteritis. Death usually occurs in 1–3 days. The intestinal form consists of fever, diarrhea, dehydration, and oral-nasal discharges and ulcerations. Lymphadenopathy can occur for 4–9 days. The head and eye or classic form is the characteristic syndrome of MCF and is typically fatal. It lasts for 7–18 days. Fever (104°–107°F) occurs along with ocular-nasal discharges that are serous and become very purulent as the disease progresses. Depression, diarrhea, enlarged lymph nodes and drooling takes place. Erosions of the lips, gums, soft and hard palates are apparent. Dyspnea occurs as the muzzle and nose become encrusted. Corneal opacity, photophobia, and conjunctival edema may cause partial to complete blindness. Incoordination, hyperesthesia, and trembling may also be noted. The skin form is characterized by encrustation on the muzzle, hyperemia, and hemorrhagic lesions of the muzzle, legs, udder, and interdigital space. The nervous form is characterized by ataxia, circling, ear twitching, aggressiveness, tremors, and a distorted gait. A latent or asymptomatic form is also seen.

9.22.7. *Treatment:* Treatment consists of supportive care and antibiotics to control secondary bacterial infections. Animals that survive MCF tend to become carriers.

9.22.8. *Prevention:* Currently, no effective vaccine is available. Cattle should be kept separate from sheep, goats, alcelaphine antelope, and wildebeest. This is especially important during calving, lambing, and kidding since MCF is most frequently spread at this time. All wild ruminants placed on game farms or in zoos should be tested for MCF. In the case of an outbreak, cattle and other susceptible ruminants should be separated from sheep and goats. Malignant catarrhal fever is a reportable disease in the United States.

9.22.9. *Control:* MCF is rapidly inactivated by sunlight and most disinfectants. It is susceptible to freezing. It survives in cells at 4°–5°C for up to 30 days.

9.22.10. *Zoonotic potential:* Humans are not susceptible to MCF.

9.23. Menangle (Menangle Virus)

9.23.1. *Agent:* Menangle virus is an RNA virus in the Paramyxoviridae family that can infect pigs. It was first identified in 1997 in Menangle, New South Wales, Australia. It causes mummification, stillborn pigs, decreased litter size, and abortion.

9.23.2. *Affected species:* Menangle appears to affect primarily the fetus and newborn pigs. Humans are susceptible to the disease. Various species of fruit bats (flying foxes) appear to serve as a reservoir for this disease (Table 9.23).

Table 9.23. Menangle.

| Disease Severity in Potentially Affected Species S = Severe D = Moderate M = Mild | | | | | | | | |
Dogs	Horses	Cattle	Sheep	Goats	Pigs	Cats	Birds	Other Animals
					S			

9.23.3. *Incubation period:* Unknown, probably 10–14 days in pig.

9.23.4. *Transmission:* Unknown but may be oral-fecal route or oral-urinary route.

9.23.5. *Occurrence:* Only known cases to date were found in Menangle, New South Wales, Australia, at a large piggery in 1997.

9.23.6. *Predominant clinical signs:* Mummified and autolyzed fetuses along with stillborn pigs were seen. Some normal pigs were born and at the initial outbreak dropped to 27% of normal expected live pigs. Some of the pigs had deformities, especially of the skeletal or nervous system. Abortion was occasionally noted. Postnatal animals showed no sign of disease. Delayed return to estrus in some infected sows occurred.

9.23.7. *Treatment:* None. No vaccine is available.

9.23.8. *Prevention:* No vaccine is available.

9.23.9. *Control:* Control or prevent contact between pigs and fruit bats. Confinement operations should be located where bats do not have access or house pigs away from fruit or flowering trees that may attract these bats. Pigs 10–16 weeks in an endemic should be removed to protect them. The other option is to euthanize all exposed animals, disinfect the premises, and repopulate.

9.23.10. *Zoonotic potential:* Humans are susceptible to Menangle and should take precautions when handling suspected cases. It is unknown at this time as to how transmission from pigs to humans occurs. Two workers at separate locations (one at the affected piggery, the other performed necropsies without protective gear) had unknown flu-like illness. The workers experienced illness for 10–14 days, flu-like symptoms, malaise, sweating, a rash, and headache. Both workers had been closely associated with the pigs over a period of time. They both tested positive for the Menangle virus.

9.24. Nairobi Sheep Disease (NSD)

9.24.1. *Agent:* NSD is viral disease of sheep and goats in the Bunyaviridae family that is spread by the brown tick *Rhipcephalus appendiculatus*. It is an extremely pathogenic disease that causes hemorrhagic gastroenteritis, fever, and abortion. NSD has high morbidity and mortality. The virus is similar to the Ganjam virus in India which is carried by ticks and infects sheep, goats, and humans. The virus is also similar to the Dugbe virus in West African cattle.

9.24.2. *Affected species:* Sheep and goats seem to be the most susceptible. The African field rat is possibly the reservoir for this disease (Table 9.24).

Table 9.24.　Nairobi Sheep Disease.

Disease Severity in Potentially Affected Species S = Severe D = Moderate M = Mild								
Dogs	Horses	Cattle	Sheep	Goats	Pigs	Cats	Birds	Other Animals
			S	S				

9.24.3. *Incubation period:* The incubation period is 4–15 days after being bitten by a tick.

9.24.4. *Transmission:* Only transmitted by ticks and is therefore considered noncontagious. *R. appendiculatus* is the primary vector for NSD. It is also the only known tick species which transmits the disease transovarially. There is possibly another *Rhipcephalus* species in Somalia that may be able to transmit transovarially. Adult ticks, without being fed, can transmit disease for more than two years.

9.24.5. *Occurrence:* NSD is mostly found in east Africa. It has also been reported in Kenya, Somalia, Uganda, Ethiopia, Tanzania, Mozambique, and Botswana.

9.24.6. *Predominant clinical signs:* A fever (104°–106°F) along with depression is initially seen. The fever drops and a thin, watery diarrhea develops. There is a blood-stained mucopurulent nasal discharge that is prominent and breathing may be elevated. As the disease progresses, the feces have more blood and mucus in them. Less severely affected animals may show anorexia, weakness, and a slower onset of disease. These animals develop diarrhea and may become recumbent. Abortions may be seen. In the hyperacute infections, a fever suddenly develops that drops within 3–6 days. These animals shortly become prostrate and die within 12 hours of the fever drop.

9.24.7. *Treatment:* Supportive care and good nutrition may help.

9.24.8. *Prevention:* Animals that recover from NSD are immune for life. It is thought that this protection can be passed on to the lambs and kids. Animals in endemic areas have good immunity because of the constant exposure to the infected ticks. A modified-live vaccine is available but is generally not recommended because of adverse effects with it and inconsistency in some breeds to respond to it.

9.24.9. *Control:* Weekly dipping and spraying of susceptible sheep and goats are recommended. Avoid movement of animals that are endemic for NSD. Bury or incinerate dead animals. Transmission is not through contact, so quarantine in endemic areas is not essential. Bunyaviridae virus is susceptible to hypochlorite and phenolic solutions. NSD is reportable in the United States.

9.24.10. *Zoonotic potential:* Humans may be susceptible to NSD. Individuals should use caution with the aerosol spread of this virus. Rarely, a mild influenza-like illness has been described.

9.25. Ovine Progressive Pneumonia (OPP) (Progressive Pneumonia, Maedi-Visna, Maedi, Marsh's Progressive Pneumonia, Montana Progressive Pneumonia, Chronic Progressive Pneumonia, La Bouhite, Graaff-Reinet Disease, Zwoegersiekte)

9.25.1. *Agent:* OPP or maedi-visna (meaning "dyspnea"—"wasting") is a lentivirus in the Retroviridae family that causes chronic disease in sheep. Progressive dyspnea and neurological signs develop and are fatal. Caprine arthritis-encephalitis is a similar disease in goats.

9.25.2. *Affected species:* Sheep are affected with Finnish breeds, Texel, and Border Leicester being more susceptible. Suffolk, Rambouillet, and Columbia breeds appear more resistant. Goats may also be affected to a lesser degree (Table 9.25).

Table 9.25. Ovine Progressive Pneumonia.

Disease Severity in Potentially Affected Species S = Severe D = Moderate M = Mild								
Dogs	Horses	Cattle	Sheep	Goats	Pigs	Cats	Birds	Other Animals
			S	M				

9.25.3. *Incubation period:* The incubation period is long and most commonly seen in sheep greater than 3–4 years of age and not likely to occur under 2 years of age. OPP is a slow, progressive disease.

9.25.4. *Transmission:* The oral route via contaminated colostrum or milk is the most common form of transmission for OPP. Aerosol transmission via close contact may also occur. Rarely, intrauterine infection happens.

9.25.5. *Occurrence:* It occurs in the United States, Canada, Europe, Great Britain, South Africa, India, Kenya, Israel, Myanmar, southern parts of the former USSR, and Peru. The lentiviral infection rate of sheep in the United

States ranges from 9%–49% depending on the region of the country. The western part of the United States has a higher percentage, while the northeastern part is lower in prevalence. Other countries show similar disparity in prevalence.

9.25.6. *Predominant clinical signs:* Because this is a slow progressive disease, signs are not seen immediately. Most animals are asymptomatic. The maedi (dyspnea) form is the most common and is deadly. Weight loss is evident and dyspnea is progressive. Death results from secondary bacterial infections and hypoxia. Other signs that may be noted include depression, fever, mastitis, severe lameness, and coughing. The visna (neurologic) form may exhibit circling, ataxia, loss of condition, muscle tremors, weakness in the hind legs, paresis, and paralysis. This progression of disease may go on for up to a year.

9.25.7. *Treatment:* None, except supportive care.

9.25.8. *Prevention:* No vaccine is available.

9.25.9. *Control:* Testing for positive animals and humanely euthanizing them. Testing should be done at least one to two times yearly. Lambs that are from seropositive ewes should be removed from the ewes and fed colostrum and milk that is seronegative for the virus or fed heat-inactivated colostrum and milk. Milk replacer may also be used to raise the lambs. OPP is vulnerable in hot, dry situations and only survives for a few days in the environment. Most common disinfectants deactivate lentiviruses. OPP is reportable in the United States.

9.25.10. *Zoonotic potential:* Humans are not susceptible to OPP.

9.26. Pest of Small Ruminants (PPR) (Peste Des Petits Ruminants, Pest of Sheep and Goats, Pseudorinderpest of Small Ruminants, Kata, Stomatitis-Pneumoenteritis Syndrome or Complex, Pneumoenteritis Complex, Goat Plague, Contagious Pustular Stomatitis)

9.26.1. *Agent:* PPR is an acute or subacute contagious disease of sheep and goats caused by the Morbillivirus in the Paramyxodiridae family. PPR causes necrotic stomatitis, fever, gastroenteritis, and pneumonia. PPR is closely related to rinderpest in cattle.

9.26.2. *Affected species:* Goats are more susceptible than sheep to PPR. The gemsbok, dorcas gazelle, Nubian ibex, and Laristan sheep are susceptible. The American white-tailed deer is thought to be susceptible to PPR. Although cattle and pigs are susceptible, they do not show clinical signs of PPR and do not spread it to other animals (Table 9.26).

Table 9.26. Pest of Small Ruminants.

| | | | Disease Severity in Potentially Affected Species S = Severe D = Moderate M = Mild | | | | | |
Dogs	**Horses**	**Cattle**	**Sheep**	**Goats**	**Pigs**	**Cats**	**Birds**	**Other Animals**
		M	S	S	M			D Gemsbok, dorcas gazelle, Nubian ibex, Laristan sheep American white-tailed deer?

9.26.3. *Incubation period:* The incubation period of PPR is generally 4–5 days, but it can range from 3 to 10 days.

9.26.4. *Transmission:* Transmission of PPR is by close contact with oral, nasal, or ocular secretions or excretions. Aerosolization of the virus through coughing and sneezing is the main source of infection. Feces and fomites also serve as an indirect source of infection. The mortality, depending on the form of the virus, varies from 20% to 90%. Morbidity is nearly 100%. There are no carrier animals.

9.26.5. *Occurrence:* The disease has been reported from the Sahara to the Equator of central Africa, the Middle East, and India.

9.26.6. *Predominant clinical signs:* The acute form is most commonly seen. A high fever (104°–106°F) is the first sign seen and lasts about 5–8 days. Decreased appetite, depression, dull coat, restlessness, and a dry muzzle are seen. Classic symptoms of PPR include ocular and nasal discharges that are at first serous and then gradually become mucopurulent. These exudates crust over the eyes, nose and lips, breathing becomes difficult, and sneezing occurs. Oral and nasal mucous membranes may have necrotic areas. The gum surrounding the incisors, the end of the tongue, the dental pad, the papillae and cheeks, and the hard palate may have areas of erosion and necrosis. Profuse nonhemorrhagic diarrhea occurs and results in dehydration, weight loss, respiratory distress, hypothermia, and death within 5–10 days. Coughing is a result of bronchopneumonia. Abortion can occur in pregnant animals. Younger animals are more severely affected by PPR. Sheep more frequently develop the subacute form of the disease. There is a longer incubation period and course of the disease. Signs of fever and nasal discharge are less severe. Oral erosions tend to reappear. Diarrhea is sporadic with most animals recovering from the subacute form.

9.26.7. *Treatment:* There is no specific treatment for PPR. Antibiotics and antiparasitics can be used symptomatically to help decrease mortality.

9.26.8. *Prevention:* Eradication by quarantine, test, and slaughter is recommended over vaccination when PPR appears in new areas. Proper disposal of carcasses and decontamination of fomites is also necessary. Restrictions on importation of sheep and goats from affected areas should be followed. PPR is a reportable disease in the United States and is an OIE List A Disease.

9.26.9. *Control:* PPR is a fragile virus. It is sensitive to heat and sunlight. It survives outside the host for only a few hours. PPR is susceptible to ether, chloroform and most common disinfectants (3% bleach, 2% lye, Virkon-S, 1% One Stroke Environ).

9.26.10. *Zoonotic potential:* Humans are not susceptible to PPR.

9.27. Parafilariasis

9.27.1. *Agent:* Parafilariasis is caused by the nematode *Parafilaria bovicola* and is spread by vector to cattle and buffalo. Hemorrhagic nodules ("bleeding spots" or "bleeding points") are present on the skin. It is of economic importance in the cattle industry due to the damage to the hide and underlying tissues and control of the vector and parasite.

9.27.2. *Affected species:* Cattle and buffalo are the most susceptible (Table 9.27).

Table 9.27. Parafilariasis.

Disease Severity in Potentially Affected Species S = Severe D = Moderate M = Mild								
Dogs	Horses	Cattle	Sheep	Goats	Pigs	Cats	Birds	Other Animals
		S						S Buffalo

9.27.3. *Incubation period:* The incubation period is about 240 days after the female nematode penetrates the skin and lays her eggs.

9.27.4. *Transmission:* Flies feed on infected lesions of cattle and consume the eggs of the parasite. The *Parafilaria* develops and becomes the infective third stage larvae in the fly. The larvae infected fly then feeds on ocular secretions and wounds on naïve animals or bleeding spots on infected animals. Licking flies of the *Musca* species (*M. xanthomela, M. lusoria, M. nevilli*) carry the *P. bovicola*. The potential exists that *M. autumnalis*, the face fly found in the United States, also can transmit *P. bovicola*. This is very much a concern to the cattle industry in the United States, not only as a parasite, but the damage it causes to the carcass. The European face fly also can carry the *P. bovicola*. Most cases of disease appear to be the result of intraconjuntival inoculation versus subcutaneous. Introduction of parafilariasis into unaffected areas can occur by active vector movement into those areas, carriage on animals, or the movement of infected animals to area.

9.27.5. *Occurrence:* Parafilariasis has been reported in most regions of the world except for Australia and South America. It was first reported in the Philippines. It is thought that Charolais cattle from France introduced the disease in both Sweden and Canada. Native Canadian cattle were not infected with the disease. To date, parafilaraisis has not been reported in the United States.

9.27.6. *Predominant clinical signs:* Clinical signs are usually mild and distinctive. The female *P. bovicola* lives in the subcutaneous layer of the skin. The eggs are deposited on the skin by burrowing through the dermal and epidermal layer of skin. Once the female penetrates the outer skin layer, blood can be seen dripping from the sight. The result is a painful hemorrhagic nodule or "bleeding spot" that develops. In the northern hemisphere these nodules are most prominent from December until mid-year. The cutaneous bleeding points will start about February and last until about mid-year. In the southern hemisphere, the seasonal cycle occurs from about June through January.

9.27.7. *Treatment:* Ivermectin has proven to be very effective in treating parafilariasis. Levamisole, fenbendazole, and nitroxynil have also been used successfully to treat parafilariasis.

9.27.8. *Prevention:* There is no vaccine available.

9.27.9. *Control:* In endemic areas, good vector control has had limited success because of the large areas occupied by the flies and the short time they spend on animals. Continuous vector control (sprays, ear tags, spot-ons, dust bags, or oilers) will help control the number of vectors. Animals imported from endemic areas should be serotested before entering *P. bovicola*–free countries such as the United States. Parafilariasis should be reported in the United States.

9.27.10. *Zoonotic potential:* Humans are not susceptible to parafilariasis.

9.28. *Psoroptes ovis* (Sheep Scab, Sheep Scab Mite, Psoroptic Mange)

9.28.1. *Agent:* Sheep Scab is caused by the *Psoroptes ovis* mite. The disease is characterized by large scabs and intense pruritus.

9.28.2. *Affected species:* Sheep and cattle are primarily affected. The mite has also been found on llamas, goats, and alpacas (Table 9.28).

Table 9.28. Psoroptes ovis.

Disease Severity in Potentially Affected Species S = Severe D = Moderate M = Mild								
Dogs	**Horses**	**Cattle**	**Sheep**	**Goats**	**Pigs**	**Cats**	**Birds**	**Other Animals**
		D	D					

9.28.3. *Incubation period:* The life cycle of *P. ovis* is 10–12 days. The *P. ovis* is a one-host mite where all stages (larvae, nymph, and adult) feed on the host.

9.28.4. *Transmission:* Transmission is by direct contact with infected animals and fomites. *Psoroptes* is more often seen during the winter months. Under ideal environmental conditions all stages of the mite can survive for 10 days, while adult females can survive for up to 3–6 weeks. Sheep may be asymptomatic of disease. They can spread *Psoroptes* to other animals and infrequently to cattle.

9.28.5. *Occurrence:* Worldwide. Present in cattle in the United States in Colorado, Kansas, Nebraska, New Mexico, Oklahoma, and Texas. *P. ovis* has not been found in sheep in the United States since 1970.

9.28.6. *Predominant clinical signs:* The mites survive at the base of the hairs and introduce toxic saliva, which is extremely irritating. Severe pruritis, yellow crusts, heavy scabs lichenification, and excoriation occur in cattle. Generally the lesions are first noted on the head and rump. If severe enough, the disease will spread to the rest of the body and secondary bacterial infections may result. Weight loss, susceptibility to other infections, mortality in untreated calves, and decline in milk production are all serious economic losses as a result of *Psoroptes* infection. In sheep, the lesions are primarily on the wooly regions of the body. They also develop crusty, scaly lesions that are extremely pruritic. If left untreated, weight loss and anemia can occur.

9.28.7. *Treatment:* Ivermectin and dips such as coumaphos, toxaphene, phosmet, and hot lime sulfur may be used to control the mite. Infested animals should be quarantined until treatment is complete to prevent exposure to naïve animals.

9.28.8. *Prevention:* No vaccine is available.

9.28.9. *Control:* Fly populations, especially houseflies, should be controlled to prevent spread of the disease. *Psoroptes ovis* is reportable in the United States in cattle and sheep.

9.28.10. *Zoonotic potential:* Humans are not susceptible to *Psoroptes ovis*.

9.29. Rabbit Hemorrhagic Disease (RHD) (Viral Hemorrhagic Disease of Rabbits, Rabbit Hemorrhagic Disease Syndrome, X Disease, Necrotic Hepatitis of Rabbits, Rabbit Calicivirus Disease)

9.29.1. *Agent:* RHD is a peracute to acute caliciviral disease of rabbits (*Oryctolagus cuniculus*). RHD causes necrosis of the liver, intestines, and lymphoid tissues. As the disease progresses, there is extensive coagulopathy and hemorrhage in the organs. Mortality rates can approach 90%–100%. RHD is used in Australia and New Zealand as a biological control agent to manage free-range rabbits, as they are major pests in these countries.

9.29.2. *Affected species:* The domestic rabbit and the European rabbit are most affected. The Eastern cottontail, volcano rabbit, black-tailed jackrabbit, hares, and the European brown hare do not appear to be susceptible (Table 9.29).

Table 9.29. Rabbit Hemorrhagic Disease.

Disease Severity in Potentially Affected Species S = Severe D = Moderate M = Mild								
Dogs	**Horses**	**Cattle**	**Sheep**	**Goats**	**Pigs**	**Cats**	**Birds**	**Other Animals**
								S Domestic rabbit, European rabbit

9.29.3. *Incubation period:* The incubation period is from 24 hours after oral exposure to 3 days.

9.29.4. *Transmission:* RHD is spread by direct contact with infected animals or indirect contact with contaminated fomites (food, water, cages, clothing, rabbit products, frozen rabbit carcasses). Mechanical transmission occurs through rodents, biting insects, vehicles, and birds. Most exposures are thought to be through the fecal-oral route. Exposure occurs through conjunctival or nasal secretions and experimentally through intravenous, subcutaneous, and intramuscular methods. Acutely infected rabbits that survive the disease may become persistently infected and shed the virus in the feces and urine for 4 weeks or longer. Transmission by aerosol does not seem to be important.

9.29.5. *Occurrence:* The People's Republic of China is where RHD was first reported. It has since spread to other countries including the United States, Europe, Australia, New Zealand, Morocco, Cuba, and Mexico (Mexico City). It was eradicated from Mexico through testing and slaughter.

RHD in the United States first occurred in Denison, Iowa, in 2000. It has since occurred in Illinois, New York, and Utah in 2001 and Indiana in 2005. All cases occurred in small groups of animals.

9.29.6. *Predominant clinical signs:* Rabbits less than 5–7 weeks can be infected with RHD, but typically do not show any signs of illness. Rabbits older than 7 weeks of age will have a fever (up to 105°F) within 16–48 hours. Sudden death can occur 6–36 hours after clinical signs are seen. There may be few signs prior to death in peracute cases. Oftentimes a final squeal may be heard preceding collapse and death. Rabbits with acute disease may often have vague signs. They may show depression, diarrhea or constipation, anorexia, and dyspnea. As the disease progresses, there may be neurological signs noted (opisthotonos, paddling, incoordination, and excitement). A foamy, bloody, serosanguineous nasal discharge has been noted in 20% of RHD-infected rabbits. Rabbits that survive are often persistently infected and will shed the virus for 4 weeks or more.

9.29.7. *Treatment:* There is currently no treatment for RHD as most rabbits die from the peracute disease.

9.29.8. *Prevention:* An inactivated vaccine is available and is protective within 5–10 days. Rabbits must be revaccinated every 6 months. Rabbits that survive RHD may shed the virus.

9.29.9. *Control:* Strict restriction of rabbits, frozen rabbit carcasses, angora-rabbit wool, and raw rabbit pellets should be enforced from endemic countries. The challenge in the United States is that healthy rabbits (unknown carrier state) can be imported without testing, restriction, or quarantine. All imported rabbits and the introduction of new animals to a rabbit facility should be quarantined a minimum of 7 days. RHD is stable in blood for at least 9 months if kept cooled and much longer if frozen. In countries where RHD is endemic, test and slaughter, strict sanitation, vaccination, and maintaining closed colonies of rabbits should be performed. Deactivation of the calicivirus may be done using 10% household bleach, 1%–1.4% formalin, 10% sodium hydroxide or 2% One-stroke Environ. Chloroform and ether are ineffective against RHD. RHD is a reportable disease in the United States and is an OIE List B Disease.

9.29.10. *Zoonotic potential:* Humans are not susceptible to RHD.

9.30. Rabies (Lyssa, Hydrophobia)

9.30.1. *Agent:* Rabies is a highly fatal virus that causes acute encephalomyelitis. It is a Lyssavirus in the Rhabdoviridae family that can infect all mammals, but *primarily* carnivores and insectivorous bats. Once clinical signs are seen, it is almost always fatal.

9.30.2. *Affected species:* All warm-blooded animals are susceptible to rabies (Table 9.30). Humans are also susceptible.

Table 9.30.   Rabies.

								Disease Severity in Potentially Affected Species S = Severe D = Moderate M = Mild

Dogs	Horses	Cattle	Sheep	Goats	Pigs	Cats	Birds	Other Animals
S	S	S	S	S	S	S		S Bats, raccoons, skunks, foxes, coyotes, jackals, mongooses

9.30.3.   *Incubation period:* The rabies incubation period is inconsistent, ranging from 15 to 80 days. The incubation period may be less or longer than listed. One man incubated the disease for almost 7 years.

9.30.4.   *Transmission:* Infections are usually established following introduction of virus-infected saliva into tissues, either through a bite or scratch. Infected tissue fluids in contact with fresh wounds or intact mucous membranes (oral) have the ability to introduce the disease. Animals can also be infected by the nasal (olfactory) route. Bat-infested caves may produce infectious aerosols. Nonbite transmission (aerosols) has been reported in a number of animal species, including humans.

9.30.5.   *Occurrence:* Worldwide. It is found in most of Europe, throughout Africa, the Middle East, and most of Asia and the Americas. The UK, Ireland, parts of Scandinavia, Japan, much of Malaysia, Singapore, Australia, New Zealand, Papua New Guinea, and the Pacific Islands are free of rabies.

9.30.6.   *Predominant clinical signs:* The clinical signs of rabies are usually related to a change in behavior. Paralysis of unknown origin is commonly seen. The disease is divided into three phases: prodromal, excitative, and paralytic. Signs are extremely variable in expression and length. The prodromal phase (lasting 1–3 days) consists of indistinct neurological signs, which become progressively worse. The excitative phase or "furious form" occurs when sporadic episodes of rage are the primary sign seen. A normally lively and sociable dog may become anorexic, withdrawn, irritable, or restless. This behavior may suddenly change, with the animal becoming highly affectionate. The dog may try repeatedly to lick the hands and face of its owner or handler. As the disease progresses, the animal appears to have difficulty swallowing, as if a bone were caught in its throat. Any attempt to alleviate the problem manually exposes the handler to considerable risk, either through a bite or the deposition of virus-infected saliva on mucous membranes, or minor scratches. The dog's bark becomes high pitched and hoarse, indicating the onset of paralysis. Saliva drools from the dog's mouth. Convulsive seizures and muscular incoordination become apparent, followed by progressive paralysis, usually terminating in death within 7–10 days of the onset of symptoms. In about 25%–50% of cases, apparently as a result of limbic lobe dysfunction, dogs with rabies develop the furious form of the disease. Affected animals may eat abnormal objects, lose all fear, and, during paroxysms of rage, will attack almost anything. The paralytic phase or "dumb" phase is evidenced as little change in behavior, but there is an early progressive paralysis. The first signs noted are inability to swallow, drooling, and dropped lower jaw, as a result of paralysis of the muscles. Typically these animals are not vicious and make no attempt to bite. The paralysis will be progressive and is followed by coma and death. Despite the phase or form exhibited from an infected animal, death is invariably the result. Regardless of the species involved, a change in behavior and paralysis of unknown origin are present.

I.   Cattle will attack with the furious form. These animals are overly alert to their surroundings. Bellowing sounds will change and milk production will stop in dairy animals.

II.   Horses and mules may appear as if they have colic, may be very agitated, and may attack or bite. Many times they will have self-inflicted wounds present. Any horse with neurological signs should be considered as possible exposure to rabies.

III.   Foxes and coyotes will enter yards and attack people and other animals.

IV.   Skunks and raccoons generally show no fear of man and are discovered out during the day despite the fact that they are nocturnal animals. They may or may not show neurological signs and will readily attack humans and other animals.

V.   Bats may be out during the day despite that they are also nocturnal animals. They may be seen flying, found on the ground, and may also attack humans and animals.

VI   Rodents and lagomorphs (rabbits, hares) are not considered a source of rabies, but should be handled as any rabies suspect animal is handled until a diagnosis has been confirmed.

9.30.7.   *Treatment:* There is no treatment available for animals. Once a virulent strain of rabies virus has established itself in the central nervous system of an infected animal or human, the outcome is almost always death. Supportive care is given to humans with rabies. Rarely, have humans survived rabies after the onset of clinical disease.

9.30.8.   *Prevention:* Rabies vaccination is recommended for dogs and cats. There are several vaccines available: killed, modified-live, and attenuated. Modified-live is not used in the United States. Vaccine for ferrets, horses, cattle, and sheep is also available. Currently, no vaccine is approved in wildlife and is not recommended until efficacy can be demonstrated. An oral vaccine is available for wildlife in Canada and Europe which appears to be effective. A vaccinia-rabies glycoprotein recombinant vaccine is under investigation in the United States. Humans who have been exposed to rabies are given a series of vaccinations along with immunoglobulin. Humans who may be exposed to suspect animals should be vaccinated, checked regularly for a rabies titer, and revaccinated as needed. These individuals may still need to be vaccinated after exposure to a rabid animal. Rabies is a reportable disease in the United States and is an OIE List B Disease.

9.30.9. *Control:* Any animal that receives a bite from a possible infected bat or infected wildlife is treated as exposed to rabies. In addition, if the rabies status of the biting animal cannot be determined, the bitten animal is to be treated as a possible exposure to rabies. The current recommendation is that any unvaccinated cat, dog, stock animal, or ferret that has been exposed to rabies must be euthanized. If the owner is reluctant to euthanize their pet, the animal is placed under strict quarantine for 6 months and monitored. Some states may require direct veterinary supervision. The quarantined animal is to have no contact with humans or other animals and must be kept inside a facility that prevents other animals from entering. One month prior to release of the quarantined animal, a rabies vaccination will be given. Some states may require the animal be vaccinated prior to quarantine and 1 month before release from quarantine. All vaccinated animals that have been exposed to rabies should be vaccinated at once and then monitored for the next 45 days. The wound should be thoroughly washed and debrided as necessary to decrease the presence of rabies virus. Animals that are presumed to have rabies should be humanely euthanized and the brain submitted for testing. The rabies virus is not very stable outside the body for any length of time. It does survive at room temperature in carcasses or refrigerated for up to 48 hours. Rabies is readily inactivated by 45%–75% ethanol, formaldehyde, 1% sodium hypochlorite, quaternary ammonium compounds, heat, 2% glutaraldehyde, ultraviolet light, and iodine.

9.30.10. *Zoonotic potential:* Humans, as well as all warm-blooded animals, are susceptible to rabies.

9.31. *Rhipicephalus appendiculatus* (Brown Ear Tick)

9.31.1. *Agent: Rhipicephalus appendiculatus* is a tick that is found in the ears of livestock such as cattle, ruminants, and carnivores. The tick can cause serious injury to the ears as well as carry other infectious diseases.

9.31.2. *Affected species:* Cattle, antelope, sheep, goats, carnivores, and sometimes rodents (Table 9.31).

Table 9.31. *Rhipicephalus appendiculatus* (Brown Ear Tick).

				Disease Severity in Potentially Affected Species S = Severe D = Moderate M = Mild				
Dogs	**Horses**	**Cattle**	**Sheep**	**Goats**	**Pigs**	**Cats**	**Birds**	**Other Animals**
		S	S	S				S Antelope, carnivores

9.31.3. *Incubation period:* Experimentally the incubation period is 5–6 days before hatching into larvae.

9.31.4. Life Cycle: *R. appendiculatus* is a three-host tick. Cattle are the primary host for these ticks. So for large numbers of *R. appendiculatus* to occur, cattle must be present.

9.31.5. *Transmission:* Direct contact. The immature and adult ticks feed on the ears of cattle and other ruminants. When infestations are particularly severe, ticks may be found on other parts of the body. Carnivores, small antelope, and sometimes rodents will serve as a host for the immature ticks.

9.31.6. *Occurrence: R. appendiculatus* is found in southern Sudan, South Africa, and eastern Zaire to Kenya. The tick can be found from as low as sea level to greater than 8000 feet. It is a major problem in areas that tend to be shrubby, cool, woody, or shaded savannas. The tick is mostly seasonal, in that it is associated with rain and temperature.

9.31.7. *Predominant clinical signs:* The tick causes damage to the ears of infected cattle, which can be quite serious with heavy infestations. The infected animals can also have a decreased resistance to other infections and occasionally a fatal toxemia. Transmission of other diseases by *R. appendiculatus* tick include Nairobi sheep disease, Corridor disease, East Coast Fever, Thogoto virus, Zimbabwe malignant theileriosis, *Theileria taurotragi, Rickettsia conorii,* and *Ehrlichia bovis.*

9.31.8. *Treatment:* The use of acaricides (pyrethrins, carbamates, synthetic pyrethroids, fipronil, imidacloprid, malathion) will greatly decrease the number of ticks on animals.

9.31.9. *Control:* These three-host ticks spend nearly 90% or more of their lifecycle off the animal. For maximal control of these ticks, the environment and the animal must be treated. *R. appendiculatus* is a reportable disease in the United States.

9.31.10. *Zoonotic potential:* Humans are susceptible to tick typhus caused by *Rickettsia conorii* that is carried by *R. appendiculatus.*

9.32. Rinderpest (RP) (Cattle Plague)

9.32.1. *Agent:* Rinderpest is a contagious single-stranded RNA Morbillivirus in the Parmyxoviridae family. It causes disease in cattle, domestic buffalo, and some species of wildlife. It most likely infects all cloven-hoofed animals. Morbidity can be as high as 100% and the mortality approaches 90%.

9.32.2. *Affected species:* Most domestic and wild cloven-hoofed animals are thought to be susceptible. European pigs and hippopotami have subclinical infections, while Asiatic pigs and warthogs are very susceptible. Moderate infections of RP occur in the East African zebus and wildebeest. Mild infections of RP exist in the small domestic ruminants and gazelle. Pigs, sheep, goats, and wild ungulates may also show signs of disease (Table 9.32).

Table 9.32. Rinderpest.

			Disease Severity in Potentially Affected Species **S = Severe D = Moderate M = Mild**					
Dogs	**Horses**	**Cattle**	**Sheep**	**Goats**	**Pigs**	**Cats**	**Birds**	**Other Animals**
		S	S	S	D Hippos, warthog			S Buffalo, wildlife, giraffes, camels, wild suidae, tragelaphinae

9.32.3. *Incubation period:* The incubation period varies from 3 to 15 days, but it is usually 4–5 days.

9.32.4. *Transmission:* Transmission is either through direct or indirect contact. Ocular-nasal and fecal secretions are important in transmission. RP infected animals are most contagious (due to high levels of virus) primarily 1–2 days before a fever develops and for at least the first 8–9 days of the clinical disease.

9.32.5. *Occurrence:* The disease is found only in the Indian subcontinent, the Near East, and sub-Saharan Africa. Countries bordering endemic areas: East, North, and West Africa, parts of Asia, and parts of the Near East have had outbreaks of RP due to poor control.

9.32.6. *Predominant clinical signs:* Four clinical forms of RP have been reported: peracute, acute, subacute, and atypical. The peracute form is seen in the young and very susceptible animals. Fever (104°–107°F), congested mucous membranes, and death occur 2–3 days after the fever. The acute or classic form has a fever (104°–106°F) with serous ocular and nasal secretions that become mucopurulent. Depression and anorexia may also occur. Drooling may be profuse as a result of the oral lesions.

Diarrhea is often watery with or without blood, mucus, and mucous membranes in it. Dehydration, weight loss, abdominal pain, and dyspnea may be present. Death usually occurs 6–12 days after the initial onset of signs. If the animal survives RP, recovery is slow and these animals are almost always immunocompromised. The subacute form is characterized by one or two of the classic signs and a lower mortality rate. The atypical form is characterized by an intermittent fever and little to no diarrhea. The four Ds to remember for this disease are as follows: Depression, Diarrhea, Dehydration, and Death.

9.32.7. *Treatment:* No treatment is available. Supportive care may be given. Immunity is thought to be lifelong.

9.32.8. *Prevention:* Vaccination (an attenuated cell culture) is given to cattle and buffalo greater than 1 year of age in endemic areas. If an outbreak occurs, the area should be quarantined. Both infected and exposed animals are slaughtered, disposal is by burial or burning, and ring vaccination should be considered. Rinderpest is a reportable disease in the United States and it is an OIE List A Disease.

9.32.9. Decontamination: It remains present in frozen tissues for at least a year. Direct sunlight, heat, frequent freezing and thawing of blood and tissue will inactivate the virus. pH 12.0 and pH 2.0 will inactivate RP after 10 minutes. Most regularly used disinfectants can be used to inactivate the virus.

9.32.10. *Zoonotic potential:* Humans are not susceptible to Rinderpest.

9.33. Sarcoptic Mange (Scabies, Cutaneous Acariasis, Mite Infestation, Itch Mite)

9.33.1. *Agent:* Scabies is an extremely contagious parasite caused by the *Sarcoptes scabiei* spp. mite (Fig. 9.4). Although scabies tends to be host specific, it can reside on other animals, including humans. Scabies causes severe pruritus, and hair is lost due to continuous scratching.

9.33.2. *Affected species:* Dogs (*Sarcoptes scabiei var canis*), cattle (*Sarcoptes scabiei var bovis*), horses (*Sarcoptes scabiei var equi*), sheep (*Sarcoptes scabiei var ovis*), goats (*Sarcoptes scabiei var caprae*), pigs

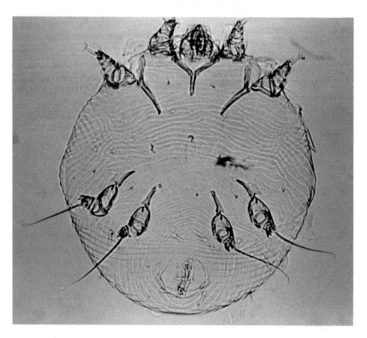

Figure 9.4. Scabies is an extremely contagious parasite caused by the *Sarcoptes scabiei* mite. (Source: Public Domain. Image #6301. http://phil.cdc.gov/phil/details.asp.)

(*Sarcoptes scabiei var suis*), wild canids (coyotes, foxes [*Sarcoptes scabiei var vulpis*], etc), cats (*Notoedres cati*), ferrets, rabbits, and other warm-blooded animals are considered susceptible to scabies (Table 9.33). Humans are also susceptible to this mite.

Table 9.33. Sarcoptic Mange.

Disease Severity in Potentially Affected Species S = Severe D = Moderate M = Mild								
Dogs	**Horses**	**Cattle**	**Sheep**	**Goats**	**Pigs**	**Cats**	**Birds**	**Other Animals**
S	S	S	S	S	S	D		S Most warm-blooded animals

9.33.3. *Incubation period:* At 3–5 days after the female mite lays eggs, the six-legged larvae hatch and can burrow into the skin. The incubation period on dogs is anywhere from 10 days to 8 weeks depending on how many mites are present, the site where they affix, and susceptibility of the individual animal.

9.33.4. *Life Cycle:* The entire life cycle, approximately 17–21 days, of the *Sarcoptes* mite is on the host animal. The female mite burrows into the skin and lays as many as 40–50 eggs (or 3–5 eggs daily). Once the eggs hatch in 3–5 days, they are six-legged larvae. These larvae can then roam the skin or remain burrowed under the skin. Burrowed larvae molt into the eight-legged nymph, which eventually becomes the adult mite.

9.33.5. *Transmission:* Direct and indirect contact.

9.33.6. *Occurrence:* Worldwide.

9.33.7. *Predominant clinical signs:* In most species, affected animals are extremely pruritic. Scabies is a burrowing mite that causes irritation. It is thought that the pruritus is a result of the actual bite of the mite and toxic or allergic substances produced by the mite. Dogs may have a severe pruritus. Papules may be present and a thickened yellow crust results due to the intense scratching by the affected dog. Lesions are most commonly found on the ventral abdomen, ears, legs, and elbows. These lesions may extend to the rest of the body if not treated. Secondary bacterial infections are often present. In chronic conditions, there is skin keratinization, seborrhea, loss of weight, peripheral lymphadenopathy, and if severe enough, death results. There may be asymptomatic carriers. Signs are more often seen under warm conditions or at night, although scabies can occur at any time. Cattle are affected initially around the neck, shoulders, and head. There is crusting and thickening of the skin as the disease progresses. Eventually the entire body may be affected by this mite within in about 6 weeks. Scabies is more common when the weather is either cold, wet, or both partly due to huddling of animals. It is also seen with poor nutrition, crowding, or animals that are housed under inadequate conditions. As the disease progresses, there are weight loss, excessive keratinization, secondary bacterial infections, and decreased production. Abrasions or self-mutilation may be noted due to the animal constantly scratching itself. Confined animals may have increased abrasions on the teats and udder. Death may result in some animals if left untreated. Horses in the United States seldom present with scabies. When they do, scabies is the most serious mange they can acquire and it proliferates rapidly. The head, neck, and shoulders will show initial signs of the mite as well as severe pruritus. The affected animal may be seen scratching and biting at itself. Papules, vesicles, and eventually crusts will form. As the disease progresses, there is keratinization of the skin and loss of hair over the entire body. The legs and areas where long hair is present do not seem to be as affected as the rest of the body. With progression of scabies, there is weight loss, anorexia, and weakness. Scabies in horses is usually chronic and it is the most challenging mange in horses, especially when animals are in poor health or have serious infections. Sheep do not usually present with scabies in the United States. When it is seen in sheep, nonwooly areas such as the face and head are affected first. Goats have widespread hyperkeratosis, crusts, wrinkles, and reddening. Again, lesions are initially noted on the ears, nose, face, lips, and neck. As the disease progresses, there is weight loss, lymphadenopathy, and secondary bacterial infections. Pigs are usually infected with the introduction of diseased breeding animals. Scabies is again initially seen on the ears and head before spreading to the rest of the body, including the legs and tail. Pigs tend to be hypersensitive to the mite, so pruritus and rubbing can be intense. The skin becomes hyperkeratinized, there may be large folds in the skin, and grayish crusts develop. Unhealthy, decreased growth rate, or stunted pigs may be seen. Occasionally scabies may be seen as a chronic dermatitis with only some pigs afflicted. Fox and other wild canids show clinical signs similar to dogs. Cats seldom develop mange, but it is considered extremely contagious. The ear tips are initially involved, followed by the face, head, body, and legs. There is extreme pruritus, erythematous papules, hyperkeratinization, loss of hair, and yellow-gray crusts. Secondary bacterial infections and generalized lymphadenopathy may also be noted. Weight loss, anorexia, toxemia, and death are less often seen. Ferrets with scabies usually have involvement of the feet which become swollen and ulcerated. Rabbits may be infected with S. scabiei or N. cati. They are very contagious and not easily treated. Often, humane euthanasia is recommended as they can spread the disease to humans. Rabbits display signs of extreme pruritus as well as loss of hair at the base of the ears, around the nose and eyes, and on the head.

9.33.8. *Treatment:* Treatment can be done with a number of insecticides that are available as topicals, sprays, dips, pour-ons, dusts, and oral or injectable formulations. Some products that are used to treat scabies include avermectins, amitraz, lime sulfur, milbemycins, toxaphene, phosmet, coumaphos, organophosphates, lindane, malathion, and 0.25% chlordane solution to name a few. Not all of these medications are approved in each of these species or may be allowed for use in food-producing animals. In some animals, best results for scabies treatment may require bathing with antiseborrheic shampoos to facilitate removal of crusts and scabs. In addition, antibiotics should be used if secondary bacterial infections are present. Corticosteroids used short term are used to control pruritus.

9.33.9. *Prevention:* Any introduction of new animals or breeding animals should be quarantined and treated prior to introduction to the rest of the herd. If mange is already present in a group of animals, they should be routinely examined, treated and tested for mange. Infected animals should be separated from the rest of the group to help facilitate clearing the mange.

9.33.10. *Control:* Although indirect contact is minor in the spread of scabies, disinfection of equipment, instruments, pens, bedding, etc. will decrease the presence of the mite. It survives only a few days off the host and is vulnerable to desiccation. When scabies is present in a group of animals, carrier or asymptomatic animals should be identified, culled, and the remaining animals treated for mange. *Sarcoptes scabiei* is reportable in the United States and is an OIE List B Disease.

9.33.11. *Zoonotic potential:* Humans are susceptible to scabies and it is usually self-limiting. Humans will have pruritus that affects much of the body and the pruritus may be more noticeable at night. A rash is usually present on the elbows or knees, between the fingers, shoulders, or the genitals. The intense scratching can cause secondary bacterial infections. Initial signs of scabies make take 2–6 weeks (usually four weeks) before clinical signs are noticed. Subsequent exposure to the mite (due to mite sensitization), clinical signs will appear in 1–4 days. "Scabies rash" or a papule may appear in the scapular region, abdomen, and buttocks despite the female mite not being present in these areas. Immunocompromised individuals are at a higher risk and develop Norwegian scabies. This form of scabies causes vesicles and thickened crusts to form on the skin. There will be numerous mites present in these lesions, but very little itching associated with it.

9.34. Screwworm Myiasis (Mosca Verde, Gusanos, Gusano Barrendor, Gusaneras)

9.34.1. *Agent:* Myiasis is the infestation of live animals with the New World screwworm fly larvae *Cochliomyia hominivorax* and the Old World screwworm *Chrysomya bezziana*. The screwworm larvae feed on the host's dead or living tissue, body secretions, and ingested food. The larva penetrates deeply into a wound of a warm-blooded animal and subsequently feeds on the living tissue.

9.34.2. *Affected species:* All warm-blooded animals are susceptible. Birds are rarely infected (Table 9.34).

Table 9.34. Screwworm.

				Disease Severity in Potentially Affected Species S = Severe D = Moderate M = Mild				
Dogs	**Horses**	**Cattle**	**Sheep**	**Goats**	**Pigs**	**Cats**	**Birds**	**Other Animals**
S	S	S	S	S	S	S	M	S All warm-blooded animals

9.34.3.   Incubation period: Larvae hatch from the eggs in as little as 8–12 hours. It takes about 5–7 days for the larvae to mature and exit the wound.

9.34.4.   *Transmission:* Adult females lay batches of eggs (200–400 eggs) on somewhat overlapping rows in fresh wounds and to some extent in moist areas of the body. The larvae hatch after 8–12 hours and move into the wound. They then consume tissue and fluids, finishing their growth in 5–7 days. At this time, the mature larvae leaves the wound, falls to the ground and tunnels into the soil to enter into the pupal period. The larvae do not like light, hence the tunneling in the ground. The environmental temperature plays a role in the length of the pupal stage, which can last from 1 week (warmer temperatures) to 2 months (cooler temperatures). An adult female fly emerges and breeds only once in its lifetime.

   The adult male generally breeds several times. The adult female fly feeds and lays eggs in the wound. The life cycle of the screwworm can occur in as little as 21 days. Male screwworms live about 2 weeks and the female screwworm survives about a month. As a wound is invaded by screwworm larvae, they release large amounts of a malodorous discharge that further attracts the adult screwworm and other insects.

9.34.5.   *Occurrence:* New World screwworms are present in some Caribbean Islands, Mexic o, Central, and South America. Infrequently, they may be found at altitudes as high as 7000 feet. Reports of screwworms periodically in the United States have been the result of imported animals from endemic areas. Old World screwworms are found in sub-Saharan and tropical Africa, Kuwait, India, Southeast Asia, Oman, Fujaira, Muscat, and Papua New Guinea.

9.34.6.   *Predominant clinical signs:* Any wound, damage to the skin (hide) or orifice (nasal, vaginal, or anal) is optimal for screwworms to feed on. Bites from other insects, castration, cuts, dehorning, branding, viral infections (sore mouth in sheep), navels of the newborn all serve as sources for the screwworm to feed. It may take 3 or more days before a screwworm infestation is noticed. Prior to this time, minor movement may be noticed by the screwworm. After about 3 days, the wound will become much larger and cavernous. The larvae are found vertically oriented in the wound and as many as 100–200 may be present. Once the screwworm has invaded a wound, a malodorous, reddish-brown discharge is produced. This discharge attracts other screwworms and insects that further damage and enlarge the wound. Disturbed larvae tend to tunnel deeper into the tissue layers. Often a small wound will be present on the surface (skin) and a much deeper area will be affected underneath. Animals infected with screwworms will lose their appetite, have decreased milk production, and display discomfort. They will often separate themselves from the herd/flock and seek the shade. If left untreated, death occurs in these animals in 7–14 days. Death is thought to be a result of toxins produced by the screwworm, secondary infections, or a combination of both.

9.34.7. *Treatment:* A diagnosis of screwworm myiasis should be confirmed prior to treatment. Application of an approved topical larvicide is placed directly into the infested wound. Retreatment of the wound should be performed at least 2 or 3 successive days to ensure that all larvae have been removed and killed. Once the larvae have been removed, the wound heals fairly quickly.

9.34.8. *Prevention:* There is no vaccine available. Screwworm endemic areas should inspect animals every 3–4 days to avoid infestation and treat infected wounds. Breeding and calving seasons should be planned during the cooler seasons, when flies are less likely to be present. Sterile male flies have been used to eradicate screwworms from the United States. This is a reportable disease in the United States.

9.34.9. *Control:* Approved insecticides (organophosphates) are used to control screwworms. Larvicides need to be used to treat larvae in wounds. All larvae should be destroyed with alcohol or a similar solution to prevent them from maturing into adults.

9.34.10. *Zoonotic potential:* Humans are susceptible to screwworm myiasis.

9.35. Sheep Pox and Goat Pox (SGP)

9.35.1. *Agent:* Sheep pox and goat pox, in fully susceptible animals, is a highly contagious and often fatal virus caused by Capripox in the Poxviridae family. It is characterized by fever and pox. The disease ranges from acute to subacute.

9.35.2. *Affected species:* Sheep and goats are susceptible. Wild ungulates do not appear to be affected by SGP (Table 9.35).

Table 9.35. Sheep Pox and Goat Pox.

Disease Severity in Potentially Affected Species S = Severe D = Moderate M = Mild								
Dogs	Horses	Cattle	Sheep	Goats	Pigs	Cats	Birds	Other Animals
			S	S				

9.35.3. *Incubation period:* The incubation period is 4–8 days for sheep pox and 5–14 days for goat pox. Clinical signs of SGP last for 4–6 weeks and may take up to three months to completely heal.

9.35.4. *Transmission:* Transmission is by direct and indirect contact. Inhalation (aerosol, dust) is the primary means of transmission, followed by contact with skin lesions, fomites, transmission by insects, and through inoculation (SQ, IV, ID, IN). SGP can survive on contaminated premises for many months.

9.35.5. *Occurrence:* SGP is endemic in Africa, the Middle East, Turkey, and India. Sporadic cases occur in the Greek Isles.

9.35.6. *Predominant clinical signs:* The young are more severely affected, with lambs and kids (less than 1 month old) approaching 100% morbidity and 95% mortality. In older sheep and goats, morbidity runs 5%–80% and mortality is 5%–50%. Signs are very similar in both sheep and goats. The younger the animal is when exposed, the more severe the symptoms. Fever, swollen eyelids, ocular-nasal discharges, depression, and salivation are first seen. Pox lesions show up several days after the initial signs. These lesions are best seen where the hair and coat are absent or sparse. Typically, the more pox lesions that are seen, the more severe is the disease. The lesions first appear erythematous, then become a raised, edematous plaque, followed by a necrotic, depressed lesion, and then scab formation (2–4 weeks after initial signs). If the lesion is severe enough, the area will not regrow hair or a scar may be present. Secondary bacterial infections may also complicate the course of the disease. Some pox lesions can occur on the lungs, causing dyspnea and pneumonia

9.35.7. *Treatment:* No treatment is available.

9.35.8. *Prevention:* Immunity to SGP is lifelong. Modified-live vaccine is used to control SGP in endemic areas. If SGP occurs in a new area, animals should be quarantined, identified as infected or exposed animals, and slaughtered. The premises and all equipment should be cleaned and disinfected. No carrier state occurs, but the virus persists in the environment for long periods of time. SGP is a reportable disease in the United States and is an OIE List A Disease.

9.35.9. Decontamination: SGP is especially hardy to both chemical and physical agents. Sodium hypochlorite is effective at deactivating SGP.

9.35.10. *Zoonotic potential:* Humans are not susceptible to SGP.

9.36. Strangles (Distemper, Equine Distemper)

9.36.1. *Agent:* Strangles is an extremely contagious respiratory disease of equine caused by bacteria (*Streptococcus equi equi*). It is one of the oldest diseases of horses.

9.36.2. *Affected species:* Horses, mules, and donkeys are very susceptible to strangles. Younger animals (less than 5 years of age) appear to be particularly susceptible. Humans have been reported to be infected with the strangles organism (Table 9.36).

Table 9.36. Strangles.

		Disease Severity in Potentially Affected Species S = Severe D = Moderate M = Mild						
Dogs	**Horses**	**Cattle**	**Sheep**	**Goats**	**Pigs**	**Cats**	**Birds**	**Other Animals**
	S Donkeys, mules							

9.36.3. *Incubation period:* The incubation period is normally 3–10 days.

9.36.4. *Transmission:* Transmission of strangles is by inhalation (nasal discharges), ingestion (food and water containers), or fomites (grooming equipment, clothing, stomach tubes, blankets). A few equidae become carrier animals, which is important in the maintenance of strangles between outbreaks.

9.36.5. *Occurrence:* Strangles is found worldwide.

9.36.6. *Predominant clinical signs:* Morbidity can approach 100% in some naïve herds. Age, management of the herd, and immune status are important factors in morbidity. Mortality can range from 2% to 5%. Submandibular swelling (usually first seen by the owner) and fever (up to 106°F) are frequently first noted. A fever along with abscessed lymph nodes around the head and neck is nearly pathognomonic for strangles. Depression, pain, and lack of an appetite are common. There is usually a nasal discharge (serous to mucopurulent) present and there may also be an ocular discharge. Lymphadenopathy involving most of the lymph nodes around the head and neck may spread to other lymph tissues of the body. Dyspnea, dysphagia, and coughing will be noted as the swelling progresses. Hence, the term "strangles" is used to describe these animals. Signs may persist for 10–14 days or up to several months. Generally, when the abscesses begin to open and drain, recovery occurs quickly. The term "bastard strangles" relates to abscesses that arise in other parts of the body (liver, kidney, spleen, lungs, thorax, guttural pouches, joints, etc.). Peritonitis and pleuritis can result from these abscesses. These conditions are thought to happen in animals that do not have a fully developed immune system or do not develop an immune response to strangles. Metastatic abscesses cause chronic weight loss. Lactating mares often will have decreased milk production. Very rarely does purpura hemorrhagica occur, but it can be deadly. Fever, depression, hemorrhages (especially on the mucosa and skin), and peripheral edema result. Septic emboli develop in the blood vessels of the affected tissues.

9.36.7. *Treatment:* Treatment consists of quarantine, rest, and supportive care. Mild cases are usually treated with hot packs to encourage abscesses to open and drain. The use of antibiotics is controversial as to when they are needed. Animals with a tracheostomy, that are not improving, nursing foals, or animals with severe infections should be placed on antibiotics.

9.36.8. *Prevention:* Any new horse that is introduced into the herd should be quarantined for at least 30 days. If at anytime during the quarantine a nasal discharge is noted, swabs should be performed to determine it the horse has been exposed to the strangles organism. It is important to note that recovered horses should be quarantined for at least 1–2 months after recovery or exposure (even if no clinical signs are seen) to strangles. Three consecutive nasal swabs (at 4- to 7-day intervals) should be performed on an infected horse. All three swabs should be negative before introduction to other horses. Thorough cleaning and disinfection of the facilities and equipment is important to decrease the spread of the disease. Personnel must practice good hygiene to prevent the spread of disease not only to other horses, but to themselves. There are several vaccines available. These vaccines do not always prevent the disease, but will lessen the clinical signs. Annual revaccination is recommended.

9.36.9. *Control:* The strangles organism is very hardy and can survive 7–9 weeks under ideal environmental conditions. Strict cleaning and disinfection of all facilities, equipment, tack, grooming devices, food and water troughs should be performed and should not be used for at least 4 weeks.

9.36.10. *Zoonotic potential:* Humans have been known to be susceptible to the strangles organism. Flu-like symptoms are usually seen. Skin and soft tissue infections, pharyngitis, pneumonia, and sepsis have been described.

9.37. Swine Vesicular Disease (SVD)

9.37.1. *Agent:* SVD is a contagious porcine enterovirus in the Picornaviridae family. SVD may have been a result of pigs eating human feces. It is very closely related to coxsackie B5, a human virus. This disease is important because it produces lesions that are grossly indistinguishable from those of FMD. Pigs with natural disease have a favorable prognosis; however, in most countries, as soon as it is recognized, the pigs are slaughtered.

9.37.2. *Affected species:* Pigs are susceptible to SVD. Laboratory personnel have been infected with the virus. The virus has isolated in cattle and sheep, but it does not cause disease in them. Experimentally, baby mice are capable of being infected (Table 9.37).

9.37.3. *Incubation period:* The incubation period is 2–7 days with direct contact with infected pigs. If the virus is ingested (garbage, contaminated food), the incubation period is 2–3 days.

Table 9.37. Swine Vesicular Disease.

Disease Severity in Potentially Affected Species S = Severe D = Moderate M = Mild								
Dogs	Horses	Cattle	Sheep	Goats	Pigs	Cats	Birds	Other Animals
					S			

9.37.4. *Transmission:* Transmission is either through direct (feces, secretions, body fluids, infected garbage) or indirect contact (fecal contaminated vehicles and equipment).

9.37.5. *Occurrence:* SVD was originally recognized in Italy. It has since occurred in Great Britain, France, Austria, Belgium, Portugal, Malta, Germany, Poland, the Netherlands, Greece, Spain, and Switzerland. It still occurs occasionally in parts of Asia. SVD has not occurred in North America.

9.37.6. *Predominant clinical signs:* Morbidity is 25%–60% and mortality is extremely low except in baby pigs. SVD cannot be distinguished from FMD and other vesicular diseases. The symptoms are often so mild, that they may go unnoticed. Signs of SVD comprise of fever, reluctance to eat, and vesicles or erosions on the mouth, nose, and feet. Seldom are neurological signs seen due to SVD. If so, it is usually a result of encephalitis which may cause lameness, jerking, unsteady gait, or shivering. Recovery from SVD usually takes 2–3 weeks with little to no long term effects.

9.37.7. *Treatment:* No treatment, other than symptomatic.

9.37.8. *Prevention:* No vaccine is available. Preventive measures should include restriction of animals imported from infected areas. Garbage from international aircraft and ships should be sanitized. Eradication is done through quarantine, identification of infected animals and premises, and slaughter and disposal of infected and exposed pigs. Thorough cleaning and disinfecting of infected premises, vehicles, and equipment should be performed. SVD is a reportable disease in the United States and is an OIE List A Disease.

9.37.9. *Control:* SVD is very resistant to disinfectants and is hardy in most environments. It remains active in meat, meat byproducts, and treated meat products (salted, smoked, and dried meat) for up to 2 years. It remains active from pH 2.5 to 12.0 and in frozen meat. It is inactivated by temperatures of 157°F and disinfectants such as 3% bleach, 1% Virkon S, and 2% lye.

9.37.10. *Zoonotic potential:* Humans are susceptible to SVD. It has been reported in laboratory personnel working with the virus. Caution should be used when around SVD-infected tissues, garbage, equipment, etc.

9.38. Theileriases (Theileriosis, East Coast Fever, Corridor Disease, January Disease, African Coast Fever, Zimbabwean Tick Fever)

9.38.1. *Agent:* The Theileria species is a protozoan that causes tick-borne diseases. The most important of these protozoans are *T. parva* and *T. annulata*, which may cause death in cattle.

9.38.2. *Affected species:* Cattle in endemic areas and young cattle appear to be somewhat more resistant to disease. Cattle, especially introduced cattle and Indian water buffalo are susceptible *T. parva*. African buffalo and waterbucks serve as reservoirs for *T. parva*. Cattle, buffalo, and yak may be infected with *T. annulata*. Buffalo have a milder disease with *T. annulata* (Table 9.38).

Table 9.38. Theileriases.

Disease Severity in Potentially Affected Species S = Severe D = Moderate M = Mild								
Dogs	Horses	Cattle	Sheep	Goats	Pigs	Cats	Birds	Other Animals
		S Indian water buffalo						D Yak, buffalo

9.38.3. *Incubation period:* The incubation period may be as little as 8–12 days to greater than 3 weeks depending on conditions for the tick.

9.38.4. *Transmission:* Transmission is primarily done by the *R. appendiculatus* tick from one stage to the next and not transovarial. Infected ticks are able to survive for up to two years on pasture depending on proper environmental conditions. Adult ticks survive longer than the nymphs. Hot weather is less favorable to the tick, especially the nymph. The tick attaches to the host for several days to feed, which allows the Theileria sporozoite to mature in the saliva of the tick. When the weather is especially hot, the sporozoite may mature in the tick while it is on the ground. If this happens, cattle can become infected within hours of attachment of the tick.

9.38.5. *Occurrence: T. parva* is found in central and east Africa; from southern Sudan to South Africa and west to Zaire. *T. annulata* is known as Mediterranean or tropical theileriosis and is found in the Mediterranean coastal area, the Middle East, North Africa, Asia, India, and the former USSR.

9.38.6. *Predominant clinical signs:* Signs of theileriasis occurs usually 7–15 days after the infected tick has attached to the host. Swelling and draining of the parotid lymph nodes are usually noted first, as they are near the infected ears. Superficial widespread lymphadenopathy usually follows. A fever (103°–106°F) generally occurs fairly quickly and remains throughout the disease process. There is loss of appetite and condition. Other clinical signs that may be seen prior to death include nasal discharge, corneal opacity, lacrimation, diarrhea, and respiratory distress. Death occurs 18–30 days after initial exposure. The animal has difficulty breathing, decreased temperature, and is recumbent. Nearly 100% of susceptible animals will die from theileriasis. Depending on multiple factors such as infestation, the strain of the disease, etc, a chronic wasting may occur. "Turning sickness" is a fatal neurological condition that affects the capillaries in the brain by blocking them. Cattle often show little to no signs of disease with theileriasis and are carriers. A few that have recovered from theileriasis may have long lasting affects of the disease and have low productivity or be stunted. Tropical theileriosis can cause death losses up to 90%. Affected animals also have swollen superficial lymph nodes and fever. Loss of weight is evident. Jaundice, anemia, pale mucous membranes, as well as hemoglinuria may occur.

9.38.7. *Treatment:* Three medications can be used: parvaquone, buparvaquone, and halofuginone lactate. All three medications are expensive, which may be difficult for the typical African farmer to afford. In addition, diagnosis must be made quickly for therapy to be effective.

9.38.8. *Prevention:* Another method is to vaccinate by "infection and treatment." The animal is exposed to a heavy dose of ticks and treated with one of the medications and/or tetracyclines with them. Depending on the strain of *T. parva* (no cross-protection between strains), immunity can last for up to 3.5 years. *T. annulata* does cross-protect.

9.38.9. *Control:* Use of medications and vaccinations works best. Acaricides work well but need to be applied weekly or more frequently, depending on the tick season. The acaricides can be very expensive and there is the risk of tick resistance if the products are used too much. Pasture rotation, selecting breeds resistant to ticks, fencing, and pasture management will help control the level of ticks. Theileriosis is a reportable disease in the United States.

9.38.10. *Zoonotic potential:* Humans are not susceptible to *T. parva* or *T. annulata*.

9.39. Transmissible Spongiform Encephalopathies (TSE)

9.39.1. *Agent:* Unknown, but appears to be a prion, which is a folded, propagated protein.

9.39.2. *Affected species:* Cattle (bovine spongiform encephalopathy, BSE, mad cow disease); sheep, goats, Moufflon, rodents, monkeys (scrapie); white-tailed deer, elk, black-tailed deer, mule deer, moose (chronic wasting disease, CWD); mink (transmissible mink encephalopathy, TME); cats (feline spongiform encephalopathy, FSE); and exotic ruminants (spongiform encephalopathy of exotic ruminants, SEER) (Table 9.39).

Table 9.39. Transmissible Spongiform Encephalopathies.

				Disease Severity in Potentially Affected Species S = Severe D = Moderate M = Mild				
Dogs	**Horses**	**Cattle**	**Sheep**	**Goats**	**Pigs**	**Cats**	**Birds**	**Other Animals**
		S	S	S		S		S Deer, mink, elk, rodents, monkeys, gemsbok, bison, kudu, Arabian oryx, scimitar-horned oryx, eland, nyala, ankole

9.39.3. *Incubation period:* The incubation period is months to years for many of these diseases.

9.39.4. *Transmission:* For many of these diseases the transmission is thought to be oral. BSE is found in the nervous tissue. Spongiform encephalopathy of exotic ruminants may also occur parenterally. Feline spongiform encephalopathy, in wild cats in zoos, is transmitted orally, through infected carcasses. In domestic cats it is the cattle offal in pet food. CWD is unknown transmission, but it may be through direct or indirect contact.

9.39.5. *Occurrence:* BSE was first recognized in Great Britain in 1986. It has been reported in numerous other countries including the United States and Canada. Scrapie is found worldwide. CWD is endemic in the United States. TME is found in the United States, Canada, Germany, Finland, and Russia. Both FSE and spongiform encephalopathy of exotic ruminants occurred in Great Britain and have declined since BSE has been controlled. There was one report of a cat in Norway with FSE.

9.39.6. *Predominant clinical signs:* Progression of disease is slow and usually involves the nervous system. CWD is mainly a wasting disease, where there is loss of weight over time. All of these diseases are progressive and cause death.

9.39.7.   *Treatment:* No treatment other than supportive. The diseases are fatal.

9.39.8.   *Control:* Both scrapie and TME are contagious, so quarantine may be needed. BSE is controlled by not allowing nervous tissue into feed. The other transmissible spongiform encephalopathy diseases do not appear to be spread laterally.

9.39.9.   *Prevention:* It is known that scrapie is very resistant to heat, disinfectants, ultraviolet radiation, formalin, and ionizing radiation. Sodium hypochlorite and sodium hydroxide are good disinfectants. Sodium hypochlorite with 2% chlorine or 2N sodium hydroxide need to be applied for at least 1 hour at 20°C to be effective. Disinfect any equipment overnight for best results. Autoclaving for a minimum of 18 minutes at 134°–138°C is very effective at controlling scrapie. Therefore, infective tissue needs to be autoclaved or incinerated. BSE, TME, FSE, and spongiform encephalopathy of exotic ruminants is reportable in the United States. Scrapie and CWD although endemic in the United States, may still be reportable in many states. A scrapie eradication program has been established to eliminate scrapie in the United States by 2010.

9.39.10.   *Zoonotic potential:* Creutzfeldt-Jakob disease (CJD) is thought to be related to consuming BSE contaminated tissue. The disease is progressive and fatal. There is no treatment other than supportive. Care should be used when handling any animal suspected of having BSE. Scrapie does not appear to infect humans.

9.40. Trypanosomiasis (Tsetse-Transmitted Trypanosomiasis, Trypanosomosis, Tsetse Disease, Tsetse Fly Disease, Nagana)

9.40.1.   *Agent: Trypanosoma* is a protozoan that can infect all domestic animals and many wild animals. The most important species that cause infection are *T. brucei brucei, T. congolense, T. simiae,* and *T. vivax. Trypanosoma* causes chronic, subacute or acute infections and even death in animals. Cattle are the most affected species.

9.40.2.   *Affected species: T. congolense* is most important in cattle, sheep, and goats. It also causes infection in pigs, horses, and dogs. *T. vivax* is next in importance in cattle, sheep, and goats. *T. brucei brucei* also infects cattle, sheep, and goats as well as cats, dogs, horses, pigs, and camels. *T. simiae* is important in pigs, while *T. brucei* is important in cats and dogs. Other animals that may be infected by trypanosomes include rabbits, guinea pigs, mice, rats, and monkeys. Animals that are carriers for the disease include lions, leopards, ruminants, wild pigs, and wild Equidae. Animals may also be infected with more than one trypanosome species. Sleeping sickness in humans is caused by *T. brucei rhodesiense* and *T. brucei gambiense* (Table 9.40).

Table 9.40. Trypanosomiasis.

			Disease Severity in Potentially Affected Species S = Severe D = Moderate M = Mild						
Dogs	**Horses**	**Cattle**	**Sheep**	**Goats**	**Pigs**	**Cats**	**Birds**	**Other Animals**
S	S	S	S	S	S	S		S Camels, monkeys

9.40.3. *Incubation period:* The incubation period is 4–24 days for *T. congolense*, 4–40 days for *T. vivax*, and 5–10 days for *T. brucei brucei*.

9.40.4. *Transmission:* The tsetse fly is primarily responsible for carrying *T. congolense*, *T. vivax* and *T. brucei brucei*. This protozoan reproduces in the tsetse fly and is introduced to the host animal by the saliva of the tsetse fly. Three tsetse fly species of importance are *Glossina fusca* (high, thick-wooded areas), *G. morsitans* (wide open woodland of the savanna), and *G. palpalis* (shaded areas near lakes and rivers). Trypanosomes may also be transmitted by other biting flies. Infected blood can be carried by biting flies and tsetse flies from one animal to the next causing the mechanical transfer of these protozoa. In addition, fomites such as surgical instruments, syringes, and needles can serve as a source of infection. *T. vivax* has an unidentified vector in Central America, South America, and the Caribbean, which do not have the tsetse fly.

9.40.5. *Occurrence:* Latitude 15° N to Latitude 20° S in Africa (southern part of the Sahara desert and including Zimbabwe, Angola, and Mozambique). In the Western Hemisphere, *T. vivax* is present in approximately 10 countries excluding North America.

9.40.6. *Predominant clinical signs:* Multiple infections can occur with trypanosomes along with other diseases such as *Babesia* spp., *Anaplasma* spp., *Ehrlichia* spp., and *Theileria* spp. Therefore, it is often difficult to determine clinical signs for a particular disease. The condition the animal is in at the time of infection as well as nutrition status, and stress to the animal are important. In animals with minimal stress, no clinical signs may occur. Anemia is one of the generally accepted signs of disease with trypanosomes. In addition, weight loss, intermittent fever, and edema may be seen. Abortion may occur as well as decreased fertility in females and males. Immunosuppression is common with these protozoa. Cattle, goats, sheep, camels, and horses infected with *T. congolense* may have a peracute, acute, or chronic infection. Dogs will tend to have a chronic infection whereas pigs may only have a mild infection. Fever, weight loss, weakness, depression, anemia, lethargy, salivation, nasal discharge, or lacrimation may be seen. The hair color usually lightens as the disease progresses. *T. vivax* is less pathogenic in cattle, but can still cause death losses up to 50%. It is mostly responsible for disease in cattle, sheep, and goats in West Africa. Horses have a mild disease whereas in dogs the disease tends to be chronic. *T. brucei brucei* causes serious and often fatal disease in cats, dogs, horses, and camels. Cattle, goats, sheep, and pigs can have subclinical, mild, or chronic disease. Horses tend to have a fever that can come and go. Their appetite may be good despite losing weight and being weak. Anemia, ventral edema, and icterus may be seen. Death can occur weeks to months after exposure to the protozoa.

9.40.7. *Treatment:* There are several medications that can be used to treat trypanosomiasis. Unfortunately, the trypanosomes tend to develop resistance to many of these medications somewhat quickly. Currently, there is no vaccine available.

9.40.8. *Prevention:* Maintaining low levels of tsetse flies will help decrease further infections from occurring. In addition, blood transfer between animals should be not permitted. Trypanosomiasis is spread by an arthropod vector; therefore, cleaning and disinfecting is not effective for this disease.

9.40.9. *Control:* Spraying and dipping animals on a regular basis, clearing bushes, spraying breeding areas, etc. can help to control or eliminate the tsetse fly. Prophylactic use of medications in endemic areas is also useful. Perhaps the most effective way to protect cattle is to use breeds that tend to be resistant to trypanosomes. Many of these African cattle have been in the region for more than 5000 years and include the N'Dama and various West African short-horned cattle. Trypanosomiasis is a reportable disease in the United States.

9.40.10. *Zoonotic potential:* Humans are not susceptible to *T. congolense*, *T. vivax*, and *T. brucei brucei*. However, humans are susceptible to *T. b. gambiense* and *T. b. rhodesiense* which causes sleeping sickness and is closely related to *T. b. brucei*. Sleeping sickness can be serious and often fatal to humans. Domestic animals may serve as a source of infection for humans.

9.41. Vesicular Exanthema of Swine (VES)

9.41.1. *Agent:* VES is a highly contagious viral disease of pigs in the Caliciviridae family. It is important because it cannot be distinguished from FMD or other vesicular diseases. VES first occurred in pigs in Orange County, California, in 1932 and was mistaken for FMD. San Miguel sea lion virus disease was discovered in 1972 to be identical to VES. It can be isolated from California sea lion pups, northern elephant seal pups, and northern fur seal pups. It has also been identified from other marine mammals.

9.41.2. *Affected species:* VES only occurs in pigs. Marine mammals, other mammals (dogs, mink, calves, reptiles, seals, and chimpanzees), and Pacific Ocean fish have similar caliciviruses (Table 9.41).

Table 9.41. Vesicular Exanthema of Swine.

				Disease Severity in Potentially Affected Species S = Severe D = Moderate M = Mild				
Dogs	**Horses**	**Cattle**	**Sheep**	**Goats**	**Pigs**	**Cats**	**Birds**	**Other Animals**
					S			

9.41.3. *Incubation period:* The incubation period of VES is 18–72 hours.

9.41.4. *Transmission:* Transmission is either through direct contact with an infected pig, secretions, or eating uncooked, contaminated garbage or uncooked fish.

9.41.5. *Occurrence:* It occurred in the United States from 1932 to 1959, when it was eradicated. The United States is now considered VES free.

9.41.6. *Predominant clinical signs:* Morbidity may approach 100% and mortality is very low. VES is very similar in signs to FMD and other vesicular diseases. It is characterized by fever, followed by vesicle formation on the mouth, nose, and feet. Lameness, decreased appetite, and a reluctance to move are seen. Decreased milk production, abortion, and mild encephalitis may occur. VES lesions are commonly deeper than seen with other vesicular diseases.

9.41.7. *Treatment:* Treatment is symptomatic, but more often animals will be humanely euthanized.

9.41.8. *Prevention:* When found in an area, animals should be quarantined, identified as exposed or infected, slaughtered and disposed of properly. The premises should be cleaned and disinfected. VES is reportable in the United States and is an OIE List B Disease.

9.41.9. Decontamination: VES is very resistant to lipid solvents and survives well at 4°C and in 15°C sea water. VES is unstable at pH 3 and at 50°C. Disinfectants used to deactivate VES include 3% bleach, 2% lye, or 1% Virkon S.

9.41.10. *Zoonotic potential:* Humans are not susceptible to VES.

9.42. Vesicular Stomatitis Virus (VSV)

9.42.1. *Agent:* VSV is a contagious viral disease in the Rhabdoviridae family. It causes disease in cattle, horses, and pigs. Two serotypes occur: New Jersey and Indiana.

9.42.2. *Affected species:* Species infected include horses, mules, donkeys, cattle, pigs, and humans. South American camels, raccoons, deer, monkeys, and bobcats will develop disease. Sheep and goats are fairly resistant to VSV (Table 9.42).

Table 9.42. Vesicular Stomatitis Virus.

| Disease Severity in Potentially Affected Species S = Severe D = Moderate M = Mild | | | | | | | | |
Dogs	Horses	Cattle	Sheep	Goats	Pigs	Cats	Birds	Other Animals
	S	S	M	M	S			D South American camels, raccoons, deer, monkeys, bobcats

9.42.3. *Incubation period:* The incubation of VSV is 1–8 days or longer. In humans, the incubation is 1–2 days.

9.42.4. *Transmission:* Transmission is thought to be primarily by the black fly and sand fly. Movement of infected animals, infected fomites (food and water containers), and equipment (milking machines) can also transmit VSV. Humans are infected by aerosol or direct contact.

9.42.5. *Occurrence:* The disease is reported in North and Central America and the northern part of South America. In recent years, there have been outbreaks in the United States.

9.42.6. *Predominant clinical signs:* Excessive drooling is often the first sign seen. Fever is usually present (104°–106°F) and lesions can be found around the mouth, in the mouth, on the tongue (horses), muzzle, and nose. Lesions may be noted on the coronary bands of the feet, which may cause lameness (pigs). Lesions may also be found on the teats of dairy cattle causing a decrease in milk production. VSV is very similar to FMD and other vesicular diseases. Secondary bacterial infections often occur, such as mastitis, causing more economic losses. Most animals recover in about 2 weeks. Clinical disease is usually 4–7 days.

9.42.7. *Treatment:* Treatment is symptomatic—use of mild antiseptics and astringents on the mucosa of the mouth. Antibiotics are used to prevent secondary bacterial infections.

9.42.8. *Prevention:* A vaccine is available in some Latin American countries. Infected and exposed animals should be identified and quarantined for a minimum of 30 days after the last lesion is seen. Healthy animals should be separated from VSV infected animals. Infected animals should be stabled or housed to prevent insect transmission and insect control should be performed. Equipment must be disinfected and this is especially important in milking cows (with healthy animals milked before infected animals). VSV is a reportable disease in the United States and is an OIE List A Disease.

9.42.9. *Control:* VSV is readily inactivated by lipid solvents and heat (58°C for at least 30 minutes). Disinfectants that inactivate VSV include 1% formalin (minimum 10 minutes contact), 1% Virkon S, 4% lye (sodium hydroxide), 2% sodium carbonate, 2% iodophore, 1:1000 Roccal, 1:50 hexachlorophene septisol, and chlorine dioxide. Lye 2% does not inactivate the virus after 2 hours. VSV survives in soil (4°–6°C) for several weeks. It is resistant to pH 2–11.

9.42.10. *Zoonotic potential:* Humans are susceptible to VSV. They have flulike symptoms, which include headache, fever, blister formation in the mouth (not common, but similar to herpesvirus), and sore muscles. The Indiana and New Jersey subtypes (occur in the United States) typically cause flulike symptoms. Other VSV subtypes (Piry, Isfahan, and Chandipura do not occur in the United States) cause more disease in humans.

Suggested Reading

Cats contract avian influenza virus. 2006. www.avma.org/0nlnews/javma/apr06/060415a.asp.

Center for Emerging Issues: Menangle virus, Australia, November 1998, Emerging Disease Notice. www.aphis.usda.gov/vs/ceah/cei/tag/emergingdiseasenotice.

Center for Food Security & Public Health, Iowa State University, Nairobi sheep disease, last updated August 5, 2005. www.cfsph.iastate.edu/Factsheets/pdfs/nairobi_sheep_disease.pdf.

Centers for Disease Control and Prevention. Scabies. www.dpd.cdc.gov/dpds/HTML/Scabies.htm.

Committee on Foreign Animal Diseases of the United States Animal Health Association. 1998. Foreign animal diseases. In *The Gray Book*. Richmond, VA, Pat Campbell & Associates and Carter Printing Company, 1998.

Control of Canine Influenza in Dogs. Questions, Answers, and Interim Guidelines. 2005. www.avma.org/public_health/influenza/canine_guidelines.asp.

Dog dies of avian influenza. 2006. JAVMA News. www.avma.org/onlnews/javma/dec06/061215c.asp.

Fraser CM, editor. *The Merck Veterinary Manual*, ed 6. Editor, Rahway, NJ, Merck and Co, Inc., 1986.

Goodly L. Rabbit hemorrhagic disease. Compend Small Anim Pract 2001;23:249–254.

Howard JL, editor. *Current Veterinary Therapy: Food Animal Practice*, ed 2, Philadelphia: WB Saunders, 1986.

Influenza Updates from the AVMA, 2006, Backgrounder Avian Influenza. www.avma.org/public_health/influenza/avinf_bgnd.asp.

Influenza Updates from the AVMA, Backgrounder: Canine influenza. 2007. www.avma.org/public_health/influenza/canine_bgnd.asp.

Kahn CM, editor. *The Merck Veterinary Manual*, ed 8. Whitehouse Station: Merck and Company, Inc., 2005.

Mackenzie JS. Emerging viral diseases: An Australian perspective. Emerg Infect Dis 1999;5(1).

Menangle virus, Australia, November 1998. Emerging Disease Notice. Center for Emerging Issues. www.aphis.usda.gov. 1998.

Morgan RV, editor. *Handbook of Small Animal Practice*, ed 3. Philadelphia: WB Saunders, 1997.

Mueller B. African horse sickness. In *Horse Sickness Fever to Peracute Dyspnea and Death, Lumpy Skin and Sheep and Goat Pox: Out of Africa, Malignant Catarrhal Fever: A Vesicular Disease Differential Diagnosis*. IVERT Training & Homeland Security Seminar June 17–18, 2004, Boise, Idaho.

Philbey AW, Kirkland PD, Ross AD, et al. An apparently new virus (family Paramyxoviridae) infectious for pigs, humans, and fruit bats. Emerg Infect Dis 1998;4(2).

Senne DA. Avian influenza and Newcastle disease. IVERT Training & Homeland Security Seminar, June 17–18, 2004, Boise, Idaho.

Spickler AR, Roth JA, editors. *Emerging and Exotic Diseases of Animals*, ed 3. Ames, Iowa State University College of Veterinary Medicine, 2006.

Waladde SM, Ochieng SA, Gichuhi PM. Artificial membrane feeding of the ixodid tick, Rhipicephalus appendiculatus, to repletion. Exp Appl Acarol 1991;11:297–306.

White WR. African swine fever & classical swine fever, avian influenza, contagious bovine pleuropneumonia, foot and mouth disease, Newcastle disease, peste des petits ruminants, Rinderpest, swine vesicular disease, vesicular exanthema of swine, vesicular stomatitis virus. Idaho Veterinary Emergency Response Team (IVERT) Training & Homeland Security Seminar, June 17–18, 2004, Boise, Idaho.

Whiteman CE, Bickford AA. Avian Disease Manual, ed 2. Kennett Square, The American Association of Avian Pathologists, 1983.

CHAPTER 10
VETERINARY EUTHANASIA

Wayne E. Wingfield, MS, DVM

It is our responsibility as veterinarians and human beings to ensure that if an animal's life is to be taken, it is done with the highest degree of respect, and with an emphasis on making the death as painless and distress free as possible. Euthanasia techniques should result in rapid loss of consciousness followed by cardiac or respiratory arrest and ultimately the loss of brain function. In addition, the technique should minimize distress and anxiety experienced by the animal prior to loss of consciousness.

10. Euthanasia

10.1. What Is Euthanasia?

10.1.1. Euthanasia is the act of inducing humane death in an animal. Euthanasia is derived from the Greek terms *eu* meaning "good" and *thanatos* meaning "death." A good death is one that occurs with minimal pain and distress.

10.1.2. As disaster workers, it is our responsibility to ensure that if an animal's life is to be taken, it is done with the highest degree of respect, and with an emphasis on making the death as painless and free of distress as possible.

10.1.3. Euthanasia techniques should result in rapid loss of consciousness followed by respiratory and cardiac arrest and ultimately the loss of brain function. In addition, the technique should minimize distress and anxiety experienced by the animal prior to loss of consciousness.

I. Unfortunately, we cannot always assure that alleviation of pain and distress are achieved but they should always be minimized. If in doubt, you should always seek a veterinarian with training and expertise for that species to ensure proper procedures are followed.

10.2. Role of Pain

When discussing euthanasia we need to also discuss the *role of pain* in the procedure.

10.2.1.   Pain is the sensation (perception) that results from nerve impulses reaching the cerebral cortex via ascending neural pathways. For pain to be experienced, the cerebral cortex and subcortical structures must be functional.

10.2.2.   If the cerebral cortex is nonfunctional because of hypoxia (decreased blood oxygen levels), depression by drugs, electric shock, or concussion, pain is not experienced. Therefore, the choice of euthanasia agent or method is less critical if it is to be used on an animal that is already unconscious, provided the animal does not regain consciousness prior to death.

10.2.3.   Identification of pain in animals is difficult but some of the following factors will help define the animal that is:

I.   Vocalization may indicate pain; however, it is an insensitive and non-specific indicator. Pain is frequently associated with abnormal activity, which may appear as either an increase or a decrease in activity. Some animals may appear restless, agitated, or even delirious. At the other end of the spectrum, other animals may be lethargic, withdrawn, dull, or depressed. These animals may not pay attention to environmental stimuli. Animals may bite, lick, chew, or shake painful areas.

II.   Painful animals may adopt abnormal body postures in an attempt to relieve or cope with pain in a given area. For example, dogs with abdominal pain may assume a posture with a rigid torso and arched back. Animals with thoracic pain may be reluctant to lie down in spite of obvious exhaustion. Disuse or guarding of a painful area is a fairly reliable indicator of pain. The animal's gait may be abnormal or may appear much more rigid than normal.

III.   Interactive behaviors are frequently changed in the painful animal. Some animals may become more aggressive and resist handling or palpation. In contrast, they may become more timid than usual and seek increased contact with care-givers. Although most animals do not have the same degree of motor control over their facial muscles as do primates, changes in facial expression can be used in some to detect pain. Animals may hold their ears back or in a down position. The eyes may be wide open with dilated pupils, or partially closed with a dull appearance. Many animals will display a "fixed stare" into space, apparently oblivious to their surroundings. Some may display a type of grimace uncharacteristic when not painful.

IV.   Occasionally, the outwardly recognizable clinical signs of pain are masked by the underlying cause of the pain. Trauma and other causes may blunt an animal's behavioral response to pain. Lack of overt signs of pain (vocalizing, thrashing, etc.) does NOT confirm the animal is not painful. A good rule of thumb is to recall that the greater the amount of trauma, the more intense the pain.

V.   Tachypnea, tachycardia, hypertension, dilated pupils, and salivation are physiological signs suggestive of pain. Tachypnea, tachycardia, and hypertension are less likely to be observed in an unconscious patient that is painful.

10.3. One Must Also Be Cognizant of Differentiating Stress From Pain

10.3.1.   Stress is defined as the effect of physical, physiological, or emotional factors (stressors) that induce an alteration in an animal's homeostasis or adaptive state. The response of an animal to stress represents the adaptive process that is necessary to restore the baseline mental and physiological state.

10.3.2.   An animal's response to stress varies according to its experience, age, species, breed, and current physiological and psychological state.

10.3.3.   There are three phases of stress in an animal.
  I.   *Eustress* results when harmless stimuli initiate adaptive responses that are beneficial to the animal.
  II.   *Neutral stress* results when the animal's response to stimuli causes neither harmful nor beneficial effects to the animal.
  III.   *Distress* results when an animal's response to stimuli interferes with its well-being and comfort.

10.4. Proper Handling

Proper handling is vital to minimize pain and distress in animals, to ensure safety of the person performing euthanasia, and often, to protect other people and animals. Some methods of euthanasia require physical handling of the animal. The amount and kind of restraint will be determined by the animal's species, breed, size, state of domestication, degree of taming, presence of painful injury or disease, degree of excitement, and method of euthanasia.

10.4.1.   INAPPROPRIATE handling techniques prior to euthanasia.
  I.   Electric prods or whips should not be used to encourage movement of animals. Instead, properly designed chutes and ramps should be used.
  II.   Placing the animal in a painful position should NOT be allowed.
  III.   Inducing undue stress on the animal is not condoned.

10.4.2.   Several animal behavioral considerations that should be followed prior to euthanasia include the following:
  I.   Gentle restraint, careful handling, and talking during euthanasia often have a calming effect on animals that are used to being handled.
  II.   Sedation and/or anesthesia may assist in achieving the best conditions for euthanasia.
  III.   Observers of the euthanasia should be aware of what is to take place.
  IV.   Show compassion towards the animal, the animal owner, and other professionals involved with the euthanasia.
    A.   Euthanasia of wild, feral, injured, or already distressed, diseased animals may differ from what occurs with well-cared-for animals. These animals are already distressed and methods of pre-euthanasia handling may not be effective. Because handling may stress animals unaccustomed to human contact,

the degree of restraint required to perform euthanasia should be evaluated prior to the procedure. When handling these animals, calming may be accomplished by minimizing visual, auditory, and tactile stimulation.

  1. Because struggling during capture or restraint may cause pain, injury, or anxiety to the animal or danger to the rescuer, the use of tranquilizers, analgesics, and/or anesthetics may be necessary.

  B. The most common human psychological response to euthanasia of animals is *grief* at the loss of life.

10.5. Actions of Euthanasia

10.5.1. There are three main methods in which euthanatizing agents cause death:

I.   Hypoxia, direct and indirect.
II. Direct depression of neurons necessary for life function.
III. Physical disruption of brain activity and destruction of neurons necessary for life.

10.5.2. The loss of consciousness should precede loss of motor activity (muscle movement) in order to assure death is painless and distress-free.

I.   The loss of motor activity does NOT equate with the loss of consciousness and the absence of distress.

  A   There are agents that induce muscle paralysis without the loss of consciousness and these agents should NOT be used as sole agents for euthanasia. Examples of these unacceptable euthanasia drugs include depolarizing and non-depolarizing muscle relaxants, strychnine, nicotine, and magnesium or potassium salts.

10.6. Physical Techniques of Euthanasia

10.6.1. Physical destruction of brain activity, caused by concussion, direct destruction of the brain, or electrical depolarization of neurons, induces rapid loss of consciousness. Death occurs because of destruction of midbrain centers controlling cardiac and respiratory activity or as a result of adjunctive methods (e.g., exsanguination) used to kill the animal.

10.6.2. See Tables 10.1 and 10.2 for acceptable methods and agents of euthanasia.

10.6.3. See Table 10.3 for conditionally acceptable methods and agents for euthanasia.

I.   What are some of the physical methods of euthanasia?
  A. Captive bolt
  B. Gunshot
  C. Cervical dislocation
  D. Decapitation
  E. Electrocution

Table 10.1. Agents and Methods of Euthanasia by Species[a] (Refer to Table 10.4 for Unacceptable Agents and Methods).

Species	Acceptable* (refer to Table 10.2 for details)	Conditionally Acceptable[†] (refer to Table 10.3 for details)
Amphibians	Barbiturates, inhalant anesthetics (in appropriate species), CO_2, CO, tricaine methane sulfonate (TMS, MS 222), benzocaine hydrochloride, double pithing	Penetrating captive bolt, gunshot, stunning and decapitation, decapitation and pithing
Birds	Barbiturates, inhalant anesthetics, CO_2, CO, gunshot (free-ranging only)	N_2, Ar, cervical dislocation, decapitation, thoracic compression (small, free-ranging only), maceration (chicks, poults, and pipped eggs only)
Cats	Barbiturates, inhalant anesthetics, CO_2, CO, potassium chloride in conjunction with general anesthesia	N_2, Ar
Dogs	Barbiturates, inhalant anesthetics, CO_2, CO, potassium chloride in conjunction with general anesthesia	N_2, Ar, penetrating captive bolt, electrocution
Fish	Barbiturates, inhalant anesthetics, CO_2, tricaine methane sulfonate (TMS, MS 222), benzocaine hydrochloride, 2-phenoxyethanol	Decapitation and pithing, stunning and decapitation/pithing
Horses	Barbiturates, potassium chloride in conjunction with general anesthesia, penetrating captive bolt	Chloral hydrate (IV, after sedation), gunshot, electrocution
Marine mammals	Barbiturates, etorphine hydrochloride	Gunshot (cetaceans <4 meters long)
Mink, fox, and other mammals produced for fur	Barbiturates, inhalant anesthetics, CO_2 (mink require high concentrations for euthanasia without supplemental agents), CO, potassium chloride in conjunction with general anesthesia	N_2, Ar, electrocution followed by cervical dislocation
Nonhuman primates	Barbiturates	Inhalant anesthetics, CO_2, CO, N_2, Ar
Rabbits	Barbiturates, inhalant anesthetics, CO_2, CO, potassium chloride in conjunction with general anesthesia	N_2, Ar, cervical dislocation (<1 kg), decapitation, penetrating captive bolt
Reptiles	Barbiturates, inhalant anesthetics (in appropriate species), CO_2 (in appropriate species)	Penetrating captive bolt, gunshot, decapitation and pithing, stunning and decapitation

*Acceptable methods are those that consistently produce a humane death when used as the sole means of euthanasia.
[†]Conditionally acceptable methods are those that by the nature of the technique or because of greater potential for operator error or safety hazards might not consistently produce humane death or are methods not well documented in the scientific literature.
[a]http://www.avma.org/issues/animal_welfare/euthanasia.pdf (2007).

Table 10.2. Acceptable Agents and Methods of Euthanasia.

Agent	Classification	Mode of Action	Rapidity	Ease of Performance	Safety for Personnel	Species Suitability	Efficacy and Comments
Barbiturates	Hypoxia attributable to depression of vital centers	Direct depression of cerebral cortex, subcortical structures, and vital centers; direct depression of heart muscle	Rapid onset of anesthesia	Animal must be restrained; personnel must be skilled to perform IV injection	Safe except human abuse potential; DEA-controlled substance	Most species	Highly effective when appropriately administered; acceptable IP in small animals and IV
Benzocaine hydrochloride	Hypoxia attributable to depression of vital centers	Depression of CNS	Very rapid, depending or dose	Easily used	Safe	Fish, amphibians	Effective but expensive
Carbon dioxide (bottled gas only)	Hypoxia attributable to depression of vital centers	Direct depression of cerebral cortex, subcortical structures, and vital centers; direct depression of heart muscle	Moderately rapid	Used in closed container	Minimal hazard	Small laboratory animals, birds, cats, small dogs, rabbits, mink (high concentrations required), zoo animals, amphibians, fish, some reptiles, swine	Effective, but time required may be prolonged in immature and neonatal animals

Method	Mode of action	Mechanism	Onset	Equipment	Safety	Species	Comments
Carbon monoxide (bottled gas only)	Hypoxia	Combines with hemoglobin, preventing its combination with oxygen	Moderate onset time, but insidious so animal is unaware of onset	Requires appropriately maintained equipment	Extremely hazardous, toxic, and difficult to detect	Most small species including dogs, cats, rodents, mink, chinchillas, birds, reptiles, amphibians, zoo animals, rabbits	Effective; acceptable only when equipment is properly designed and operated
Inhalant anesthetics	Hypoxia attributable to depression of vital centers	Direct depression of cerebral cortex, subcortical structures, and vital centers	Moderately rapid onset of anesthesia, excitation may develop during induction	Easily performed with closed container; can be administered to large animals by means of a mask	Must be properly scavenged or vented to minimize exposure to personnel	Some amphibians, birds, cats, dogs, furbearing animals, rabbits, some reptiles, rodents and other small mammals, zoo animals, fish, free-ranging wildlife	Highly effective provided that subject is sufficiently exposed; either is conditionally acceptable
Microwave irradiation	Brain enzyme inactivation	Direct inactivation of brain enzymes by rapid heating of brain	Very rapid	Requires training and highly specialized equipment	Safe	Mice, rats	Highly effective for special needs
Penetrating captive bolt	Physical damage to brain	Direct concussion of brain tissue	Rapid	Requires skill, adequate restraint, and proper placement of captive bolt	Safe	Horses, ruminants, swine	Instant loss of consciousness, but motor activity may continue

Table 10.2. *Continued.*

Agent	Classification	Mode of Action	Rapidity	Ease of Performance	Safety for Personnel	Species Suitability	Efficacy and Comments
2-Phenoxyethanol	Hypoxia attributable to depression of vital centers	Depression of CNS	Very rapid, depending on dose	Easily used	Safe	Fish	Effective but expensive
Potassium chloride (intracardially or intravenously in conjunction with general anesthesia only)	Hypoxia	Direct depression of cerebral cortex, subcortical structures, and vital centers secondary to cardiac arrest	Rapid	Requires training and specialized equipment for remote injection anesthesia, and ability to give IV injection of potassium chloride	Anesthetics may be hazardous with accidental human exposure	Most species	Highly effective, some clonic muscle spasms may be observed
Tricaine methane sulfonate (TMS, MS 222)	Hypoxia attributable to depression of vital centers	Depression of CNS	Very rapid, depending on dose	Easily used	Safe	Fish, amphibians	Effective but expensive

ᵃ http://www.avma.org/issues/animal_welfare/euthanasa.pdf (2007).

Table 10.3. Conditionally Acceptable Agents and Methods of Euthanasia[a].

Agent	Classification	Mode of Action	Rapidity	Ease of Performance	Safety for Personnel	Species Suitability	Efficacy and Comments
Blow to the head	Physical damage to brain	Direct concussion of brain tissue	Rapid	Requires skill, adequate restraint, and appropriate force	Safe	Young pigs <3 weeks old	Must be properly applied to be humane and effective
Carbon dioxide (bottled gas only)	Hypoxia due to depression of vital centers	Direct depression of cerebral cortex, subcortical structures and vital centers; direct depression of heart muscle	Moderately rapid	Used in closed container	Minimal hazard	Nonhuman primates, free-ranging wildlife	Effective, but time required may be prolonged in immature and neonatal animals
Carbon monoxide (bottled gas only)	Hypoxia	Combines with hemoglobin, preventing its combination with oxygen	Moderate onset time, but insidious so animal is unaware of onset	Requires appropriately maintained equipment	Extremely hazardous, toxic, and difficult to detect	Nonhuman primates, free-ranging wildlife	Effective; acceptable only when equipment is properly designed and operated
Cervical dislocation	Hypoxia due to disruption of vital centers	Direct depression of brain	Moderately rapid	Requires training and skill	Safe	Poultry, birds, laboratory mice, rats (<200 g), rabbits (<1 kg)	Irreversible; violent muscle contractions can occur after cervical dislocation
Chloral hydrate	Hypoxia from depression of respiratory center	Direct depression of brain	Rapid	Personnel must be skilled to perform IV injection	Safe	Horses, ruminants, swine	Animals should be sedated prior to administration

277

Table 10.3. *Continued.*

Agent	Classification	Mode of Action	Rapidity	Ease of Performance	Safety for Personnel	Species Suitability	Efficacy and Comments
Decapitation	Hypoxia due to disruption of vital centers	Direct depression of brain	Rapid	Requires training and skill	Guillotine poses potential employee injury hazard	Laboratory rodents; small rabbits; birds; some fish, amphibians, and reptiles (latter 3 with pithing)	Irreversible; violent muscle contraction can occur after decapitation
Electrocution	Hypoxia	Direct depression of brain and cardiac fibrillation	Can be rapid	Not easily performed in all instances	Hazardous to personnel	Used primarily in sheep, swine, foxes, mink (with cervical dislocation), ruminants, animals >5 kg	Violent muscle contractions occur at same time as loss of consciousness
Gunshot	Hypoxia due to disruption of vital centers	Direct concussion of brain tissue	Rapid	Requires skill and appropriate firearm	May be dangerous	Large domestic and zoo animals, reptiles, amphibians, wildlife, cetaceans (<4 meters long)	Instant loss of consciousness, but motor activity may continue
Inhalant anesthetics	Hypoxia due to disruption of vital centers	Direct depression of cerebral cortex, subcortical structures, and vital centers	Moderately rapid onset of anesthesia; excitation may develop during induction	Easily performed with closed container; can be administered to large animals by means of a mask	Must be properly scavenged or vented to minimize exposure to personnel; ether has explosive potential and exposure to ether may be	Nonhuman primates, swine; ether is conditionally acceptable for rodents and small mammals; methoxyflurane is conditionally acceptable for rodents and small mammals	Highly effective provided that subject is sufficiently exposed

Method	Mode of action	Mechanism	Rapidity	Ease of performance	Safety for personnel	Species	Efficacy and comments
Nitrogen, argon	Hypoxia	Reduces partial pressure of oxygen available to blood	Rapid	Used in closed chamber with rapid filling	Safe if used with ventilation	Cats, small dogs, birds, rodents, rabbits, other small species, mink, zoo animals, nonhuman primates, free-ranging wildlife	Effective except in young and neonates; an effective agent, but other methods are preferable
Penetrating captive bolt	Physical damage to brain	Direct concussion of brain tissue	Rapid	Requires skill, adequate restraint and proper placement of captive bolt	Safe	Dogs, rabbits, zoo animals, reptiles, amphibians, free-ranging wildlife	Instant loss of consciousness but motor activity may continue
Pithing	Hypoxia due to disruption of vital centers, physical damage to brain	Trauma of brain and spinal cord tissue	Rapid	Easily performed but requires skill	Safe	Some ectotherms	Effective, but death not immediate unless brain and spinal cord are pithed
Thoracic compression	Hypoxia and cardiac arrest	Physical interference with cardiac and respiratory function	Moderately rapid	Requires training	Safe	Small- to medium-sized free-ranging birds	Apparently effective
Maceration	Physical damage to brain	Direct concussion of brain tissue	Rapid	Easily performed with properly designed, commercially available equipment	Safe	Newly hatched chicks and poults, and pipped eggs only	Effective when equipment is properly designed and operated

[a]http://www.avma.org/issues/animal_welfare/euthanasia.pdf (2007).

    F. Kill traps
    G. Thoracic compression
    H. Exsanguination
    I. Stunning
    J. Pithing
II. From the list above which physical methods of euthanasia are NOT recommended as a sole means of euthanasia?
    A. Exsanguination
    B. Stunning
    C. Pithing
III. See Table 10.4 for UNACCEPTABLE means and agents of euthanasia.

Table 10.4. Some *Unacceptable* Agents and Methods of Euthanasia[a].

Agent or Method	Comments
Air embolism	Air embolism may be accompanied by convulsions, opisthotonos, and vocalization. If used, it should be done only in anesthetized animals.
Blow to the head	Unacceptable for most species.
Burning	Chemical or thermal burning of an animal is not an acceptable method of euthanasia.
Chloral hydrate	Unacceptable in dogs, cats, and small mammals.
Chloroform	Chloroform is a known hepatotoxin and suspected carcinogen and, therefore, is extremely hazardous to personnel.
Cyanide	Cyanide poses an extreme danger to personnel and the manner of death is aesthetically objectionable.
Decompression	Decompression is unacceptable for euthanasia because of numerous disadvantages. (1) Many chambers are designed to produce decompression at a rate 15 to 60 times faster than that recommended as optimum for animals, resulting in pain and distress attributable to expanding gases trapped in body cavities. (2) Immature animals are tolerant of hypoxia, and longer periods of decompression are required before respiration ceases. (3) Accidental recompression, with recovery of injured animals, can occur. (4) Bleeding, vomiting, convulsions, urination, and defecation, which are aesthetically unpleasant, may develop in unconscious animals.

Table 10.4. *Continued.*

Agent or Method	Comments
Drowning	Drowning is not a means of euthanasia and is inhumane.
Exsanguination	Because of the anxiety associated with extreme hypovolemia, exsanguination should be done only in sedated, stunned, or anesthetized animals.
Formalin	Direct immersion of an animal into formalin, as a means of euthanasia, is inhumane.
Household products and solvents	Acetone, quaternary compounds (including CCl_4), laxatives, clove oil, dimethylketone, quaternary ammonium products*, antacids, and other commercial and household products or solvents are not acceptable agents for euthanasia.
Hypothermia	Hypothermia is not an appropriate method of euthanasia.
Neuromuscular blocking agents (nicotine, magnesium sulfate, potassium chloride, all curariform agents)	When used alone, these drugs all cause respiratory arrest before loss of consciousness, so the animal may perceive pain and distress after it is immobilized.
Rapid freezing	Rapid freezing as a sole means of euthanasia is not considered to be humane. If used, animals should be anesthetized prior to freezing.
Smothering	Smothering of chicks or poults in bags or containers is not acceptable.
Strychnine	Strychnine causes violent convulsions and painful muscle contractions.
Stunning	Stunning may render an animal unconscious, but it is not a method of euthanasia (except for neonatal animals with thin craniums). If used, it must be immediately followed by a method that ensures death.
Tricaine methane sulfonate (TMS, MS 222).	Should not be used for euthanasia of animals intended as food.

*Roccal D Plus, Pharmacia & Upjohn, Kalamazoo, Michigan.
[a]http://www.avma.org/issues/animal_welfare/euthanasia.pdf (2007).

IV.   Since most physical means of euthanasia involve trauma, there is inherent risk for animals and humans. Extreme care and caution must be practiced. Skill and experience of personnel is essential. If the method is not correctly performed, animals and personnel may be injured.

V.   Euthanasia by a blow to the head must be evaluated in terms of anatomic features of the species on which it is to be performed. A blow to the head can be a humane method of euthanasia for neonatal animals with thin craniums. The blow to the head of all animals must be delivered with sufficient force to the central skull bones to produce immediate depression of the central nervous system and destruction of brain tissue.

VI.   Euthanasia Using Either a Captive Bolt or Gunshot.

  A.   Aesthetic concerns

    1.   Both gunshot and penetrating captive bolt are aesthetically displeasing procedures. Euthanasia by either technique results in involuntary movements, and occasionally vocalization, that may be inaccurately interpreted as painful to an inexperienced person. Therefore, when and where possible, it is recommended that such procedures be performed in areas out of the public view.

  B.   Anatomical landmarks

    1.   Horses may be euthanized by gunshot or penetrating captive bolt.

    2.   Use of the captive bolt requires good restraint so that the device may be held in close contact with the skull when fired.

    3.   The site for entry of the projectile is described as a point slightly above the intersection of two diagonal lines each running from the inside corner of the eye to the base of the opposite ear (Figs. 10.1 and 10.2). The optimum site in the horse is slightly above the intersection of these two lines.

VII.   Confirmation of death,

  A.   Regardless of the method of euthanasia used, death must be confirmed before disposal of the animal. The following should be used to evaluate consciousness or confirm death:

    1.   Absence of a heartbeat.

      a.   The presence of a heartbeat can best be determined with a stethoscope placed under the left elbow. Please note that a pulse is usually not palpable under such circumstances and palpation should not be used to confirm death.

    2.   Absence of respiration.

      a.   Movement of the chest indicates respiration; however, respiration rates may be very erratic and slow in unconscious animals. Therefore, one must be cautious in the interpretation of respiration for confirmation of death.

    3.   Absence of a corneal reflex.

      a.   One may test for evidence of a corneal reflex by touching the surface of the eyeball. Normal or conscious animals will blink when the eyeball is touched. Absence of a corneal reflex, failure to detect respiration, and absence of a heartbeat for a period of more than 5 minutes should be used to confirm death.

  B.   An alternative is to observe the animal over a period of several hours. Lack of movement and absence of a heartbeat, respiration, or corneal reflex over an extended period of time provides further confirmation of death.

  C.   A physical blow to the head is an unacceptable technique of euthanasia in neonatal foals.

VIII.   A properly placed gunshot can cause immediate insensibility and humane death. In some cases, gunshot may be the only practical method of euthanasia. Shooting should be performed only by highly skilled personnel trained in using

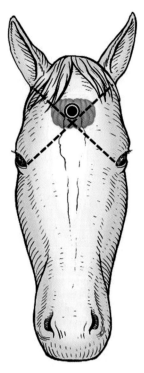

Figure 10.1. The site for entry of the projectile is described as a point slightly above the intersection of two diagonal lines each running from the inside corner of the eye to the base of the opposite ear. Note that contrary to that described for cattle, the optimum site in the horse is slightly above the intersection of these two lines. (Information and figures used with permission from the following. This document is modified from VM152, one of a series of the Veterinary Medicine—Large Animal Clinical Sciences Department, Florida Cooperative Extension Service, Institute of Food and Agricultural Sciences, University of Florida. Original publication date April, 2007. Visit the EDIS Web Site at http://edis.ifas.ufl.edu; Jan K. Shearer, DVM, Professor, and Paul Nicoletti, DVM, Professor, College of Veterinary Medicine—Large Animal Clinical Sciences, Cooperative Extension Service, University of Florida, Gainesville, FL 32611.)

appropriate caliber firearms. Personnel, public, and nearby animal safety should be of paramount importance. The procedure should only be performed outdoors and away from public access.

IX. Electrical activity in the brain persists for 13 to 14 seconds following cervical dislocation or decapitation.

X. Electrocution, using alternating current, induces death by ventricular fibrillation, which causes cerebral hypoxia. However, animals do not lose consciousness for 10 to 30 seconds after the onset of ventricular fibrillation. It is imperative that animals be unconscious before being electrocuted.

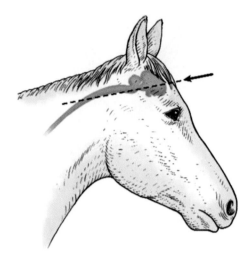

Figure 10.2. Direct the projectile parallel to the neck of a horse during euthanasia. (Information and figures used with permission from the following. This document is modified from VM152, one of a series of the Veterinary Medicine—Large Animal Clinical Sciences Department, Florida Cooperative Extension Service, Institute of Food and Agricultural Sciences, University of Florida. Original publication date April, 2007. Visit the EDIS Web Site at http://edis.ifas.ufl.edu; Jan K. Shearer, DVM, Professor, and Paul Nicoletti, DVM, Professor, College of Veterinary Medicine—Large Animal Clinical Sciences, Cooperative Extension Service, University of Florida, Gainesville, FL 32611.)

10.7. Mass Euthanasia Techniques Used in Disease Eradication and Natural Disasters Provide Limited Options

10.7.1. The most appropriate technique minimizes human and animal health concerns. These options include, but are not limited to, CO_2, and physical methods such as gunshot, penetrating captive bolt, and intravenous administration of euthanasia solutions.

Suggested Reading Websites

AVMA panel on euthanasia (2007). http://www.avma.org/issues/animal_welfare/euthanasia.pdf.

Blackmore DK. Energy requirements for the penetration of heads of domestic stock and the development of a multiple projectile. Vet Rec 1985;116:36–40.

http://www.vetmed.ufl.edu/lacs/HumaneEuthanasia/acrobat/brochureEng.pdf.

http://www.vetmed.ufl.edu/lacs/HumaneEuthanasia/acrobat/wallchart.pdf.

Longair JA, Finley GG, Laniel M-A, et al. Guidelines for euthanasia of domestic animals by firearms. Can Vet J 1991;32: 724–726.

Not Between the Eyes! Humane Euthanasia Procedures for Sick, Injured, and/or Debilitated Livestock. University of Florida College of Veterinary Medicine and University of Florida Institute of Food and Agricultural Sciences.

Operational Guidelines, Euthanasia. National Animal Health Emergency
   Management. Systems Guidelines. USDA, January 2004.
Shearer JK, Nicoletti P. Procedures for Humane Euthanasia for Sick, Injured or
   Debilitated Livestock. University of Florida College of Veterinary Medicine.
The emergency euthanasia of horses. Sacramento: California Department of Food and
   Agriculture and Davis, Calif: University of California's Veterinary Medical
   Extension, 1999.

EMERGENCY RESPONSE CONTACTS DIRECTORY

Wayne E. Wingfield, MS, DVM

Key Federal Government Agency Web Sites

Centers for Disease Control and Prevention (CDC)
http://www.cdc.gov/
Department of Agriculture (USDA)
http://www.usda.gov/
Department of Defense (DOD)
http://www.defenselink.mil/
Department of Energy (DOE)
http://www.energy.gov/
Department of Health and Human Services (HHS)
http://www.hhs.gov/emergency/
Department of Homeland Security (DHS)
http://www.dhs.gov/
Department of the Interior
http://www.doi.gov/
Department of Transportation (DOT)
http://www.dot.gov/
Disaster Medical Assistance Teams (DMAT)
http://www.dmat.org/
Disaster Mortuary Operational Response Teams (DMORT)
http://www.dmort.org/
Environmental Protection Agency (EPA)
http://www.epa.gov/
Federal Aviation Administration
http://www.faa.gov/
Federal Bureau of Investigation (FBI)
http://www.fbi.gov/
Federal Emergency Management Agency (FEMA)
http://www.fema.gov/
Food and Drug Administration (FDA)
http://www.fda.gov/
International Medical Surgical Response Team (IMSURT)
http://www.imsurtwest.com/

National Animal Health Emergency Management System (NAHEMS)
http://emrs.aphis.usda.gov/nahems.html
National Disaster Medical System (NDMS)
http://www.hhs.gov/aspr/opeo/ndms/index.html
National Institutes of Health (NIH)
http://www.nih.gov/
National Interagency Fire Center
http://www.nifc.gov/
National Medical Response Team (NMRT)
http://www.nmrtcentral.com/
National Response Center
http://www.nrc.uscg.mil/nrchp.html
National Veterinary Response Teams (NVRT or VMAT)
http://www.vmat.org/
Naval Maritime Forecast Center/Joint Typhoon Warning Center
http://metocph.nmci.navy.mil/
Nuclear Regulatory Commission (NRC)
http://www.nrc.gov/
Office of Preparedness and Emergency Operations
http://www.hhs.gov/aspr/opco/index.html
Ready.Gov (from the U.S. Department of Homeland Security)
http://www.ready.gov/
Substance Abuse and Mental Health Services Administration (SAMHSA)
http://www.samhsa.gov/
U.S. Army Corps of Engineers
http://www.usace.army.mil/
U.S. Army Veterinary Command
http://vets.amedd.army.mil/vetcom/
U.S. Coast Guard Command Center
http://www.uscg.mil/hq/commandcenter/
U.S. Geological Society Volcano Center
http://volcanoes.usgs.gov/
U.S. Geological Survey Earthquake Hazards Program
http://earthquake.usgs.gov/

Important Topical Web Sites

Agency for Toxic Substances and Disease Registry (ATSDR)
http://www.atsdr.cdc.gov/
American Association of Equine Practitioners
http://www.aaep.org/
American Cat Fanciers Association
http://www.acfacats.com/
American Humane
http://www.americanhumane.org/site/PageServer
American Kennel Club
http://www.akc.org/
American Quarter Horse Association

http://www.aqha.com/
American Red Cross
http://www.redcross.org/
American Society for the Prevention of Cruelty to Animals (ASPCA)
http://www.aspca.org/site/PageServer
American Veterinary Identification Devices (AVID)
http://www.avidid.com/
American Veterinary Medical Association
http://www.avma.org
Animal and Plant Health Inspection Service (APHIS)
http://www.aphis.usda.gov/
Animal Blood Bank
http://www.animalbloodbank.com/
Animal Blood Bank and Restore Health Center
http://www.hemopet.org/
Animal Poison Control Center
http://www.aspca.org/
Animal Rescue
http://www.code3associates.org/
http://hspca.convio.net/site/PageNavigator/homepage_new
Biological Agents
http://www.bt.cdc.gov/agent/agentlist.asp
BioSense
http://www.syndromic.org/pdf/work3-JL-BioSense.pdf
Bureau of Explosives
http://boe.aar.com/
Chem/Bio Terrorism Links
http://www.chem-bio.com/links/misc.html
Chemical Agents
http://www.bt.cdc.gov/chemical/
Chemical Spills
http://www.chemicalspill.org/EPCRA-facilities/ehs.html
CHEMical TRansportation Emergency Center (ChemTrec)
http://www.chemtrec.org/Chemtrec/
Colorado Veterinary Medical Reserve Corps
http://cosart.org/COVMRC.htm
Control of Communicable Diseases Manual. James Chin.
http://www.amazon.com/Control-Communicable-Diseases-Manual-James/dp/087553242X
County Animal Response Teams
http://cosart.org/county_animal.htm
Days End Farm Horse Rescue
http://www.defhr.org/
Delta Society
http://www.deltasociety.org/
Emergency Response Guidebook 2008
http://www.labelmaster.com/ERG/
Epidemic Information Exchange (Epi-X)
http://www.cdc.gov/epix/
Epidemic Intelligence Service (EIS)
http://www.cdc.gov/eis/

Euthanasia Guidelines (AVMA)
http://www.avma.org/onlnews/javma/sep07/070915b.asp
First Responder's Field Guide to Hazmat & Terrorism Response by Jill Meryl Levy.
  2006 Edition
http://www.amazon.com/Responders-Hazmat-Terrorism-Emergency-Response/dp/0965151697
Foodborne Diseases Active Surveillance Network (FoodNet)
http://www.cdc.gov/foodnet/
Health Alert Network (HAN)
http://www.phppo.cdc.gov/han/
HomeAgain Microchip
http://www.homeagainid.com/
Humane Euthanasia of Sick, Injured, and/or Debilitated Livestock
http://lacs.vetmed.ufl.edu/HumaneEuthanasia/
Humane Society of the United States (HSUS)
http://www.hsus.org/
InfoPet Microchip
http://www.infopet.biz/
International Pet Travel Microchip Information
http://www.pettravel.com/passports_pet_microchip.cfm
International Wildlife Rehabilitation Council
http://www.iwrc-online.org/
Jane's Mass Casualty Handbook: Pre-hospital
http://catalog.janes.com/catalog/public/index.cfm?fuseaction=home.
  ProductInfoBrief&product_id=84857
Laboratory Response Network (LRN)
http://www.bt.cdc.gov/lrn/
National Animal Control Association
http://www.nacanet.org/
National Association for Search and Rescue (NASAR)
http://www.nasar.org/nasar/
National Association of Wildlife Rehabilitators
http://www.nwrawildlife.org/home.asp
National Disaster Medical System (NDMS)
http://ndms.dhhs.gov/
National Hurricane Center
http://www.nhc.noaa.gov/
National Response Plan (NRP)
http://www.dhs.gov/nrp/
National Response Team (NRT)
http://www.nrt.org/
National Weather Service (NOAA)
http://www.nws.noaa.gov/
NIOSH Pocket Guide to Chemical Hazards
http://www.cdc.gov/niosh/npg/
Pandemic Influenza
http://www.pandemicflu.gov/
Pesticide Hotline
http://chppm-www.apgea.army.mil/ento/hotken.htm
Radiological Agents
http://www.bt.cdc.gov/radiation/

Rocky Mountain Poison and Drug Center
http://www.rmpdc.org/
Safe Drinking Water Hotline
http://www.epa.gov/ogwdw/drinklink.html
Severe Acute Respiratory Syndrome (SARS)
http://www.cdc.gov/ncidod/sars
State Animal Response Teams (SART)
http://nc.sartusa.org/
http://cosart.org/
Strategic National Stockpile (SNS)
http://www.bt.cdc.gov/stockpile/index.asp
United Animal Nations
http://www.uan.org/
Veterinary Emergency and Critical Care Society (VECCS)
http://www.veccs.org/
West Nile Virus (WNV)
http://www.cdc.gov/ncidod/dvbid/westnile/index.htm

Animal Control Equipment and Supplies

Aazel Corporation (animal control equipment)
http://www.aazelcorp.com
Animal Care Equipment & Services, Inc. (animal control equipment & supplies)
http://www.animal-care.com
Ark Shelter Software (shelter software)
http://www.arksoftware.com
Business Computing (shelter software)
http://www.youramerica.net
Crawford Industrial Group, LLC (Animal Cremation and Incineration Systems)
http://www.crawfordequipment.com
http://www.animal-cremation.com
Critter Control (animal facts/wildlife trivia)
http://www.crittercontrol.com/?doc=resources
C Specialties, Inc. (small animal products, animal control equipment)
http://www.cspecialties.com
Deerskin Manufacturing, Inc. (animal transport units)
http://deerskinmfg.com
Harford Systems (animal transport units)
http://www.harfordsystems.com
HDL Software (Licensing Software)
http://www.hdlcompanies.com
Jones Trailer Company (animal transport units)
http://www.jonestrailers.com
Ketch-All Company—The Original Animal Control Pole
http://www.Ketch-All.com
Matthews Cremation Division (Animal Cremation and Incineration Systems)
http://www.matthewscremation.com
Mavron, Inc. (animal transport units)
http://www.mavron.com

PetData (animal licensing)
http://www.petdata.com
Petfinder.com (Free Online Service for Shelters)
http://www.Petfinder.com
RoseRush Services, LLC (Animal Control and Shelter software)
http://www.ShelterPro.com/
Swab Wagon Company (animal transport bodies)
http://www.swabwagon.com
T-Kennel (animal housing, cages)
http://www.T-Kennel.com
Tomahawk Live Trap Company (traps, animal control equipment)
http://www.livetrap.com
Wildlife Control Supplies (wildlife control & animal handling)
http://www.wildlifecontrolsupplies.com/
Wolfe Pack Press, Inc. (Publications)
http://www.wolfepackpress.com
Wolverine Coach (animal transport units)
http://www.wolverinecoach.com

Index

Chlorhexidine diacetate solution 2%,
  wound care for horse and use of,
  46t, 47
Chlorhexidine solution
  for decontamination purposes, 111
  working dogs and, 13
Chlorhexidine surgical scrub, contagious
    equine metritis treatment and, 211
Chlorine (Cl), 126
  concentrations of, and effect on
    animals, 127t
  exposure to, 127
Chlorine dioxide, vesicular stomatitis
    virus inactivation and, 266
Chloroacetophenone (tear gas or mace),
    129
Chloroform, as unacceptable form of
    euthanasia, 280t
Choking (pulmonary) agents, 115,
    126–128
  aftercare, 128
  clinical signs with exposure to, 127
  decontamination after exposure to,
    128
  supportive care and, 128
  treatment following exposure to,
    127–128
  triage guidelines for animals exposed
    to, 128t
  types of, 126–127
Cholinesterase enzymes, nerve agents and
    inhibition of, 113, 114
Chronic forms of disease
  African swine fever, 196
  contagious bovine pleuropneumonia,
    209
  equine infectious anemia, 214
  hog cholera, 225
  progressive pneumonia, 235
Chronic wasting disease, 185, 186,
    188–189, 260
  agent responsible for, 188
  clinical signs in species affected by,
    189
  decontamination and, 189
  disease severity in species affected by,
    188t
  incubation period for, 188
  occurrence of, 260
  prevention of, 189

  route of transmission of, 188–189
  transmission of, 188
  treatment of, 189
Chrysomya bezziana, 251
CI. See Canine influenza
Ciloxin, horses and use of, 49
Ciprofloxacin, anthrax exposure
    treatment and, 152
Ciprofloxacin Ophthalmic Solution,
    horses and use of, 49
Circulatory system, explosive-related
    injuries and, 97t
CJD. See Creutzfeldt-Jakob disease
Classical swine fever, 224
Clostridium botulinum, 177
Clostridium botulinum C + D antitoxin,
    179
Clostridium perfringens toxins, 180–181
  clinical signs in animals and humans,
    180–181
  decontamination and, 181
  disease severity in species affected by,
    180t
  incubation period for, 180
  prevention of, 181
  route of transmission of, 180
  transmission of, 180
  treatment of, 181
Cloth muzzles, 4
  for large-breed dog, 5
Cobalt (Co), 140–141
Coban, 49, 51, 54
Cochliomyia hominivorax, 251
Coffin bone, 66
Coggins disease, 213
Coggins test, 214
Cold water founder, 66
Colera porcina, 224
Colic
  clinical signs of, 73
  in horses
    atropine administration and, 118
    first aid for, 72–73
Collars, decontamination of, after
    biological toxins exposure, 109
Colorado Veterinary Medical Reserve
    Corps, web site for, 289
ComboPen autoinjector, 119
Concussion founder, 66
Conform, 49